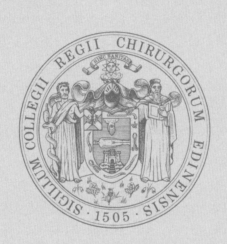

# 'A Famous and Flourishing Society'

The History of the
Royal College of Surgeons of Edinburgh,
1505–2005

HELEN M. DINGWALL

EDINBURGH UNIVERSITY PRESS

© The Royal College of Surgeons of Edinburgh, 2005

Edinburgh University Press Ltd
22 George Square, Edinburgh

Typeset in Century Schoolbook by
Pioneer Associates, Perthshire, and
printed and bound in Singapore by
Tien Wah Press (Pte) Ltd

A CIP record for this book is available from the British Library

ISBN 0 7486 1567 9 (hardback)

# Contents

# Subscribers

Professor Frank **Abbas**, Groningen, The Netherlands

Mirza M. **Abbas**, Sutton in Ashfield, England

Edward Maurice **Absoud**, Boston, England

Maged Awni **Abu-Ramadan**, Gaza, Palestine

Ian Victor **Adair**, Belfast, Northern Ireland

William **Adair**, Leicestershire, UK

Alexander **Adam**, Aberdeen, Scotland

Alistair D. **Adams**, Edinburgh, Scotland

Vida **Adib**, London, England

Patricio Manuel **Aduriz-Lorenzo**, Gijon, Spain

E. Andreas **Agathos**, Athens, Greece

Maryam M. S. **Ahmad**, Cairo, Egypt

Mirza Mubashar **Ahmad**, Rabwah, Pakistan

Tariq **Ahmad**, Cambridge, England

Mohamed **Ahmad Shukri**, Kuala Lumpur, Malaysia

Gamal Eldeen Hamed **Ahmed**, Port Said, Egypt

Ziauddin **Ahmed**, New Jersey, USA

Samir Raja **Akel**, Beirut, Lebanon

Akintunde **Akin-Deko**, Ibadan, Nigeria

Hiroshi **Akiyama**, Tokyo, Japan

Abubaker Ibrahim A. **Al-Aieb**, Tripoli, Libya

Mohammed Majeed **Alam**, Ranchi, India

Temitope Oluwagbenga **Alonge**, Ibadan, Nigeria

Mohammad Hunidel Abdulrahman **Al-Sharood**, Riyadh, Kingdom of Saudi Arabia

Nada Hassan **Al-Yousuf,** Manama, Kingdom of Bahrain

Eric G. **Anderson**, Glasgow, Scotland

John **Anderson**, Cumbria, UK

Matthew Philip **Armon**, Norwich, England

Godwin Toyin **Arotiba**, Lagos, Nigeria

Puraviappan **Arunasalam**, Selangor, Malaysia

Peter **Atkinson**, Darlington, England

Michael William **Austin**, Swansea, Wales

Abdul Lateef Issa **Babata**, Ilorin, Nigeria

Sir John **Baird**, Ely, England

Roger **Baird**, Bristol, UK

**Balakrishnan** Ratnam, Ipoh, Malaysia

Manickavasagar **Balasegaram**, Kuala Lumpur, Malaysia

Graham Harold **Barker**, Kingston upon Thames, UK

Professor Hugh **Barr**, Gloucester, England

Professor Bruce **Barraclough** AO, Australia

Professor Aires A. B. **Barros D'Sa**, Belfast, UK

Alban Avelino John **Barros D'Sa**, Coventry, England

Ian James **Barros D'Sa**, Coventry, England

Sonia Helen **Barros D'Sa**, Coventry, England

William G. **Bartlett**, Tampa, USA

El Fatih Mahmoud **Bashir**, Doha, State of Qatar

Thomas Firth **Baskett**, Halifax, Nova Scotia, Canada

Allan **Basson**, Wynyard, Australia

Arthur Wynyard **Beasley**, Wellington, New Zealand

Frank Howard **Beddow**, Liverpool, England

Richard Clayton **Bennett**, Melbourne, Australia

Michael **Beverly**, London, UK

Harikant **Bhanushali**, Thane, India

William H. **Bisset**, Edinburgh, Scotland

Duncan Arthur **Black**, Dundee, Scotland

Anthony **Bleetman**, Solihull, England

Vladimir **Bobic**, Chester, England

George C. **Borthwick** CBE, Edinburgh, Scotland

Patrick Stewart **Boulter**, Edinburgh, Scotland

John Graham **Bradley**, Scarborough, UK

John Ewart Dawson **Bramley**, Stafford, UK

David N. **Bremner**, St Boswells, Scotland

Jason **Brockwell**, Hong Kong

Bazil Ricardo **Brown**, Kingston, Jamaica

John E. **Buck**, Bexleyheath, England

Joseph A. **Buckwalter**, Iowa City, USA

Steve R. **Budhooram**, San Fernando, Trinidad/Tobago

Juliusz Jan **Buras**, Victoria, Australia

Professor Anthony **Busuttil**, Edinburgh, Scotland

Neil **Buxton**, Ormskirk, England

Richard Anthony, **Buxton**, Fife, Scotland

Peter Dudley **Byrne**, Tusmore, South Australia

Christopher M. **Caddy**, Sheffield, England

Professor James **Calnan**, Berkhamstead, England

Neil **Cartwright**, London, UK

Francis Dominic **Cavallo**, Maryborough, Queensland, Australia

Randolph George **Cesareo**, Perth, Western Australia

Pradip Kumar **Chakrabarti**, Allentown, Pennsylvania, USA

John **Chalmers**, Edinburgh, Scotland

John **Chamberlain**, Newcastle upon Tyne, UK

Shailesh **Chaturvedi**, Westhill, Scotland

Chatenya Amritlal **Chauhan**, Southend on Sea, UK

Jack C. Y. **Cheng**, Hong Kong

Anelechi Barnabas **Chukuezi**, Umudim, Nigeria

Rosemary **Chukwulobelu**, Birmingham, UK

The City of Edinburgh Council

W. B. **Clark**, Brisbane, Australia

David John **Clarke**, Comrie, Scotland

Forrester **Cockburn**, Glasgow, Scotland

John Calvin **Coffey**, Cork, Ireland

Ivan **Coll**, Natal, South Africa

Brian Patrick Danvers **Colquhoun**, Saskatoon, Canada

John **Colville**, Belfast, Northern Ireland

Professor John E. **Connolly** FRCSEd (Hon), Newport Beach, California, USA

William A. **Copland**, Edinburgh, Scotland

Stephen William Valentine **Coppinger**, Shrewsbury, England

David Logan **Cross**, Glasgow, Scotland

Gale **Curtis**, Queensland, Australia

Christopher James **Cutting**, Taunton, UK

Saleem Ahmed **Dahduli**, Riyadh, Kingdom of Saudi Arabia

Danish Surgical Society

Pradip Kumar **Datta**, Wick, Scotland

Paul Adrian **Davey**, London, England

Gareth Rhys **Davies**, Australia

Leo J. **de Souza**, Minneapolis, USA

Alan **Dean**, North Berwick, Scotland

Toshio **Deguchi**, Nagoya, Japan

William James **Dempster**, Lockerley, UK

Sharayu **Desai**, Karnatak, India

Binay K. **Desarkar**, Chattishgarh, India

Alexander A. **Deutsch**, Kfar Sava, Israel

Visist **Dhitavat**, Bangkok, Thailand

J Rüdiger **Döhler**, Plau am See, Germany

Nanjappachetty Velaswamychetty **Doraiswamy**, Glasgow, Scotland

JohnLindsay **Douglas**, Glasgow, Scotland

Douglas Marshall **Druitt**, Melbourne, Australia

Hugh Arnold Freeman **Dudley**, Huntly, Scotland

John L. **Duncan**, Inverness, Scotland

Robert Buchan **Duthie** CBE, Shipton, England

Peter **Edmond**, Pickering, North Yorkshire

Michael Harpur **Edwards**, Darlington, UK

Spencer **Efem**, Calabar, Nigeria

Pianto Idonbagha **Egberipou**, Kolokuma-Kaiama, Nigeria

Asaad Abdusalam Mohamed **Elfighi**, Tripoli, Libya

Abdelrahman Abdelkarim **Elwasila**, Khartoum, Sudan

Oleg **Eremin**, Lincoln, England

Anthony Thomas **Ethell**, Sydney, Australia

Christine Mary **Evans**, Llanarmon-Yn-Ial, Wales

John Dillwyn **Evans**, Sale, Great Britain

András **Ézsiás**, Hungary

Richard Grey **Faber**, Berkshire, UK

Patrick Eniola **Fadero**, Lagos, Nigeria

Richard E. T. **Fan**, Republic of Singapore

Ridzuan **Farouk**, Reading, England

Richard Keith **Faulkner**, Perth, Western Australia

David H. **Felix**, Glasgow, Scotland

Lawrence Donald **Finch**, Liverpool, England

Geoffrey Raymond **Fisk**, Cambridge, England

Michael **Fogarty**, Melbourne, Australia

Alastair John Winter **Fordyce**, California, USA

James Richard Charles **Foster**, Edinburgh, Scotland

Hugh Jonathan **Fox**, Winchester, UK

John N. **Fox**, Beverley, England

David M. A. **Francis**, Melbourne, Australia

Lennox Stanley Brian **Francis**, Kingston, Jamaica

Matthew Hamilton **Fraser**, Glasgow, Scotland

Louis Kuo-Tai **Fu**, Hong Kong

David Peter **Gale**, Melbourne, Australia

John Millie Dow **Galloway**, Hull, England

Shanmugam **Ganesan**, Coimbatore, India

Professor O. James **Garden**, Edinburgh, Scotland

Dugald Lindsay **Gardner**, Edinburgh, UK

Geoghegan & Co., Edinburgh, Scotland

Iain Edward **Gibb**, London, UK

Norman Otway Knight **Gibbon**, Liverpool, UK

Ewen Walford **Gillison**, Brushford, UK

Hugh Montgomery **Gilmour**, Edinburgh, Scotland

Aik Hong **Goh**, Eastleigh, England

Jacob Henry **Goldin**, Birmingham, UK

Shivkumar **Gopal**, Bhopal, India

Harry **Gordon**, London, England

Malcolm William George **Gordon**, Bearsden, Scotland

Henry H. **Gossman**, Plymouth, UK

John Ferguson **Gould**, Edinburgh, Scotland

Fiona **Graham**, Cork, Ireland

Alistair Duncan **Grassie**, Isle of Arran, Scotland

Anthony William **Griffin**, Uriarra, Australia

Rimino **Guerriero**, Adelaide, South Australia

Battagodage Rohan **Gunaratne**, Nugegoda, Sri Lanka

Alexander Anton **Gunn**, Kelso, Scotland

Alan **Hair**, East Kilbride, Scotland

Ernest Graham **Hale**, Hemswell, UK

Richard **Halley-Stott**, Johannesburg, South Africa

David Lawrence **Hamblen**, Glasgow, Scotland

Timothy Bruce **Hargreave**, Edinburgh, Scotland

Douglas R. **Harper**, Aberdeen, UK

N. J. **Harris**, Leeds, UK

Phillip **Harris**, Edinburgh, Scotland

Moinul **Hassan**, Burdwan, West Bengal

Peter J. **Hayward**, West Chiltington, England

J. Michael **Henderson**, Cleveland, USA

Wilson Stephen **Hendry**, Stirling, Scotland

Efren **Herrera-Martinez**, Puebla, Mexico

Anthony David **Hockley**, Birmingham, England

Raymond Carter **Hodge**, Abergavenny, Wales

George Charol **Hoffman**, Norfolk, Virginia, USA

John Daniel **Hooley**, Hong Kong

Geoffrey **Hooper**, Edinburgh, UK

Lutz **Hostert**, Leeds, UK

Graham Peter **Howell**, Bath, England

Robert Anthony **Howell**, Liverpool, England

Shoou-Chyuan **Huang**, Singapore

Alan R. **Hudson**, Toronto, Canada

Sean Patrick Francis **Hughes**, London, England

Nilufar **Imam**, Gillingham, England

John Walker Sinclair **Irwin**, Belfast, Northern Ireland

Sherif Mouneir **Isaac**, Minia, Egypt

ISIS Asset Management plc, Edinburgh, Scotland

Daniel **Iya**, Jos, Nigeria

Sir Barry **Jackson**, London, England

Peter **Jackson**, UK

Salman Asghar **Jaffery**, Lahore, Pakistan

Michael J. **Jane**, Helensburgh, Scotland

Robert James Terry **Jarvis**, Ludham, UK

Khalid **Javed**, Lahore, Pakistan

Benjamin L. **Jenkins**, Manchester, England

Dr Ajaya Nand **Jha**, Delhi, India

Charles Finlay **Jones**, Newcastle, Australia

David John **Jones**, Manchester, England

Mel W. **Jones**, Menai Bridge, Wales

Jonathan William Morris **Jones**, Peterborough, England

**Kannan** Shanmugasigamani, Madras (Chennai), India

Sean M. **Kelly**, Inverness, Scotland

Dawn D. **Kemp**, Whittingehame, Scotland

Anthony Joseph **Keniry**, Bures St Mary, England

Mr Kamran **Khalid**, Bahawalpur, Pakistan

Iftikhar Ahmed Rasheed **Khan**, Faisalabad, Pakistan

Omar **Khan**, Rochester, England

M. I. Mohammad Nasim Sobhani **Khondker**, Dhaka, Bangladesh

Espeed **Khoshbin**, Leicester, UK

Donald Henderson **King**, Whangarei, New Zealand

Philip Allan **King**, Perth, Western Australia

William Howard **Kingston**, Bundaberg, Australia

Yusuf **Kodwaywala**, Nairobi, Kenya

Dimitrios **Kombogiorgas**, Sparta, Hellas

Mohan Gopal **Koppikar**, Mumbai, India

James **Kyle**, Aberdeen, Scotland

Thomas Chuen Fung **Lam**, Sydney, Australia

Osafo **Lartey**, Ghana

Graham Tansley **Layer**, Cobham, England

John **Leach**, Oxford, UK

William M. **Ledingham**, Aberdeen, Scotland

**Lee** Yiu-Ting, Hong Kong, China

Alex Chi Hang **Lee**, Hong Kong

Andrew Clayton **Lee**, Hong Kong, China

Hai Liang Darren **Lee**, Stoke on Trent, UK

John Siu-Man **Leung**, Hong Kong, China

Lewis Mark **Levitz**, Johannesburg, South Africa

Ernest R. **Levy**, Cooperstown, New York, USA

Albert Linton **Liburd**, Nevis, West Indies

Joo Kiong **Lim**, Kuching, Malaysia

Kok Bin **Lim**, Singapore

B. Sepiso **Linyama**, Mongu-Barotseland, Southern Africa

James **Lister**, Hownam, Scotland

Adrian **Litton**, Cambuslang, Scotland

Peter B. **Lockhart**, Charlotte, North Carolina, USA

John Robert Cunningham **Logie**, Inverness, Scotland

John Duncan Ott **Loudon**, Edinburgh, Scotland

John Henry **Lowry**, Saintfield, Northern Ireland

Michael **Mace**, Lytham St Annes, UK

John Robert **Macfarlane**, Kirkcaldy, Scotland

Neil **MacGillivray**, Edinburgh, Scotland

Iain **Macintyre**, Edinburgh, Scotland

Iain Ferguson **MacLaren**, Edinburgh, Scotland

Donald A. D. **Macleod**, Ettrick, Scotland

Stephen P. R. **MacLeod**, Minneapolis, USA

Roderick N. M. **MacSween**, Glasgow, Scotland

Patrick Kok Kheong **Mah**, Kuala Lumpur, Malaysia

Robert **Mansel**, Cardiff, Wales

Averil **Mansfield**, London, England

Victor S. **Mar**, Melbourne, Australia

Robert Charles **Mason**, London, England

Alastair H. B. **Masson**, Edinburgh, Scotland

Thomas Swan **Matheson**, York, England

Mohammad Abdul **Matin**, Bogra, Bangladesh

Hugh John Dennis **Mawhinney**, Helen's Bay, Ireland

Margaret Joyes **Mavell**, Nottingham, England

Philip James **McCahy**, Saltwood, England

John St C. **McCormick** OBE, Castle Douglas, Scotland

James P. **McDonald**, Edinburgh, Scotland

John Cummack **McGregor**, Edinburgh, Scotland

Jamie **McKenzie**, Bath, England

Shireen Natasha **McKenzie**, Leeds, England

Dermot William **McKeown**, Edinburgh, Scotland

George Campbell **McKinlay**, Glasgow, Scotland

John Winton **McNab**, Perth, Scotland

Gordon Herbert Dargavel **McNaught**, Hartlepool, UK

Donald Cragg **McNeill**, Salisbury, England

Murray Clyde **Meikle**, Dunedin, New Zealand

James Edward **Metcalfe**, Telford, England

John William **Metcalfe**, Liverpool, England

David Russell **Millar**, Sheffield, UK

Marion Conway **Miller**, Dundee, Scotland

Alistair George **Mills**, Ardross, Australia

Bhagwat **Misra**, Lubbock, USA

Meenakumari **Mithrakumar**, Colombo, Sri Lanka

Shankar **Mitra**, Calcutta, India

Colin Campbell Marshall **Moore**, Sydney, Australia

Arthur MacGregor **Morris** OBE, St Andrews, Scotland

Gordon W. **Morrison**, Adelaide, Australia

**Munuswamy** Punyakoti Naresh Kumar, Chennai, India

Douglas Stewart **Murray**, Abberley, England

Saravanamuthu **Muthulingam**, Jaffna, Sri Lanka

Sadasivam **Muthurajan**, Coimbatore, India

Bhalchandra Vasudeo **Nabar**, Neath, Wales

Dave Nigel **Nanan** and Donna M. **Nanan**, Florida, USA

Bashir Ahmed **Naz**, Kotli Loharan East, Pakistan

Roderick **Nelson**, Edinburgh, Scotland

Ham Koung **Ng Lung Kit**, Reduit, Mauritius

Mohammad Hossein **Niayesh**, Esfahan, Iran

Udofot Philip **Ntia**, Palm Springs, California, USA

Desmond A. **Nunez**, Bristol, England

John **Older**, London, England

Christopher W. **Oliver**, Edinburgh, Scotland

Professor Ridwaan **Omar**, Cape Town, South Africa

Clement Alaba **Omotola**, Oka-Akoko, Nigeria

Lindsay **Ong-Tone**, Regina, Saskatchewan, Canada

Keiran **O'Rourke**, Dublin, Ireland

John Douglas **Orr**, Edinburgh, Scotland

Cyril **Pallewela**, Sri Lanka

Trevelyan Edward **Palmer**, New York, USA

Michael **Parker**, Westerham, UK

Professor Thomas George **Parks**, Belfast, Northern Ireland

Murthi S. N. **Pasumarthi**, Hyderabad, India

Sivathanu Subramania **Pillai**, Nagercoil, Tamilnadu, India

Professor Hiram C. **Polk**, Louisville, USA

Thangarajo **Ponnusamy**, Selangor, Malaysia

John **Potter**, Newcastle upon Tyne, UK

Arvind Dattatray **Pradhan**, Dombivli, India

Krishnapada **Pradhan**, Kolkata, India

Arunasalam Pillay **Puraviappan**, Selangor, Malaysia

Abu Sayeed Mohammad Mahmudur **Rahman**, Dhaka, Bangladesh

Motior **Rahman**, Dhaka, Bangladesh

Tarak M. A. **Ramadan**, Ezawia, Libya

K. K. **Ramalingam**, Chennai, India

Andrew Harold **Ramsay**, Coffs Harbour, Australia

Juergen Ralph **Rayner-Klein**, Clifton, England

Myrddin **Rees**, Basingstoke, UK

Abdul **Rehman**, Rawalpindi, Pakistan

Andrew **Reid**, Birmingham, UK

Sir William Kennedy **Reid**, Edinburgh, Scotland

Edward Franz **Reye**, Brisbane, Australia

Alvin Anthony **Ribeiro**, Rugby, England

W. D. **Roberts**, Perth, Western Australia

Derek **Robinson**, Dublin, Ireland

Professor Alan **Rodger**, Glasgow, Scotland

William Mackie **Ross**, Durham, UK

Guy Alain **Rosset**, Pietermaritzburg, South Africa

Peter Kenneth Makin **Rostron**, Ormskirk, England

Roger Godolphin **Rowe**, Sydney, Australia

Brian James **Rowlands**, Nottingham, England

Professor David I. **Rowley**, Dundee, Scotland

Sunil C. **Roy**, Edinburgh, Scotland

The Royal Bank of Scotland plc, Edinburgh, Scotland

Royal College of Physicians and Surgeons of Glasgow

Royal College of Surgeons of Edinburgh Ladies' Club

Andrew John **Rugg-Gunn**, Sidmouth, England

Timothy E. **Rutter**, Truro, UK

Samuel **Sakker**, Sydney, Australia

Abdul Jabbar Mehdi **Salih**, Al-Najaf, Iraq

Manzar **Salim**, Karachi, Pakistan

Khalil M. **Salman**, Jeddah, Saudi Arabia

John A. **Sandiford**, Virginia, USA

**Saw**, Khay Chee, Malaysia

Alastair Duncan **Scotland**, London, England

Anne M. **Scott**, Edinburgh, Scotland

John **Scott**, Cambridge, UK

Honnett S. **Searwar**, Georgetown, Guyana

Amin A. **Seraj**, Jeddah, Saudi Arabia

Abdul-Aziz Z. **Shaalan**, Riyadh, Saudi Arabia

Tarig Ezzeldin **Shah**, Khartoum, Sudan

Zameer A. **Shah**, London, UK

Hamad **Shams**, Manama, Kingdom of Bahrain

John Ewen Greig **Shand**, Carlisle, England

William Stewart **Shand**, London, England

Palaniappa G. **Shanmugaraiu**, Croydon, UK

Andrew David **Shaw**, Ballymena, Northern Ireland

Jobn Fraser **Shaw**, Edinburgh, Scotland

Redmond S. P. **Sheedy**, Glenside, Australia

Shepherd and Wedderburn WS, Edinburgh, Scotland

Sir Robert **Shields**, West Kirby, Wirral, UK

Harwant **Singh**, Petaling Jaya, Malaysia

Grish Mohan **Singhal**, Muzaffarnagar, India

**Sinnamohideen** Jamal, Thanjavur, India

Group Captain John **Skipper**, Gosport, UK

Professor Frederick Charles **Smales**, Hong Kong

Adam N. **Smith**, Edinburgh, Scotland

John A. R. **Smith**, Sheffield/Edinburgh, UK

Marianne **Smith**, Edinburgh, UK

William A. **Souter**, Edinburgh, Scotland

Lucas **Souvlis**, Sydney, Australia

Alastair Andrew **Spence** CBE, Kilmacolm, Scotland

A. Lindsay **Stewart** OBE, Edinburgh, Scotland

Simon **Stewart**, UK

James Christopher Marnan **Strachan**, Harwich, UK

Jack **Strahan**, Enniskillen, Northern Ireland

Russell W. **Strong**, Brisbane, Australia

Simon Richard **Stubington**, Nantwich, England

Robert **Sturrock**, Dundee, Scotland

Om Prakash **Sudrania**, Mumbai, India

Peter George Herbert **Summers**, Kerikeri, New Zealand

Alasdair **Sutherland**, Aberdeen, Scotland

Adedayo Oluyomi **Tade**, Ijebu Igbo, Nigeria

Mostafa Ali **Tawfik**, Dammam, Saudi Arabia

Professor Sir John Graham **Temple**, Birmingham, UK

Sellappan **Thangavelu**, London, England

Professor David **Thomas**, Wolverhampton, UK

Philip **Thomas**, Victoria, Australia

Alistair Graham **Thompson**, Birmingham, UK

Alastair Mark **Thompson**, Auchterarder, Scotland

Matthew P. **Thomson**, Portadown, UK

Professor Sandie Rutherford **Thomson**, Congella, South Africa

Ravindranath **Tiruvoipati**, Leicester, England

David Anthony **Tolley**, Edinburgh, Scotland

Naeem **Toosy**, Oxshott, England

Paulo Sergio Da Silva **Torres**, Newcastle upon Tyne, UK

Hamish Moray Andrew **Towler**, Aberdeen, Scotland

Douglas George **Townsend**, Glenunga, Adelaide, Australia

Michael Joseph **Troy**, Melbourne, Australia

Jeffrey Y. S. **Tsang**, Hong Kong

James Hamilton **Tweedie**, Princes Risborough, England

University of Edinburgh

Hero **van Urk**, Rotterdam, The Netherlands

Dato Peter C. **Vanniasingham**, Penang, Malaysia

Peter Navaratnam **Vanniasingham**, Auckland, New Zealand

Cherian **Varughese**, Chengannur, India

Geoffrey **Vercoe**, Adelaide, Australia

Seema **Vishnu**, Trichur, India

Gunasekar **Vuppalapati**, Kodivalasa, India

John David **Wade**, Cambridge, England

John Patrick **Wadley**, London, England

Professor William Angus **Wallace**, Nottingham, UK

William F. M. **Wallace**, Belfast, UK

Eldred Wright **Walls**, Edinburgh, Scotland

Michael Edward **Walsh**, Leeds, England

Douglas **Wardlaw**, Aberdeen, Scotland

Achuthan **Warrier**, Nambucca Heads, New South Wales, Australia

Richard Wyndham **Watson**, Adelaide, Australia

Edward **Whitehead**, Brough, East Yorkshire, England

Robin **Wild**, St Boswells, Scotland

Ian Edward **Willetts**, Nottingham, England

Leslie Arnold **Williams**, Cardiff, Wales

Robert Guy **Williams**, Calgary, Canada

Professor Janet Ann **Wilson**, Newcastle upon Tyne, UK

Nairn Hutchison Fulton **Wilson**, London, UK

William **Wilson**, Glasgow, Scotland

Chi-tak Danny **Wong**, Hong Kong

Dr Hok-Leung **Wong**, Hong Kong

Tak Hing Bill **Wong**, Hong Kong, China

Professor B. Michael **Wroblewski**, Wrightington Hospital, UK

Kenneth W. C. **Wu**, Hong Kong

Romesh D. **Yagnik**, Hull, UK

Junkoh **Yamashita**, Kanazawa, Japan

Hon Hung Stephen **Yau**, Hong Kong

Aprim Yousif **Youhana**, Swansea, Wales

Dominic Shu Lok **Yu**, London, England

Paul Yue Hung **Yung**, Hong Kong

Syed Aftab **Zaman**, Nottingham, England

Bassem Salti **Zeidan**, Anjara-Ajlun, Jordan

# Acknowledgements

This book has been many years in the making, and consequently many individuals and institutions have assisted in its preparation over the years. I owe a major debt to Professor A. G. D. Maran, who was the prime mover in initiating the project almost fifteen years ago, and who has been a welcome support ever since, particularly during his period as President of the College. I am grateful to Professor Patrick Boulter, Professor Sir Robert Shields, Professor Sir John Temple and Mr John Smith, all of whom have supported the history during their presidencies. Mr I. F. Maclaren has offered encouragement and welcome suggestions for many years, as has Dr A. H. B. Masson, Honorary Archivist to the College and author of two magnificent works on the College's collections of art, silver, furniture and ephemera. Mr Maclaren, Dr Masson, Mr D. A. D. Macleod, Miss Caroline Doig, Dr P. R. Geissler, Mr J. Foster and Ms Marianne Smith have all read and commented usefully on sections of the manuscript. Their helpful comments and suggestions have been much appreciated, though, of course, errors of fact or interpretation which remain are entirely my own. Mr Macleod has been of particular support in the latter stages of preparation and I am very grateful for this.

The late Sir Michael F. A. Woodruff, the late Professor James Lister, Miss A. B. Sutherland, Mr P. Walbaum, Mr J. F. Shaw, the late Mr D. W. Lamb and Mr J. E. Newsam provided me with notes on the evolution of their specialties, and these are preserved within the College archive. Similarly, for the dental side of the College, considerable help was received from Mr L. D. Finch, Dr J. F. Gould, Dr P. R. Geissler and the late Professor Dorothy A. M. Geddes. I am also grateful to Professor D. L. Gardner, Ms Dawn Kemp and Ms Marianne Smith for valuable discussions about the College Museum, Library and Archive.

Historians rely heavily on the support and goodwill of library and archive staff, and my task has been made much easier by the efficiency of the College Library staff over the years, in particular Marianne Smith, the College Librarian, together with – at various times – Alison Stevenson, Gillian Johnstone, Steven Kerr, Simon Johnston and David Collier. My constant requests for books or manuscripts were invariably met with courtesy and cheerfulness, and this was much appreciated. I am similarly indebted to the librarians and archivists of the Edinburgh City Archive, Edinburgh University Library Special Collections Department, the National Archives of Scotland, the National Library of Scotland, the Royal College of Surgeons of England, the Royal College of Surgeons in Ireland, the Royal College of Physicians of Edinburgh, The Royal College of Physicians and Surgeons of Glasgow and the South Carolina History Society.

The staffs of the various administrative departments of the College have been consistently helpful. Miss Margaret Bean, Major Leslie Allan and Miss Alexandra Campbell were closely involved in the administration of the project in the early years. More recently Mr Jim Foster, Chief Executive, has overseen these aspects, as well as managing the arrangements with Edinburgh University Press. Miss Helen Scott, College Registrar, assisted me in elucidating the complexities of the College examinations, and Miss Violet Brown, Dental Faculty Administrator, provided me with information on the Dental examinations. Mr David Morcom, Mr Alan Watson, Senior College Officers, and their colleagues have given practical help when necessary, and this has been much appreciated.

I am most grateful to the College for funding my Research Fellowship at the University of Edinburgh between 1993 and 1995, and also to the Wellcome Trust and the Arts and Humanities Research Board for financial support which has allowed me to have an extended period of full-time research in order to complete the work.

Permission for reproduction of the illustrations was received from the College President and Council, the National Library of Scotland, John Gillingham and the Old Edinburgh Club. Considerable assistance in the collection and processing of the images was given by Marianne Smith and David Collier, who spent many hours on this task. The photographic expertise of Mr Max Mackenzie was also invaluable here.

Nicola Carr, Senior Commissioning Editor of Edinburgh University Press, has dealt calmly with my many queries and missed deadlines, and I am also grateful to Eddie Clark and Helen Johnston for their editorial expertise.

On a very personal note, I am grateful for the support I have received for a number of years from colleagues at the Department of History, University of Stirling, particularly Dr I. G. C. Hutchison, Dr R. B. McKean and Professor G. C. Peden. Professor M. Lynch and Professor C. A. Whatley have also provided encouragement over many years, as has Professor M. H. Kaufman. I am greatly indebted, for medical reasons, to Mr E. W. J. Cameron, Dr W. G. Middleton, Dr A. J. Jacob, Dr N. Grubb and Dr F. C. McRae. I wish also to acknowledge consistent family support from my sister Elizabeth, and from Bill, James, Robert and Anne.

It is hoped that the book will reflect adequately the long and distinguished history of this institution and that Fellows and Members will find something in it to strengthen their links with, and loyalty to, the College, wherever in the world they happen to practise surgery.

# Abbreviations and conventions

| | |
|---|---|
| BMA | British Medical Association |
| *BMJ* | *British Medical Journal* |
| *BOEC* | *Book of the Old Edinburgh Club* |
| *Bull. Hist. Med.* | *Bulletin of the History of Medicine* |
| *Burgh Recs* | *Extracts from the Records of the Burgh of Edinburgh, 1403–1589*, ed. J. D. Marwick; *1589–1718*, eds M. Wood et al. (Edinburgh, 1927–67) |
| CCST | Certificate of Completion of Specialist Training |
| College | Royal College of Surgeons of Edinburgh (from 1778) |
| College Business Papers | RCSEd manuscript collection, arranged chronologically |
| College Minutes | RCSEd minute books |
| DQ | Double Qualification |
| ECA | Edinburgh City Archive |
| *EMJ* | *Edinburgh Medical Journal* |
| EMS | Emergency Medical Service |
| EPGBM | Edinburgh Postgraduate Board for Medicine |
| EUL | Edinburgh University Library |
| EWTD | European Working Time Directive |
| FPSG | Faculty of Physicians and Surgeons of Glasgow (1599–1909) |
| FRCSEd | Fellow of the RCSEd |
| GDC | General Dental Council |
| GMC | General Medical Council |
| HDD RCSEd | Higher Dental Diploma of the RCSEd |
| Incorporation | The Incorporation of Barbers and Surgeons of Edinburgh (1505–1778) |
| JCHDT | Joint Committee on Higher Dental Training |
| JCHST | Joint Committee on Higher Surgical Training |
| *J. Roy. Coll. Surg. Edinb.* | *Journal of the Royal College of Surgeons of Edinburgh* |
| LHSA | Lothian Health Services Archive |
| LRCSEd | Licentiate of the Royal College of Surgeons of Edinburgh |
| MCQ | Multiple-choice question |
| *Med. Hist.* | *Medical History* |

| | |
|---|---|
| MFDS/MDS RCSEd | Member of the Faculty of Dental Surgery/Dentistry |
| MOH | Medical Officer of Health |
| MRCS | Member of the Royal College of Surgeons |
| NAS | National Archives of Scotland |
| NHS | National Health Service |
| NLS | National Library of Scotland |
| PMETB | Postgraduate Medical Education and Training Board |
| *Proc. Roy. Coll. Phys. Ed.* | *Proceedings of the Royal College of Physicians of Edinburgh* |
| RCPEd | Royal College of Physicians of Edinburgh |
| RCPEng | Royal College of Physicians of England |
| RCPSG | Royal College of Physicians and Surgeons of Glasgow (from 1962) |
| RCSEd | Royal College of Surgeons of Edinburgh |
| RCSEng | Royal College of Surgeons of England |
| RCSI | Royal College of Surgeons in Ireland |
| RFPSG | Royal Faculty of Physicians and Surgeons of Glasgow (1909–62) |
| RIE | Royal Infirmary of Edinburgh |
| SAC | Specialty Advisory Committee |
| SCPGME | Scottish Council for Postgraduate Medical Education |
| TQ | Triple Qualification |

Throughout the book quotations are given in their original form and spelling, with explanations where necessary.

All sums of money referred to in the pre-1707 period are in £Scots unless otherwise stated. £12 Scots was equivalent to £1 Sterling; one merk was two-thirds of a £Scots (13s 4d).

The year is taken as commencing on 1 January, which it did in Scotland from 1600.

# Illustrations

Unless otherwise indicated, all illustrations come from the College's collections and archives (for fuller accounts of the portraits, see Masson, *Portraits, Paintings and Busts*).

Plates (between pp. 104 and 105).

Plates (between pp. 232 and 233).

# FIGURES

# Tables

# Foreword by HRH Prince Philip, Duke of Edinburgh, Patron of the College

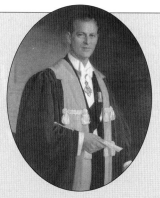

PALACE OF HOLYROODHOUSE

The Royal College of Surgeons of Edinburgh received its Seal of Cause from the Town Council in July 1505, which was then ratified by James IV in October 1506. This makes it one of the oldest surgical corporations in the world and the reason for its quincentenary celebrations. It is also the reason for this comprehensive history of the College. Its status as a 'Famous and Flourishing Society' was confirmed by the granting of a Royal Charter in 1778.

The Seal of Cause was a far-sighted document, and the Fellows continue to share the ideals and follow the aims of the founders. They were required to be literate, study anatomy and provide the best instruction for their apprentices. The purpose of the College continues to be the study of surgery and the improvement in teaching and examinations, and by adapting to the changing social, political, technological and economic circumstances, to offer the best possible service to the community.

I am sure that the general reader, as well as the 15,000 Fellows and Members, who currently operate in most countries of the world, and those who are retired, will be fascinated to read this careful analysis of how this world famous College has reacted to technical progress and social change while remaining faithful to its ideals.

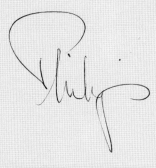

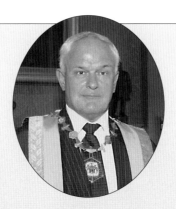

## A FAMOUS AND FLOURISHING SOCIETY

'Progress, far from consisting in change, depends on retentiveness. Those who cannot remember the past are condemned to repeat it.' Those words written by the American philosopher George Santayana around the turn of the century are as true now as they were then.

The Royal College of Surgeons of Edinburgh has adapted well to change throughout its long and distinguished history, and has been innovative in many aspects of surgical education, training and assessment. Throughout its 500 years, the College has been instrumental in maintaining and developing standards of surgical training and assessment. The visionary philosophy of the 1505 Seal of Cause ensured standards of knowledge, of competence and of discipline. Throughout its lifetime the College has continued to stay true to those principles so that standards of patient care in surgery can remain high.

Helen Dingwall has written a comprehensive and carefully researched account of the first 500 years, which provides a fascinating insight into the ways our history has influenced the present, and will inform the future. It provides us, the current Council, Fellows and Members, with the background and foundation which we need to take the College forward, to ensure that we continue to make important contributions to surgery for many years to come, and to maintain the highest standard of surgery set out by our forebears 500 years ago.

John A R Smith PhD FRCSEng PRCSEd
President

# 1

# Introduction

---

> The question of commissioning the writing of a history of the College similar to that undertaken for the Royal College of Physicians was discussed. Resolved. That the Council should commission a history of the College to be written some time before the 500th anniversary in 2005.[1]

In June 1671 the Incorporation of Surgeons and Barbers of Edinburgh decided to start awarding honorary freedoms to individuals of note, primarily of political and social note, who could help to boost the reputation of the Incorporation and assist it in political struggles. The minute of that decision describes the Incorporation as 'famous and flourishing', hence the title of this history.[2] From its first days in medieval Edinburgh the Incorporation sought incessantly to shed its craft image and become a 'learned society'.

The writing of the history of any institution has considerable inherent dangers. There is clearly a need to account for, and illustrate, the development and progress of the institution over a long time period – in this case five centuries. The most significant danger is that of producing a eulogy rather than a fully contextualised, analytical account. Most such works are commissioned by the institutions themselves, and these bodies naturally hope for their society to be portrayed in the best possible light. In the past, such accounts have often been little more than celebratory works, emphasising the key role which has been played by the institution in whatever field it happened to be. These works have not been regarded by historians as other than useful sources of factual information, as they could not have been wholly objective in their approach. This was, in some part, because many of these works were written by members of the institutions themselves, rather than by historians. This is not to claim that only professional historians can write good history – far from it – but the problem is that individuals who have had long connections with their own professional institution may have, however subconsciously, a wish to glorify that institution, whether it be school, business, hospital, charitable institution or surgical college.

General accounts of Scottish medical corporations have been produced in the past,[3] but in recent times more analytical accounts have been written on these as well as on other Scottish institutions, including histories of the Royal College of Physicians of Edinburgh, Royal Bank of Scotland and the Royal College of Physicians and Surgeons of Glasgow.[4] The present work aims to add to the academic history of surgical institutions, medicine in general, and of Scotland itself, as well as celebrating 500 years of the College's continuous existence. However erudite or elite an institution may be, it cannot divorce itself fully, or even partly, from its general context. The changing social, political, religious and economic structure of Scotland over the half-millennium had important effects on, and implications for, the future of the College. Needless to say, from 1707, the progress of Scotland was inextricably linked to that of Britain and the Empire. It is crucial, therefore, that the history of the College is embedded within this changing and influential context.

The Royal College of Surgeons of Edinburgh has had an illustrious past, both as an institution in its own right and as a body which has reacted to change in the broader context over the centuries. Its origins lay in late-medieval Scotland, in a period when surgical knowledge was limited, anatomical knowledge equally primitive, and Scotland was a relatively poor, economically backward, feudal nation with ill-defined and insecure boundaries. It was certainly not clear at that point that Scotland would wield influence within Britain and the world out of all proportion to its geographical size. The Incorporation of Barbers and Surgeons was established, not for any particularly altruistic reasons, but simply because of the nature of burgh society and structure. This was a time when as burghs became larger, groups of individuals who followed a variety of trades began to organise themselves into incorporations, mostly from the selfish motives of demarcation and protection.[5] Burgh crafts were important – perhaps not yet as politically important as merchant guilds – but their appearance reflected the early beginnings of urban demographic and economic realignment, and the growth of settlements with sufficient numbers of inhabitants to render these organisations possible or necessary.[6]

Over the ensuing half-millennium, the Incorporation of Surgeons (from 1778, Royal College) was witness to the Union of the Crowns in 1603, the Civil Wars of the mid-seventeenth century, sparked off by the signing of the National Covenant in 1638, the Union of Parliaments in 1707, the evolution of 'Great Britain', the Enlightenment, the growing influence of the state in terms of large-scale national and local government from the early nineteenth century, the building and subsequent demise of the Empire, the trauma and dislocation of two world wars, the advent of the European Union and the ongoing global conflicts of the early years of the twenty-first century, not to mention the parallel developments in medicine and surgery and the technology and politics of medicine. Throughout all of this, the Masters, Licentiates, Members and Fellows of the College have contributed both directly and indirectly to the totality of medical progress, but were themselves influenced by their contemporary context.

It is clear, therefore, that the history of this single institution cannot be constructed – or indeed deconstructed – in isolation. Context, background and, importantly, the 'Scottishness' factor were and are important in shaping the nature and direction of this and any Scottish institution. Many famous individuals helped to make the College what it has become today. Names such as Primrose, Monro, Pitcairne, Syme or Lister fall easily from the lips of those who are acquainted with the long history of surgery in Edinburgh. However individually famous, though, none of these men (and eventually women) could have made the contributions which they did without contact with, and influence from, their own times. They were all individuals of particular periods and shared the general perceptions and attitudes of their time. They may have been pioneers, but pioneers who lived and worked in a country which was at the same time influencing them and also changing and developing as a result of their own influence, in however small a way. Archibald Pitcairne, one of the most famous names of the later seventeenth century, discussed new ideas on the mechanical structure of the body and corresponded with Isaac Newton. Pictairne, though, was not at all embarrassed to try the application of live doves to the soles of a patient's feet when all attempts at cure had failed, while Newton himself never abandoned his interest in alchemy.

## APPROACH AND STRUCTURE

The history of the College is covered thematically within broad chronological periods, and falls into two main divisions, 'The Incorporation' and 'The College'. From the start it was the primary aim of the Incorporation to become a learned society. The masters may not have directly articulated the term College, but it is clear that this was the aim – to be regarded as a learned society, with all of the implications that this bore as opposed to bearing the mantle and contextual trappings of the craft organisation, however skilled. Once the political sett of the burgh had been re-drafted in 1583, allowing six craft representatives on the Town Council, the surgeons were invariably there and equally invariably named first in the Council sederunt records, tacitly, if not openly, confirming their superiority over, for example, the much larger and powerful hammermen's incorporation, some of whose members manufactured surgical instruments.

The Incorporation achieved its aim roughly half way through its current history, becoming a Royal College in 1778, in the warm glow of the Scottish Enlightenment. From that point it sought to divest itself of the trade connections it had maintained, particularly with the Town Council. This is, it must be said, just a touch ironic. The Incorporation had depended for its continued existence, not just on political and royal patronage, but also on consistent support from the Town Council, which backed its senior craft in a number of power struggles with the physicians and apothecaries. Surgeons represented the town in the Scottish parliament and at the Convention of Royal Burghs, thus giving them direct influence in local government and politics.[7] This was, though, rather forgotten, or conveniently ignored, during the 'College' phase, although links with the Town Council, which have in some ways never been wholly severed, were broken formally with the amended Royal Charter granted to the College in 1851.

In the second half of its history, the College has been able to 'flourish' in a number of ways, though progress was not without considerable problems. The backcloth of society, economy and politics was very different and changing constantly. Following the Union of Parliaments of 1707, Edinburgh and Scotland had to function politically as well as culturally, socially and economically within the context of Britain, Great or not, and even if a minority of Scots were in favour of union. The surgeons were nothing if not politically aware and astute, and the following century would see a growing utilisation of British politics and British politicians in support of College policy, particularly in the turbulent period of protracted negations towards the eventual passing of the Medical Act in 1858. The name of Henry Dundas appears in the late-eighteenth-century College records as the source of legal opinion on a number of issues. 'Harry the ninth' was considered to be both the best legal opinion on offer and the most promising politically.[8] In this period the College may be seen to have veered politically towards the Hanovarian cause – it gave one of its more dubious honorary freedoms to 'Butcher Cumberland' – but this may be to read too much into the politics of the situation rather than the practical priorities of the College, which sought to advance its own status first and foremost, and, as it had always done, attempt to gain support from individuals who, at any particular point, were most able to deliver that support.

By the turn of the nineteenth century, which saw economic depression as well as the rapid expansion of Empire, the College was accustomed to this wider view which it had been forced to take. The 'construction' of the aims and intentions of the Edinburgh surgeons owed much to general as well as to particular contextual influences. Foreign diploma candidates brought money and potential contacts and helped to develop the examining and training functions of the College. Empire afforded Edinburgh-qualified surgeons the opportunity to influence the surgical health of wider and wider concentric global circles, centred on Edinburgh. This gave important footholds in many parts of the world, footholds which would be retrod once the Empire had dissipated, and attention refocused on the more restricted but potentially lucrative area of foreign examination centres. This has continued to be the main international direction of the College and its activities.

The early part of the nineteenth century brought in big government, both at national and local levels, and this affected the ability of the medical institutions to operate independently. It would be the case increasingly that legislation would be introduced, with or without the agreement or co-operation of the surgeons, which would place restrictions on the activities and scope of the College and its Fellows and Licentiates. This legislation came about mainly in the areas of public health, medical training and registration, and ultimately a whole new raft of problems and difficulties emerged with the apparent social miracle of the National Health Service, initiated in 1948.

From that point, the activities of the College have been focused on higher surgical training and higher diplomas, the provision of modern teaching for these qualifications, the proliferation of surgical specialties, the establishment of over-seas examinations, and the embracing of the technological age with the introduction of courses in Medical Informatics, distance learning and web-based study facilities. Scotland led the way in the industrialising process and, of course, shared in its downfall, but it has also been prominent in new industry, particularly in computer-related areas. Politically, the history ends in a period of uncertainty. The effects of devolution have yet to manifest themselves fully, and in the global context the nation is perhaps a little subdued.

At the beginning of its history the Incorporation could afford to be single-minded and blinkered about its aims and functions, quite naturally, because the general context was much more simple and slower to change. By the end of the fifth century of its life, the College still has its original aims, but its ability to drive ahead to fulfil the modern equivalent of the Seal of Cause is affected, and at times severely limited, by external influences. Government Acts must be implemented; professional standards must be maintained in a public domain; political influence cannot be relied on to provide consistent support. The politics of medicine and surgery have, nowadays, rather become an end in themselves, the 'football' of political parties, which debate their respective policies heatedly rather than ensuring their rectitude and implementation. Medical people have historically relied on patronage and politics to enable progress; the relationship between the medical profession and the politicians is now much more amorphous. In terms of continued royal patronage, HRH the Duke of Edinburgh is patron of the College, but his political influence cannot be even remotely similar to that of James IV.

There are elements of continuity in history just as there are significant changes; the fascination of the history of a single institution is precisely because of its constant presence within a complex amalgam of change, continuity and causation. The College was and is at once a social club, a teaching and examining body, a source of higher surgical qualifications, a promoter of the global technology of surgical education, a leading professional institution and guardian of its heritage and history. The account which follows is an attempt to explain the evolution of a key surgical institution in context. It is, of course, in part a celebration of the achievements of 500 years of history; it is also a historical account and analysis, 'warts and all'. The long period covered here embraces a number of distinct phases and changing influences. These may be described as: establishment and consolidation; outgoing and British; outgoing and international.

A work such as this, which spans five centuries, cannot cover all of the minutiae of the events of every day or every year in its life. The aim here is to provide a structure and framework, and suggest (with apologies to postmodernists) some sort of causal relationships between and among the College, the city, the nation and the international community. The key to explaining the history of this, or any other, major institution lies in elucidating these complex and ongoing relationships. Creswell's history of the College, together with Masson's detailed works on the College portraits, furniture and artefacts, and the forthcoming account of the lives of 200 Fellows, edited by Macintyre and MacLaren, should be seen as essential complementary works.[9]


## THEORIES

Historians are nowadays pressurised increasingly to make use of theories in order to afford, apparently, a higher degree of credibility to their analysis. Relationships between historians and sociologists have in the past been strained, to say the least.

Historians are concerned about the apparently constraining nature of sociological theories and models, while sociologists accuse historians of not making enough use of exactly these things. As with most aspects of academic life, there must be room for compromise. This work is not predicated on any fixed theory or inflexible sociological or historical model, but it is useful to consider whether a little theory might just be a good thing. But what kind of theory?

There are theories, for example, about the social construction of medicine, which point out the mutual influences and inter-reactions between any individual, group or institution and the changing social, economic and political background context.[10] This certainly was the case with the College, which depended for its origins on the particular social and economic context of the late-medieval and early-Renaissance periods, coupled with the effects of urbanisation on groups of individuals following the same occupation, and for its continued existence on the evolution of medical knowledge and surgical possibility. Once the Royal Charter had been granted and Edinburgh was bathed in the intellectual glow of the Enlightenment, the focus was very much towards defending the surgical (and medical) orthodoxy which had been created against the increasing availability of knowledge, including medical knowledge, to a wider, lay audience. This fits in well with the Habermas view of the interaction between spheres of knowledge in the post-Enlightenment period, when knowledge was increasingly available to a wider public, enabled by the flourishing culture of print and the growing literacy levels of the population.[11] Habermas also claims, though, that gradually the significance of this sphere of free discussion waned once the sphere of government became more intrusive. Though there is a considerable historiography based on Habermasian theory, the emerging institutions, particularly medical institutions, have not yet featured to any great extent in this literature.[12] It may be interesting to view the shaping of the College in terms of these interacting spheres of influence. Writing on the writing of history, Michel de Certeau takes the view that institutions occupy a 'particular place in a redistribution of social space' – perhaps in this case a redistribution of potential for control and ownership of knowledge. He also focuses heavily on the relationship between knowledge and a specific place – another approach which might repay some consideration, particularly in relation to the visual symbolism of buildings.[13]

Whatever the merits or otherwise of theory, the institutional historian is always faced with the danger of lapsing into a straightforward Whiggish interpretation, because of the long-term study and the unavoidable use of words such as 'evolution', 'development' and 'progress'. It may be that for some aspects of the history of some institutions a Whiggish view is entirely acceptable, but in general the grand-sweep-of-progress view is to be treated with considerable caution.

## PROFESSIONALISATION

The professions have been the subject of a growing historiography in recent years. Many historians tend towards the view that professions did not – and could not –

come fully into being until relatively modern times, because of such factors as the structures of earlier societies, dependence on patronage and the different views on what constituted ethical behaviour. In an article outlining how historians have viewed the history of the medical profession over many centuries, Burnham claims that initially the 'profession' was simply the knowledge itself. This was superseded by the 'great doctors and places' approach, which, though rightly highlighting the contributions of significant individuals, rather neglected both the role of the medical institutions and also the influence of outside factors. Finally, Burnham assesses the less than harmonious interaction in more recent times between historians and sociologists, and asserts that these processes have produced historical concepts of professions 'on many different levels of sophistication',[14] though he questions the relevance of the whole concept of the profession in modern times. Despite these problems, though, with due acknowledgement of different discourses in different eras, it is possible to claim that the Incorporation and, subsequently, College, were working towards goals which certainly in their own times would be seen as professional. A recent contribution to the debate on professionalisation lists five main criteria or elements of the 'ideal' conception of a profession:

- special knowledge of a practical sort
- commitment to preserve and enhance that knowledge
- commitment to achieving excellence in the practice of the profession
- an intrinsic and dominant commitment to serving others on whose behalf the special knowledge is applied
- effective self-regulation by the professional group[15]

The author of that work, though, contests these criteria, claiming, for example, that altruism is selective, and that 'professions are social constructs, not facts of nature'.[16] This is a controversial view, and based to some extent on whether it is necessary to make a distinction between whether a profession exists, or if there is merely a belief on the part of the general population that it exists. Individuals in medical occupations would probably claim that they embody all or most of the criteria, and whether or not they follow them in their private lives as well may not be so relevant. In the following chapters, assessment will be made of these 'professional' elements, or constructions, and their presence in some form at all stages of the College's history (though the term profession would not have been articulated with the same nuances in earlier periods). It would seem to some extent not to matter too much whether the profession exists in reality or as a consequence of a belief system; what is important is to assess how those who followed professional occupations acted, and the role played by the institutions in shaping the work of these individuals.

An earlier assessment of the growth of the medical profession in Britain laid considerable emphasis on the relationship between professionalisation and class, and theories of structuration based on class, concluding that by the mid-twentieth century the medical profession was 'staunchly middle class'.[17] Whether or not this was the case, the College as 'collective institution' was clearly determined to be part of the changing social structure.

A claim has also been made that medical ethics were 'invented', or at least expounded in a recognisable form, by the physician John Gregory in the second half of the eighteenth century, when medicine was first described as a fiduciary profession.[18] McCullough takes the view that this 'fiduciary undertaking based on science and sympathy' was explained by Gregory in his lectures in Edinburgh in the 1760s, and that the concept of profession 'in its intellectual and moral sense' was a phenomenon of the eighteenth century.[19] Gregory emphasised that:

- the physician must be in a position to know reliably the patient's interests
- the physician should be concerned primarily with promoting the interests of the patients
- the physician should be concerned only secondarily with promoting the physician's own interests[20]

Assuming the substitution of surgeon for physician, these aspects would be somewhat more difficult to justify in a narrow sense for the earlier centuries of the College's existence. Poaching of patients from colleagues – particularly patients of high status – was not uncommon. The ethics of the seventeenth century were rather different, but the question of whether a profession can exist without a 'modern' code of ethics is difficult to assess. The evidence to be assessed in the substantive sections of the book is ambiguous at times, but not impossible to equate with ethical codes appropriate to the discourse and practices of each period.

As an example, on 18 January 1667, the College minutes note an order that:

> nather prentice nor servand sall intrud or offer to meddle or dress any patient without the master have ane lau[fu]ll call thairto by the patient or some commissionat from the patient and giff they send for two or thrie the master or servand coming first sall bruik him as his patient and nane sall offer to tak the patient out of his hands albeit the patient mak choyse of ane other (befor the first).

This was a free market, at the behest of patients, but none the less the masters and apprentices should observe the 'first come first served ethic'. The rule was there to be broken, and indeed was, and it is debatable whether this, or other acts passed against patient poaching, can be called ethics, but it was certainly in accordance with the customs of the period.

Finally, the documentation of an institution is, of course, key, but documentation is often more of an indication of intent rather than of what really happened. Important also is the changing language of documentation, in other words, the discourse of any period in the life of any longstanding instutition reflects the contemporary context, and relying on internal documentation to account for the organic development of any body is inadequate in itself, without due consideration of the general context.[21]

It is not possible in a global work of this sort to mention every individual who contributed to the life of the College over the last five centuries, nor every event. Individuals who are named are highlighted both for their own significance and, importantly, as *representative* of their contemporaries. This is particularly relevant to sections of the book which cover the modern period. The following chapters will chart the history of the College and assess the factors which shaped it and directed its actions over the last five centuries. Several major themes are covered in every chapter, though the balance of coverage reflects the particular context of each period.

In order to avoid excessive footnoting, it should be assumed that reference to the following works is implicit, where appropriate, throughout the book:

Comrie, J. D., *History of Scottish Medicine*, 2 vols (Oxford, 1932).

Craig, W. S., *History of the Royal College of Physicians of Edinburgh* (Oxford, 1976).

Creswell, C. H., *The Royal College of Surgeons of Edinburgh. Historical Notes from 1505 to 1905* (Edinburgh, 1926).

Dingwall, H. M., *A History of Scottish Medicine* (Edinburgh, 2003).

Hamilton, D., *The Healers. A History of Medicine in Scotland* (Edinburgh, 1981).

MacIntyre, I. M. C. and Maclaren, I. F., *Surgeons' Lives* (forthcoming).

Masson, A. H. B., *Portraits, Paintings and Busts in the Royal College of Surgeons of Edinburgh* (Edinburgh, 1995).

Masson, A. H. B., *A College Miscellany. An Illustrated Catalogue of Some of the Treasured Possessions of the Royal College of Surgeons of Edinburgh* (Edinburgh, 2001).

Porter, R., *The Greatest Benefit to Mankind. A Medical History of Humanity from Antiquity to the Present* (London, 1997).

## NOTES

1. College Minutes, 17 March 1978.
2. Ibid., 13 June 1671. The first recipient was Andrew Ramsay, Lord Provost of Edinburgh, on 17 October 1671.
3. These include Creswell, C. H., *The Royal College of Surgeons of Edinburgh. Historical Notes from 1505 to 1905* (Edinburgh, 1926), and Duncan, A., *Memorials of the Faculty of Physicians and Surgeons of Glasgow* (Glasgow, 1896).
4. Craig, W. S., *History of the Royal College of Physicans of Edinburgh* (Oxford, 1976); Saville, R., *The Bank of Scotland. A History* (Edinburgh, 1995); Geyer-Kordesch, J. and Macdonald, F., *Physicians and Surgeons in Glasgow. The History of the Royal College of Physicians and Surgeons of Glasgow* (Oxford, 1999); Hull, A. and Geyer-Kordesch, J., *The Shaping of the Medical Profession. The History of the Royal College of Physicians and Surgeons of Glasgow* (Oxford, 1999).
5. Lynch, M., 'Whatever happened to the medieval burgh? Some guidelines for sixteenth- and seventeenth-century historians', *Scottish Economic and Social History*, 4 (1984), pp. 5–20, discusses historical approaches to urban growth.
6. Account of early urban development in Lynch, M., Spearman, M. and Stell, G. (eds), *The*

*Scottish Medieval Town* (Edinburgh, 1988); Lynch, M. (ed.), *The Early Modern Town in Scotland* (London, 1987).

7. James Borthwick, who entered the Incorporation in 1645, represented Edinburgh at parliament in 1659–60 and in 1661; he served on the Committee for Plantation of Kirks in 1659 and on the Committee of the Estates in the same year.

8. For a recent account of Dundas, see Fry, M., *The Dundas Despotism* (Edinburgh, 1992).

9. Creswell, *Royal College of Surgeons*; Masson, A. H. B., *Portraits, Paintings and Busts in the Royal College of Surgeons of Edinburgh* (Edinburgh, 1995); Masson, A. H. B., *A College Miscellany. An Illustrated Catalogue of Some of the Treasured Possessions of the Royal College of Surgeons of Edinburgh* (Edinburgh, 2001); Macintyre, I. M. C. and MacLaren, I. F., *Surgeons' Lives* (forthcoming).

10. Jordanova, L.,'The social construction of medical knowledge', *Social History of Medicine*, 8 (3) (1995), pp. 361–83.

11. Habermas, J., *The Structural Transformation of the Public Sphere. An Inquiry into a Category of Bourgeois Society*, trans. Burger, T. (Cambridge, 1989). See also Broman, T., 'The Habermasian public sphere and "science" "in" the Enlightenment', *History of Science*, 36 (2) (1998), pp. 123–49.

12. Sturdy, S., 'Introduction: medicine, health and the public sphere', in S. Sturdy, (ed.), *Medicine, Health and the Public Sphere in Britain 1600–2000* (London, 2002), p. 4.

13. de Certeau, M., *The Writing of History*, trans. Corley, T. (New York, 1988), p. 64.

14. Burnham, J. C., 'How the concept of profession evolved in the work of historians of medicine', *Bull. Hist. Med.*, 70 (1996), p. 23.

15. Buchanan, A. E., 'Is there a medical profession in the house?', in R. G. Spece, D. S. Shimm and A. E. Buchanan (eds), *Conflicts of Interest in Clinical Practice and Research* (Oxford, 1996), p. 107.

16. Ibid., p. 109.

17. Parry, N. and Parry, J., *The Rise of the Medical Profession. A Study of Collective Social Mobility* (London, 1976), p. 255.

18. McCullough, L. B., *John Gregory and the Invention of Professional Medical Ethics and the Profession of Medicine* (London, 1998), p. 5.

19. Ibid., p. 4.

20. Ibid., p. 5. See also Torstendahl, R., 'Introduction: promotion and strategies of knowledge-based groups', in M. Burrage and R. Torstendahl (eds), *Professions in Theory and History* (London, 1980), pp. 1–10, which discusses the notion of professional bodies as 'groups based on a shared problem-solving knowledge'.

21. White, H., *The Content of the Form. Narrative Discourse and Historical Representation* (Baltimore, 1987).

2

# Origins and early years, 1505–1581

We ar and ever was of gude mynde till do this gude tovne all the staid
pleasour and seruice that we can.[1]

## GENERAL HISTORICAL BACKGROUND

The early history of the Incorporation needs to be traced deep in late-
medieval Scotland. By the start of the sixteenth century the boundaries of
the nation had been established, more or less; the Stewart dynasty had a
fairly secure grip on the throne, despite the fact that few of the incumbents managed to die in their beds; trading and cultural contacts with mainland Europe were
well established; burghs were growing in size and importance, particularly the
Royal Burghs and even more particularly Edinburgh; the highlands continued to
be a thorn in the side of Scottish kings (though highland culture was in some ways
much more sophisticated than that of the lowlands); and tensions with England
continued. Scottish society was still arranged along feudal lines and stratified into
ranks or stations in a complex hierarchy of domination, deference and dependence.
Whether or not there was any sort of cohesive view of national identity is quite
another matter, but at the time the Edinburgh barbers and surgeons made the first
moves towards incorporation, the country was relatively stable, though this would
not last long.[2] The Reformation in 1560 altered the religious profile of the country
as well as of the young Incorporation, and following the Union of the Crowns in
1603, Scotland was forced to look south as well as towards Europe. This was also
the period of the Renaissance and the emergence of humanist philosophies.[3] The
longstanding, strong cultural and trading links between Europe and Scotland
allowed the easy passage of philosophy and culture as well as wood, iron, luxury
consumer goods and exotic ingredients for medicines.[4]

### Medicine and surgery in earlier times

Medical care and treatment in medieval and early-modern Scotland were based on
the long-held humoral view of bodily functions and malfunctions as articulated in
the Western medical tradition, which evolved from the philosophy and practice of
Hippocrates and Galen, although there is evidence that elements of the Arabic
tradition of Avicenna and others were incorporated.[5] Life cycles were very much in

line with the natural cycle, and treatments based on seasonal and astrological factors as well as Galenic remedies, which themselves were derived from natural plant or animal substances. Belief in the supernatural was quite natural, and the surgeons of Edinburgh were no different. They were all individuals of their own time, shaped and influenced by factors of their own time – and this would of course be the case as times and centuries changed during the next 500 years. Extending the horizons of medical knowledge had been hampered to a great extent by the long period of influence of the medieval Roman Catholic church. Illness and disease were considered to be just reward for sin, and medical care, usually offered by monastic communities such as that at Soutra,[6] related more to symptom control and preparing the soul for death rather than assessing physical causes and cures or trying new treatments. Medieval medicine was part of medieval hospitality in its widest sense, rather than medical treatment in the more modern sense. What was required, if real progress were to be made, was separation of medicine from the sphere of the church. In other words, secularisation was a necessary precursor to change. This process gathered pace in 1163 when a Papal Bull, *Ecclesia abhorret a sanguine*, banned monks from letting blood or performing surgical procedures. From that point medicine was taught in European universities and Scottish medical students began to hollow out the path to Europe to acquire medical training, as well as for the traditional cultural experience of the gentleman.

Surgery continued to be primitive, restricted by lack of anatomical knowledge and the means to control pain and infection. It was also practised by individuals from all walks of life, from gardeners to ministers. It is difficult to make any sort of reliable claims about numbers of surgeons or other practitioners in Edinburgh, or in Scotland as a whole, before this time, but it is fairly safe to conclude that there were few, and that most of these operated in the burghs, at least in burghs which were of a sufficient size to accommodate any sort of craft element within their socio-economic structures. The accounts of the Lord High Treasurer in 1473 note the payment of 11s to 'McMwlane the barbour at the Kingis command . . . for the leichcraft done be him to the litil boys of the Chalmire';[7] while a year later 'Stephen, potinger'[8] was reimbursed for 'certane materials and potingaris deliuerit be him to the King', and apothecary William Fouler received payments from the customs revenues of Edinburgh on several occasions between 1502 and 1507.[9] The first mention of a surgical note in the burgh records came in 1451, when '. . . Aitkyne, barber [was] made burges at the instance of our Lady the Queen, without payment'.[10]

Whatever the number of Edinburgh surgeons, what they could do was both primitive and also done by many other people. Their work was concerned mainly with the effects of conflict, either in wartime or local feud, workplace accident and the ulcers and infections which resulted from many of these injuries. They had little real anatomical knowledge, few instruments, even fewer books, no hospitals (in the modern sense) and no anaesthetics (again in the modern sense, though attempts were made to numb the senses with alcohol or herbal potions). There was also no clear demarcation among surgeon, apothecary and physician, and no real difference between the treatments prescribed by 'qualified' practitioners, amateur healers, wise women or even wise men. There is considerable evidence from non-written sources that during the period of the Roman occupation of parts of Scotland, sophisticated medicine and surgery had been practised,[11] but once the Roman influence faded and grip of the medieval church took hold, there was a long period of stagnation, both in medical knowledge and the development of new treatments or secular institutions. The title of one of the chapters in Comrie's *History of Scottish Medicine* is 'Medical renaissance in the time of James IV'.[12] This title is apt, as it encapsulates two factors which influenced the foundation of the Incorporation (in addition to urbanisation) – a renewed, secular interest in medicine, science and philosophy, and royal interest in these areas.

As the population of Edinburgh grew, there were, naturally, more and more individuals carrying out manual trade occupations, and groups of these began from the third quarter of the fifteenth century to request rights of incorporation and demarcation in order to preserve their territory and status within the urban setting. Comrie describes this as the 'rise of democracy', but this is rather anachronistic, as there was little democracy in the modern sense of the term.[13] Though Comrie also claims that there was a guild of barbers in operation before 1451, citing the evidence of the burgess ticket granted to Aitkyne, this cannot be substantiated fully. The reference to the Guild may well have been the merchant guild, as it was not unknown for craftsmen to be admitted to the merchants' guild, particularly at the request of high-status patrons. Whatever the case, the hatmakers were the first to achieve incorporation, their charter being issued on 18 February 1474, and they were followed in the next few years by the skinners, wrights and masons, websters (weavers), hammermen (incorporating most metal trades), fleshers, coopers (barrel makers), waulkers (a process for softening cloth) and tailors. The surgeons and barbers were the tenth group to seek incorporation.[14] Most of these groups were formed initially as religious and friendly societies, offering support for destitute members and supporting altars in the parish church of St Giles' as well as maintaining occupational demarcation. In seeking similar status, the Edinburgh surgeons and barbers were following a trend; they may not as yet have articulated aims and objectives which would be seen nowadays as professional, but the resulting Seal of Cause was the beginning of organised surgery in Scotland. This is not necessarily to take a Whiggish view; it is not to claim that surgery ceased to be performed by individuals with no institutional affiliation; and it is not to claim that surgeons thereafter acted in ways which would now be regarded as professional; it is simply to note that from that point there has been a surgical organisation in Edinburgh. Its existence was threatened on a number of occasions, but it did survive. The early aims may not necessarily have been to further the cause of surgery – the major impetus was probably, and simply, the consequence of burgh expansion and the relationships between groups of craftsmen and those who had no training or qualification.[15] It may be seen in terms of Jordanova's views on the social construction of medicine in its widest sense – the need to organise stimulated by the wish to preserve status within the burgh environment.

It was against this general background that the surgeons and barbers of

Edinburgh began the process of incorporation. It is impossible to speculate as to how many practitioners of any branch of medicine were resident in Edinburgh before 1500; the numbers cannot have been large, but there must have been sufficient barbers and surgeons in residence to warrant an application to the Town Council for an exclusive charter, with all its attendant financial burdens as well as corporate privileges. It is fairly safe to assume that the majority of these would be barbers rather than surgeons, though there was little real distinction at that point. This chapter will, therefore, consider the important early years of the development of the Incorporation in its own context – that of late-medieval Scotland.

### Royal interest in medicine and surgery

Within the context of the trend towards the creation of exclusive trade organisations, the Edinburgh surgeons were fortunate enough to seek incorporation during the reign of James IV, a monarch well versed in many subjects and particularly interested in scientific and medical matters. A true 'Renaissance man', James' medical interests have also been ascribed to tradition by Buchanan, who stated that the king 'greedily imbibed an ancient custom of the nobility, for he was skilful in curing wounds',[16] and had allegedly performed surgical and dental operations. Accounts for the royal household contain a number of entries for payments to individuals who had received medical treatment at the instigation or under the personal knife of the monarch. One such case records payment of 2s for the cost of dressings to John Balfour's 'sair leg quhilk the King helit'.[17] It was occasionally profitable for suffering members of the public to submit themselves to royal tooth-pulling, as the king authorised payments to be made to the patients for allowing him to attend to their dental treatment; one volunteer received a monetary reward on account of his having had 'twa teeth drawen furth of his heid be the king'.[18] The king was described as 'well learned in the art of medicine and also a cunning Chirurgener that none in his realm that used that craft but would take his counsel in all their proceedings'.[19]

James IV was also alleged to have undertaken 'scientific research', with the reported instance of his sending of a dumb woman to Inchkeith with two young children, in order to ascertain 'quhat langage thir bairnis wald speik quhene they come to lauchfull aige'; while there is slightly better evidence that conjoined twins, born around 1490, were brought up in the royal court, and survived to the age of 28, when it is claimed that one died some time before the other, which was 'dollorous and heavy to the langest levar'.[20]

As well as his interests in medicine, surgery and dentistry, James had a keen interest in alchemy, a pursuit that would be continued for some time to come, and occupy the interests of Isaac Newton, the foremost 'scientist' of the seventeenth century. This interest may have been stimulated by the more practical matter of the chronic shortage of funds in the royal coffers, but whatever the case, James was well acquainted with medicine and surgery, and this would be of considerable benefit to the Edinburgh barbers and surgeons.

A number of individuals have been identified as providing some sort of medical service to the royal house around this time. These included Thomas Leich, William May, George Leich, Duncan May and James Watson (surgeon to James V) – the surname Leich taken as reflecting a family connection or association with medical treatment of some sort. There is no direct evidence that any of these individuals had Edinburgh connections, but it is likely that they spent time in the burgh during their attendance on the peripatetic royal households.[21]

What is also fairly clear from the early evidence is that surgeons were 'retained' by the Town Council to provide treatments and assessments on specific occasions, particularly in legal cases, though it is also clear that many individuals of status chose either to go abroad for treatment, or to send for a foreign surgeon or physician. In March 1580 no less than seven surgeons appeared before the Town Council to given their opinion on the wounds sustained in an attack by Robert Asbowane. It was concluded that the victim was not in mortal danger, and his assailants were freed on payment of fines of 5,000 merks.[22]

### Famous names

Although the 'names and places' or 'great doctors' approach to the history of medicine is now largely outdated, none the less each era was notable for a number of significant individuals of whom more is known than of other, more anonymous, practitioners, and it seems appropriate therefore to highlight a few of these. In the early period the first 'great name' that appears is probably that of Gilbert Primrose, who embodied many of the attributes and contextual stimuli of the sixteenth century. Ancestor of the Rosebery family, Primrose was untypical, in that he came from a relatively high social rank. He was acquainted with Peter Lowe, author of a famous surgical textbook and co-founder of the Faculty of Physicians and Surgeons of Glasgow;[23] he was deacon of the Incorporation in 1581 when the written records began; he was a royal surgeon, and indeed was in the southbound entourage of James VI in 1603, being appointed surgeon to the royal household in London.[24] Like a number of his contemporaries, Primrose's high social status and connections with royalty helped to enhance both his own prestige and, by inference, that of the Incorporation. Status and connections were invaluable assets to any aspirant surgeon. Patronage was crucial and came in many forms, directly and indirectly, and it does seem that the Edinburgh surgeons were able to secure a higher position in the early-modern medical hierarchy than did surgeons elsewhere.[25]

Primrose's contemporary, John Naysmith, was also prominent in the Incorporation as well as being surgeon to James VI, and indeed had been apprenticed to Primrose. Naysmith served as boxmaster on one occasion, and quartermaster on six, but he is perhaps more famous for his apparently pragmatic political exploits in the reigns of Mary, Queen of Scots and her son James VI. He was involved in delivering secret letters to Mary, Queen of Scots in 1575, but was apparently with the King on the occasion of the Gowrie plot in 1600.[26] At the Union of the Crowns in 1603 he travelled south and was appointed Royal Herbalist for life – which perhaps

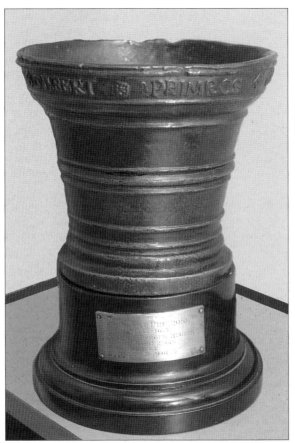

**FIG. 2.1** *Replica of mortar of Gilbert Primrose,*
*presented to the College by the*
*Rosebery family.*

explains why he only served as Deacon on one occasion.[27] During his London service, he attended Prince Henry during his fatal illness. Of more practical service to the burgh were Robert Henryson, one of a surgical dynasty of Henrysons, who was appointed to advise the Town Council on appropriate measures to deal with outbreaks of plague, and his son James, who was employed as surgeon to the poor in 1589.

It is clear then that the most prominent, or most identifiable, surgeons of the early days had strong royal connections as well as being active within the Incorporation, or were members of longstanding surgical families. The visual symbolism of an Edinburgh surgeon attending the monarch in the more refined ambience of the London court must have been powerful, and the high social rank held by some (and the literacy of all) added to this image. Whether or not this was the image held by the general population is another matter entirely. At this point there was no real repute for surgical skills, given the primitive nature and limited possibilities of late-medieval surgical practice.

## EARLIEST EVIDENCE

The earliest manuscript in the possession of the College dates from 1466, but does not have any obvious connection with the College. It is a a notarial instrument of 1 June 1466, whereby notary Richard Congilton 'notarises the lawful resignation of the superiority of land and a tenement in the constabulary of Haddington and the barony of Dirleton . . . to George Lord Haliburton'. There is no immediate link with the early history of the College, but it may have belonged to an ancestor of a future master of the Incorporation. The earliest evidence concerning plans for Incorporation appears to be a document dated 24 April 1504. This gave permission for the 'kirkmaister and ouersman [overman] of the barberis to have yr diuine service at St Mongos [Mungo's] alter of St Bryde in St Giles Kirk and St Mongow to be yr patron'.[28] This request was entirely in line with current practice. St Giles' was the parish church, and most crafts maintained altars dedicated to their respective saints and patrons, at which regular masses were offered on behalf of members and their deceased colleagues and relatives. Members of the crafts made weekly contributions towards the maintenance of the altar and the saying of the masses. This corporate religious focus was also manifested annually in Corpus Christi processions and other public religious observances and displays, at which the Incorporation banner was paraded as a mark of corporate indentity and saintly patronage. By the time of the Reformation in 1560, when such occasions were quickly outlawed, the surgeons had been incorporated for fifty-five years.

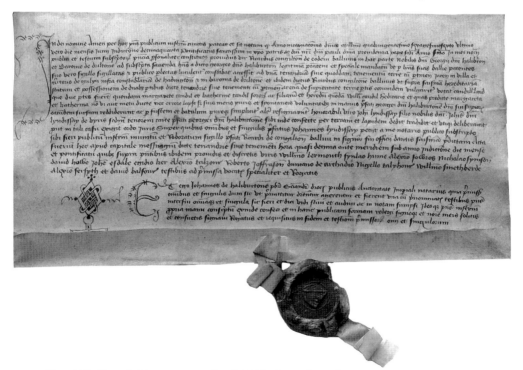

**FIG. 2.2** *Notarial instrument, dated 1466, the earliest document in the possession of the College.*

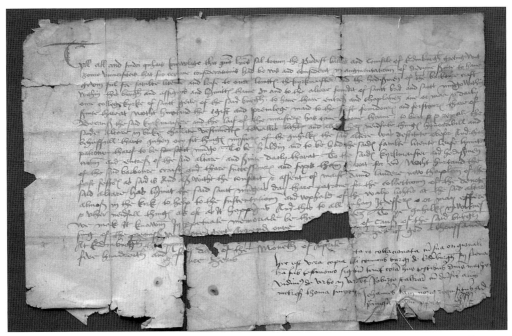

*FIG. 2.3* *Document dated 25 April 1504, giving permission for the kirkmaister and brethren to hold services at St Mungo's altar in St Giles'.*

The Reformation and its attendant upheavals were, however, in the future. On 1 July 1505, the Edinburgh Town Council considered a petition which it had received from the barbers and surgeons, craving a charter of incorporation. Following some discussion, during which the Council had been 'ryplie and distinctlie avysit [advised]',[29] perhaps by a writer (lawyer) or notary, it was decided that the document should be accepted without amendment, as the proposals it contained were deemed to contain 'na hurt to oure Soueraine Lordis hienes, vs, nor nane vtheris his leigis.' The charter was ratified by James IV the following year, the relevant entry in the Register of the Privy Seal dated 13 October 1506, stating that the King 'ratifieand and approvand ye status & rewlis maid amangst thame anent ye ser[vi]cing of ye kings leigis & upholden of yr alter in Saint Geilis Kirk' (see Appendix II for the full text of the Ratification).

### The Seal of Cause

The outcome of the petition to the Town Council was the Seal of Cause (see Appendix I for the full text), which laid out clearly the terms and conditions under which the surgeons and barbers would be allowed to operate as an incorporation. Sadly the original document no longer exists, although the text is copied in the records of the Town Council.[30] Superficially the document differs little from similar charters of incorporation issued to other groups of craftsmen. It was ordained that the altar already present in St Giles' should be maintained and that new entrants

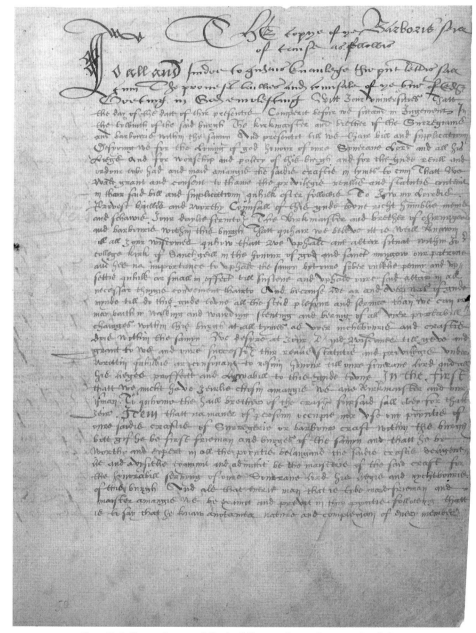

*FIG. 2.4 Part of copy of Seal of Cause, from the records of the
Town Council of Edinburgh.*

would be obliged to take the customary oath of obedience to the charter (though
post-Reformation members were not required to make such religious promises, the
stipulation being that entrants would swear to maintain the tenets of the Seal of
Cause 'excepting idolatry contenit thairintill'). However, the Seal of Cause had an
extra dimension, and three aspects must be regarded as being of particular significance: literacy, training and examinations.

Literacy would seem to be an essential prerequisite for any branch of learning. At the end of the fifteenth century, though, basic literacy levels in the general population were low; the Reformation would offer a boost to Scottish education (the *First Book of Discipline* recommending the establishment of a school in every parish in Scotland), but the inclusion of a literacy clause in the surgeons' and barbers' Seal of Cause was important.[31] The charter states that 'na maisters of the said craft sall tak ane prentis or feit man in tyme cuming to vse the Surregeane craft without he can baith wryte and reid'. If the apprentices were to benefit from an academic aspect to their training, fulfilment of this requirement was crucial. There is evidence from later minute entries that apprentices were expected to be literate not only in the vernacular, but also in Latin, and that formal testing of their abilities was carried out. Individuals with suspect competence in Latin language and grammar were ordered to be tested by the Clerk to the Incorporation, who was generally a writer and clearly well-drilled in the Latin tongue. One unprepared apprentice was remitted to his books as he was deemed 'deficient in thair pairtes of gramer',[32] and another was ordered to be re-tested as he had not demonstrated adequate abilities in 'interpretting some pairt of ane lattine authoure which is accustomed to be learned with the gramer'.[33]

This vital pre-apprenticeship qualification was never relaxed by the Edinburgh surgeons, in contrast to the situation in London, where the Company of Barber Surgeons drafted a similar rule in 1556 but within a month had rescinded the move. It was decided in July of that year that 'no barber surgeon that doth occupy the mystery of surgery in the Clothing (Company) or out of the Clothing shall take or have any prentice but that he can skill of the Latine tongue and understand the same and can write and read sufficiently'.[34] However, only a few weeks later it was decreed that a master could engage an apprentice 'though he may not be learned in the Lating tongue'.[35] The regulation was eventually reintroduced in 1727, but this seems to be one instance where it is acceptable to claim the beneficial effects of the deep-rooted Scottish regard for learning and education in all its aspects. The majority of surgical apprentices in Edinburgh were not of high social rank, and though regulations are there to be broken it does seem that most had at least a reasonable grasp of Latin and could read and write in the vernacular.

Insistence on apprenticeship literacy ensured that aspirant surgeons were able to read the books which were available, initially in the hands of the master surgeons and later in the Incorporation library, following its establishment in 1699. One very early example of the acquisition of books comes, perhaps surprisingly, from the testament of an Edinburgh physician. Dr John Chisholm stipulated in his will, dated 1577, that his medical books and instruments currently in Scotland and France should be given to one of his surgical acquaintances, William Bisset.[36] The surgeon in turn, in his own will, passed at least one of these books on to Robert Henryson, fellow member of the Incorporation.[37] This volume was, significantly, 'his greit buik of medicine callit Ambroise Parre' – the surgical techniques of the eminent French surgeon Ambroise Paré were clearly available to at least some of the surgeons of Edinburgh.[38]

The Seal of Cause also laid down requirements as to anatomical teaching, fully regulated apprenticeships, and examinations, which are considered in detail in subsequent chapters. Instructions regarding anatomical instruction and examinations were brief and vague, but the crucial factor is that they were there. The Seal of Cause granted to the FPSG in 1599 did not contain this sort of exhortation, though in 1540 the London Barbers were authorised to 'have and take without c[on]tradiction foure persons condemned adjudged and put to death for feloni . . . And to make incisione of the same deade bodies . . . for their further and better knowledge instruction in sight learning and experience in the sayd scyence or faculties of surgery'.[39] Since the revolution in anatomical studies that would be engendered by the work of Andreas Vesalius was several decades in the future (his seminal work, *De Fabrica Corporis Humani*, was not published until 1543),[40] those who drafted the Seal of Cause must be credited with a degree of foresight.

The third aspect of the Seal of Cause which set it apart from other craft charters concerned examinations. Apprentices in most crafts were obliged to submit an essay at the end of their period of employment – indeed one apprentice hammerman was asked to prepare a number of surgical instruments, including a trepan and a 'dismembering saw for the leg'[41] – but this was a little different from the oral and practical examinations undertaken by surgical trainees. Once again the terms of the Seal of Cause are vague but important; it was stipulated that each entrant master should be 'diligently and avisitly examinit and previt' in anatomy, particularly of the veins, and also astrological signs, though the claim that the Incorporation was given 'a monopoly over the study of astrological signs and observations' is a little overdrawn.[42] However vague, though, the complex examination system operated by the College in modern times owes something to these humble origins, however the dedicated postmodernist might object.

The Seal of Cause may therefore be seen as something of an early blueprint for surgical training in Edinburgh, whether or not that was one of the primary aims of the applicants. Most of the subsequent developments in organisation, training and examinations can be traced back to these apparently simple clauses in a craft charter. The highly specialised courses on surgical techniques which are organised by the College today comply fully with the view put forward five centuries ago, that each surgeon 'must knaw the nature and substance of everything that he werkes, or ellis he is negligent'. What is different in the twenty-first century is that 'everything he werkes' is specialised and detailed to an extent that could not have been imagined half a millennium ago, and shaped by very different influences.

## THE EARLY YEARS OF THE INCORPORATION

No written Incorporation records have survived before 1581 apart from a few fragments, but the minute books are continuous thereafter. It may be that the early records were lost, or that no formal minutes were kept by the founding masters; whatever the reason, any conclusions as to numbers of members or their activities can only be speculative. It is also reasonable to assume, though, that the content of any pre-1581 records would not have been so very different from the earliest surviving accounts. It would have been instructive, though, to have known the background to the exemption from bearing arms granted by Mary, Queen of Scots in 1567, a mere two months before the beginning of the end of her traumatic, difficult and historically controversial reign. This exemption excused the surgeons and barbers from taking up arms, on condition that they treated the wounded of both sides in any armed conflict. It was considered that 'cunyng men of the occupatioun and craft of chyrurgianrie ar als necessar to be within this realme as in vthir partis', and also that excusal would give them the opportunity to 'studie the perfection of the said craft and occupatioun to the vttermost of their ingynis'.[43]

Fragments of detail appear, sometimes in odd places, which give glimpses of Edinburgh surgeons and their work, but these are no more than fragments. Four surgeons were paid £12 in 1542 for 'curing of all persons that happent to be hurte be Inglis menne'; and in the same year Anthony Brussat received £20 for 'labouris done be him to the Queens grace' (Mary of Guise, mother of Mary, Queen of Scots).[44] One of the more curious examples is that of Robert Henryson, who received 20 merks in 1563 for curing 'a dead woman raised forth of the grave after she had been lying two days in the same'.[45] The high level of general background violence at this time influenced the nature of general surgery just as much as did the lack of anaesthetics or antiseptics. In February 1577, James Wauchlott was given 'the sowme of thre pundis for curing and mending of James Hendersonis leg in the townys service at the taiking of Ramsay their quha was slane in the taiking',[46] while in 1579 John Lawson 'maid faithe that Nicoll Haistie, cordiner [shoemaker] is in na daynger of his lyfe of the hurt and wound gevin him by Thomas Crawford'.[47]

Indication that the Incorporation was taking care of its right to brew aqua vitae under the terms of the Seal of Cause comes from a number of manuscript documents, including one dated 20 November 1561, which reports that 'the qlk day in presens of the provest baillies and councale comperit Jhonne Weire at the west porte and actit himself of his awin consent for Elizat Weir ye spous of Bartilmo Weire yat yai in na tyme cuming sall brew tap or sell ony aquavite within ye friedome of his burgh'. This was a potentially lucrative monopoly and it was to the advantage of the Incorporation to guard its interests well. The records say virtually nothing about the brewing operations; the minuted concerns were with demarcation in this area just as much as in surgery. There is little mention in the records thereafter about aqua vitae, and it is not clear how or when the Incorporation lost the monopoly, but it was clearly a worthwhile enterprise in the early years.

Numbers of surgeons and barbers in the early years are difficult to determine. There are no noted signatories to the petition to the Town Council for the Seal of Cause, and the main numerical evidence before 1581 comes from a list of surgeons, barbers and apprentices drawn up in 1558 at the request of the Town Council, which wished to assess the numbers of able-bodied men who could be drawn from the craft organisations to help with town defences in the event of an attack by 'our auld inemyes of Ingland'.[48] A total of twenty-seven is listed on behalf of the Incorporation, including Gilbert Primrose, but it is difficult to determine how many of these were apprentices and how many were master surgeons or barbers at that point. The figure is slightly at variance with that given by Maitland, who notes thirteen masters and twelve men. Perhaps the most salient point is that the numbers of barbers and surgeons were low as compared to other crafts, such as the total of 178 tailors, 151 hammermen, 100 bakers and even 53 bonnetmakers. Only the goldsmiths mustered fewer men than the Incorporation.[49]

There is some scattered documentary evidence that attempts were made from the beginning to stamp out unauthorised practice, both in surgery and in the potentially lucrative operation of brewing of aqua vitae. In August 1575 a general complaint was registered against the apothecaries, who 'daillie usit and exercisit yt said craft [surgery]',[50] while in 1568 a protestation was made about a barber's 'curing of certain hurt men'.[51] A few years later, in 1576, Bessie Abernethie was ordered 'to desist and ceis fra making of aquavite in all tyme coming wtout ye speciall licence of the dekyn of ye chirurgeans and barbourcraft', and on the same day sword slipper James Hunter was prohibited from 'all using or applying of emplasters salvis, medicaments or uther thinge perteinyng to ye craft of chirurgenrie under the pane of 40 shillings'.[52] It is clear that in the period before the commencement of the Incorporation's minute books, efforts were being made to preserve the new privileges and prevent any unlicensed individual practising surgery or brewing aqua vitae. This is entirely consonant with the activities of such groups, whose major purpose immediately after their foundation was to assert their newly acquired privileges and demarcations. It was not easy to persuade other individuals to cease what may well have been lucrative activities, which had been deemed acceptable by those who submitted themselves for treatment.

## EARLY ORGANISATION ELSEWHERE

Because of the need for sufficient numbers in order to sustain an incorporation of any sort, it was only in Edinburgh and Glasgow that lasting groups were able to be formed and survive in Scotland at this time. There is some evidence of an organisation of sorts in Dundee but this was not a formal grouping.[53] In Aberdeen a group of barbers and surgeons received a Seal of Cause from the Town Council in 1537, but was not recognised as one of the seven major trades in the town. After 1647, when privileges were ratified, the group appears to have contained only barbers and wigmakers, the surgeons thereafter having no formal organisation, though being obliged to take out a burgess ticket before being allowed to practise in the burgh.[54] The only other Scottish burgh with significant organisations was Glasgow, where a unique institution combining physicians and surgeons was founded in 1599 (see Chapter 3).

Incorporations were formed rather earlier elsewhere, though some were connected to universities rather than being craft guilds, and in some parts of Europe there was not such a clear distinction or demarcation between physician and surgeon. In thirteenth-century Sicily, for example, the king's licence to practise medicine could only be obtained after a lengthy course which included the study of surgery, and in Italy surgery was taught alongside medicine in the universities.[55] In Italy, although there were early universities such as Salerno, where there was a flourishing medical school in the twelfth and thirteenth centuries, to which female students and staff were admitted,[56] surgical provision and organisation by the fifteenth century were similar to those in other parts of Europe in general terms. The controlling hierarchies were distinctive, though. In the kingdom of Naples, for example, it has been shown recently that the medical marketplace was just as open and diverse as it was in Scotland, and just as the French royal surgeon would have considerable powers over surgery in general, the Neapolitan Protomedicato – a committee headed by the royal physician – controlled medical and surgical practice.[57]

The College of St Côme was founded in Paris in 1268 by Louis IX, who had a particular interest in surgery, as would James IV nearly three centuries later. Its members were divided into long-gowned and short-gowned, and only those entitled to desport the longer garment were permitted to carry out surgical procedures. By the start of the seventeenth century there was a complex interaction among the main French surgical divisions, which had been 'grouped into various legally recognised collectivities'.[58] The hybrid barber-surgeon did not feature in France to the same extent as in Scotland, England, Ireland or Germany.

By 1308 the London barbers had an organisation, and in 1446 Henry VI established the Fraternity or Guild of Barbers in Dublin (a further charter was granted to the Dublin barbers by Elizabeth 1 in 1572).[59] The key with all of these, as in Edinburgh, seems to have been royal interest and approval, though in the case of Edinburgh the royal confirmation came secondary to the Town Council charter. The first master of the London Company of Barbers was elected in 1308, at a time when Edinburgh was small in size and population and could not have supported such an organisation, even if one had been desired. Around the same time a Fellowship of Surgeons seems to have appeared in London also, but without sufficient numbers to form a guild or livery company. By 1462 the London barbers had achieved a charter of incorporation; in 1463 agreement was reached that barbers would not perform surgical procedures except pulling teeth, and in return the surgeons undertook not to offer barbering services.[60] Royal support continued, and a new charter was issued by Henry VIII, the relationship being immortalised in the famous Holbein painting of Henry with the assembled London Barbers. Finally, in 1540, some thirty-five years after the foundation of the Edinburgh Incorporation, the London barbers and surgeons united under a new charter. The Edinburgh Incorporation was therefore fairly typical of the 'British' incorporations, though different in nature from those on the continent of Europe.

The main point in all of this is that the Edinburgh Incorporation, though organised and founded rather differently from organisations in Europe, operated in the same sort of complex and open medical marketplace. The major difference, perhaps, is that the royal influence, which was just as essential in Edinburgh as elsewhere, helped to set up the Incorporation rather than direct its future operations and activities. Scotland certainly had royal surgeons, and many masters of the

Incorporation would serve successive monarchs in the royal household or on the battlefield, but they did not wield powers over the organisation and delivery of surgery in general.

## CONCLUSION

The origins of the Incorporation owed much to the general background of the period. Just as other groups had done, the barbers and surgeons wished to have exclusive rights to perform surgery and to have the powers to prosecute individuals who persisted in operating outwith these boundaries. Demarcation was difficult in an age when everyone treated his or her own diseases as far as possible, and when it was decided to consult a 'practitioner', the first choice was more likely to be an amateur healer than a 'professional' surgeon or physician. However, that was not the only initiating force. By 1505 the secularisation of medicine and medical training had begun to produce anatomical knowledge that was a little more reliable than that extrapolated from the dissection of animals. The apprenticeship system was well founded in many trades. Surgical treatises were in existence – even in the highlands of Scotland the Gaelic physicians had translations of Greek, Roman and Arabic medical texts,[61] and most of the ingredients for exclusivity were there, in however primitive a form they may have been at the time. It is difficult to assess any element of altruism or professionalism in all of this. It is true that often the reason given for the setting up of any organisation of this nature was to 'better serve the kingis liedgis', or to prevent tragedies caused by untrained practitioners, but this was only one of a number of causal circumstances. Whatever the case, by the time that its records began, the Incorporation already possessed many of the attributes and characteristics which would be sustained and developed, and, importantly, recorded in the minute books and other documentation. The next chapter will consider the major consolidation phase for the incorporation.

## NOTES

1. From the Seal of Cause granted to the barbers and surgeons of Edinburgh by the Town Council on 1 July 1505. The full text is reproduced in Appendix I.
2. For general accounts of medieval and early-modern Scotland see Barrell, A. D. M., *Medieval Scotland* (Cambridge, 2000); Mitchison, R., *Lordship to Patronage, Scotland 1603–1745* (London, 1983); Wormald, J., *Court, Kirk and Community, Scotland 1470–1625* (London, 1981).
3. For a scholarly account of humanism in Scotland see MacQueen, J. (ed.), *Humanism in Renaissance Scotland* (Edinburgh, 1990).
4. The contents of some Edinburgh apothecaries' shops are described in Dingwall, H. M., 'Making up the medicine: apothecaries in sixteenth- and seventeenth-century Edinburgh', *Caduceus*, 10 (3) (1994), pp. 121–30.
5. For a more detailed account of the emergence of Western Medicine see Porter, *Greatest Benefit*, pp. 6–8, 39–41; also Conrad, L. L. et al., *The Western Medical Tradition 800BC–1800AD* (Cambridge, 1995); Loudon, I. (ed.), *Western Medicine* (Oxford, 1997). For early Scotland see Comrie, *History*, i, pp. 25–105; Dingwall, *History of Scottish Medicine*, pp. 23–38; Hamilton, *The Healers*, pp. 1–40.

6. Moffat, B., 'SHARP practice. The search for medieval medical treatments', *Archaeology Today*, 8 (1987), pp. 22–8, discusses findings from excavations at Soutra. See also the ongoing series of reports by the Scottish Archaeoethnomorphological Group, published annually under the title *Sharp Practice*.

7. Dickson, T. and Paul, J. B. (eds), *Accounts of the Lord High Treasurer of Scotland* (Edinburgh, 1877–1916), i, p. 68.

8. 'Stephen' is also recorded as being granted a house and booth in the Bellhouse, 'sa that he may be enterit thairintil and vse the samin with his materiall and spisery'. Quoted in Comrie, *History*, i, p. 145.

9. Stuart, J. et al. (eds), *The Exchequer Rolls of Scotland* (Edinburgh, 1878–1908), xii, pp. 90, 163, 242, 464, 594.

10. *Burgh Recs*, 12 May 1451. The Queen at the time was Mary of Gueldres, whom James II had married in 1449.

11. Dingwall, *Scottish Medicine*, pp. 26–7; see also Comrie, *History*, i, pp. 33–5 for illustrations of Roman surgical instruments; Porter, *Greatest Benefit*, pp. 69–82.

12. Comrie, *History*, i, pp. 142–64.

13. Ibid., p. 145.

14. For detailed narrative of the Edinburgh incorporations see, for example, Colston, J., *The Incorporated Trades of Edinburgh* (Edinburgh, 1891).

15. For an account of early-modern Scottish burgh structures, see Lynch, *Early Modern Town in Scotland*.

16. Quoted in Comrie, *History*, i, p. 49.

17. Guthrie, D., 'The medical and scientific exploits of King James IV of Scotland', *BMJ*, 30 June 1953, p. 1191. See also Short, A. I. and Lennard, T. W. J., *James IV of Scotland, Sovereign and Surgeon*, occasional paper (The Durham Thomas Harriot Seminar) no. 7 (Durham, 1992); Short, A. I. and Lennard, T. W. J., 'James IV of Scotland: monarchy and medicine', *Journal of Medical Biography*, 1 (1993), pp. 175–85.

18. Accounts of the Lord High Treasurer, quoted in Comrie, *History*, i, p. 152. Fuller details of James's medical and scientific exploits in Comrie, pp. 151–7.

19. For a scholarly account of James IV's reign, see Macdougall, N., *James IV* (Edinburgh, 1989).

20. From Lindsay of Pitscottie's account, quoted in Comrie, *History*, i, p. 150. It was claimed that the children 'spak goode hebrew', and that the conjoined twins 'could play and sing in tuo pairtis, the on the tribill the wther the tennour quhilk was werie dulse and melodious to heir'.

21. Comrie, *History*, i, p. 165.

22. Ibid., pp. 172–3.

23. Lowe, P., *A Discourse of the Whole Art of Chirurgerie* (London, 1597) and several subsequent editions.

24. Comrie, *History*, i, pp. 175–6. In addition to his terms as Deacon, Primrose acted as quartermaster on two occasions.

25. Hamilton, *Healers*, p. 61.

26. See the account of the Gowrie plot in Lynch, *Scotland. A New History* (London, 1991), p. 232.

27. Comrie, *History*, i, pp. 176–7.

28. College Business Papers, 24 April 1504.

29. *Burgh Recs*, 1 July 1505.

30. Photograph of the copy of the Seal of Cause in the Town Council records, Comrie, *History*, i, pp. 160–1.

31. Studies of literacy in the general population include Houston, R. A., *Scottish Literacy and the Scottish Identity. Illiteracy and Society in Scotland and Northern England 1600–1800* (Cambridge, 1985).

32. College Minutes, 2 February 1643.

33. Ibid., 15 September 1664. The apprentice in question, Thomas Gibson, appears to have been a slow learner, as it is not until 19 September 1668 that the minutes record that he had been 'tryed by the clerk and found to have maid proficiencie in his learning'.
34. Company of Barber Surgeons of London, Court Minute Books, 22 July 1556.
35. Ibid., 26 August 1556.
36. NAS, Commissariot Court, Register of Testaments, CC8/8, 6 January 1577.
37. Henryson was appointed by the Town Council to advise on measures to combat plague in 1584.
38. Bisset's will was dated 6 February 1588, and included the sum of £1,600 in coin, a surprising amount in a period noted for a chronic shortage of coinage.
39. Young, S., *Annals of the Barber Surgeons of London* (London, 1890), p. 589.
40. Vesalius, A., *De Humani Corporis Fabrica Libri Septem* (Basle, 1543).
41. Colston, *Incorporated Trades*, p. 15.
42. Stott, R. M., 'The Incorporation of Surgeons and Barbers of Edinburgh and medical education in and practice in Edinburgh 1696–1755' (unpublished Ph.D. thesis, University of Edinburgh, 1984), p. 254.
43. Livingstone, M. et al. (eds), *Registrum Secreti Sigilli Regum Scotorum* (Edinburgh, 1908–), vii, no. 3515.
44. Pitcairn, R. (ed.), *Criminal Trials in Scotland, from AD 1488 to AD 1624* (Edinburgh, 1833), i, p. 25.
45. *Burgh Recs*, 6 July 1563.
46. Ibid., 9 February 1557.
47. Ibid., 11 March 1579.
48. Ibid., 10 June 1558.
49. Maitland, W., *The History of Edinburgh from its Foundation to the Present Time* (Edinburgh, 1753), p. 15.
50. College Business Papers, 20 August 1575. The penalty for each offence would be 40 shillings, half of which would go to the general burgh funds, and the rest to the Incorporation.
51. College Business Papers, 25 June 1568.
52. Ibid., October 1576.
53. Hamilton, *Healers*, pp. 32–3.
54. Lynch, M. and Dingwall, H. M., 'Elite society in town and country', in E. P. Denison, D. Ditchburn and M. Lynch (eds), *Aberdeen Before 1800. A New History* (East Linton, 2002), pp. 192–200. Aberdeen burgh records show that between 1450 and 1800 some eighty-six individuals designated surgeon became burgesses.
55. Porter, *Greatest Benefit*, p. 119.
56. Rhodes, P., *An Outline History of Medicine* (London, 1985), pp. 32–3. The famous *Regimen Sanitatem Salernitatum* continued to be published until the nineteenth century.
57. Gentilcore, D., *Healers and Healing in Early-Modern Italy* (Manchester, 1998), pp. 56–95.
58. Brockliss, L. and Jones, C., *The Medical World of Early Modern France* (Oxford, 1997), p. 8.
59. Cameron, C. A., *History of the Royal College of Surgeons in Ireland and of the Irish Schools of Medicine Including Numerous Biographical Sketches; Also a Medical Bibliography* (Dublin, 1886), p. 60.
60. Blandy, J. P. and Lumley, J. S. P. (eds), *The Royal College of Surgeons of England. 200 Years of History at the Millennium* (London, 2000), p. 4.
61. See Bannerman, J., *The Beatons. A Medical Kindred in the Classical Gaelic Tradition* (Edinburgh, 1986).

# 3

# Consolidation and organisation, 1581–1726

O Eternal God & our loving & mercifull Father in Christ Jesus. Seeing that we are conveenit heir to treat upon these things that concernis our calling, we beseik thee, O Lord, to be mercifull to us, and giff us grace to proceed thereintill without malice, grudge or partialitie; sua that the things we may do may tend to the glorie of God, the weill of our vocation & comfort of every member of the Samen; thro Jesus Christ our only Lord and Saviour; Amen.[1]

## INTRODUCTION

This chapter deals with a turbulent century in the history of Scotland, one that was significant in terms of the consolidation and development of the Incorporation and its organisation and functions. After 1680 the Incorporation would be much more heavily involved in dealing with external disputes and influences. By 1726 the early crises of numbers were over, though not entirely so, and the Incorporation participated more fully in outside matters. Quarrels about jurisdiction and demarcation were certainly not over, but by that time it was a strong force in Edinburgh society.

The seventeenth century was one of conflict for the nation following the Union of the Crowns in 1603, with subsequent civil war, the Cromwellian occupation in the 1650s, the Restoration of the monarchy in 1660 and the early Jacobite conflicts following the accession of William and Mary in 1689.[2] By this time the burgh system was expanding more rapidly and Glasgow was emerging as a town which would eventually overtake Edinburgh in terms of population size and trading activities. By the time of the still-controversial Union of Parliaments in 1707,[3] Edinburgh was the seat of Scots Law, parliament, the General Assembly and the remnants of the royal court, and it boasted the Royal College of Physicians and Advocates Library as well as the Incorporation and the University, founded in 1583. It was in this complex milieu that Scottish lowland culture, intellect and institutions flourished, and would do so even more actively in the Enlightenment period. Edinburgh and Scotland were now, like it or not, part of Great Britain, and this had far-reaching implications for the future of the Incorporation just as much as for Edinburgh itself. The feudal system had largely gone, the professions were flourishing and scientific knowledge widening, and by 1726 the Medical School at Edinburgh University had opened its doors. The Scottish economy, though, was not in quite such good shape, and at several points in the seventeenth century was in crisis, particularly during the 'ill-years' of the 1690s. The general medical market-place was still primarily one of opportunism and unregulation, and it was in the interests of the Incorporation to continue its attempts to mark out a territory and defend it. The need to find more permanent accommodation became more intense, and by the end of the seventeenth century the Incorporation had acquired its first purpose-built hall in which to hold meetings and house the library and museum collections (see Chapter 7). This chapter is therefore concerned with these major processes of consolidation and challenges for the Incorporation.

## GENERAL INCORPORATION MATTERS

Early entries in the first minute book are brief. Sixteen masters are listed at the beginning of the book: Gilbert Primrose (Deacon), Noyer Brussat, Robert Henryson, Alexander Bruce, James Lindsay, John Woddal, James Craig, Alexander Tweedie, Patrick Martine, Henry Blyth, John Lowson, Henry Lumsden, Michael Bassentyne, Alexander Fiddas, John Libertoun and Jacob Brun (Brown). Thenceforth the Incorporation sederunts listed members in order of seniority after the Deacon, so that, apart from Primrose, Brussat seems to have been the longest-serving member at that time. A second list of names, dated 7 November 1591, contained a number of additions, including James Cranston, Thomas Campbell (already a barber, who became a surgeon in June 1588), Symeon Henryson, son of Robert Henryson, and Andrew Scott. The latter was apprenticed to Henry Lumsden in February 1583, 'to remain with hym for the space of sex years'.[4] Since Scott was not admitted as a surgeon until June 1593, with the stated purpose of certifying him fit to be surgeon to the king, he may have qualified initially as a barber before 1591. This cannot be verified from the records, though in the early period it was fairly common for individuals to acquire a dual qualification, first as barber and then as full surgeon.

Scrutiny of these very early records reveals concern with organisation, behaviour, money, and the three elements already identified from the Seal of Cause as being of particular significance: literacy, training and examinations. The Incorporation was typical of the trade incorporations of the time and, in organisational terms, unremarkable, at least at the start. The matter of electing trustworthy officials was important, and on 3 May 1582 the first note of annual elections appeared – 'the quhilk day the haill brethren of chirurgeins convenit in the dykyne hous hes choissine Gilbert Primross dykain for this yeir to come'.[5] Henryson, Bruce, Blyth and Craig were chosen as the 'four maisters' or quartermasters, while Craig had the additional responsibility of keeping the (money) box, together with Henry Lumsden, and John Lawson was entrusted with the keys of the kist, or locked chest, which contained charters, banners, bonds for lent money and other items of importance to the Incorporation. The kist may also have contained the

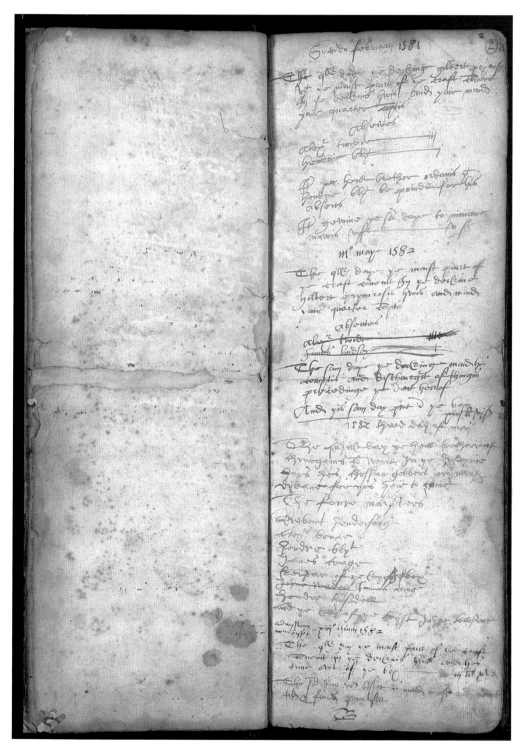

**FIG. 3.1** *First page of earliest surviving minute book, the date of the first entry being 2 February 1581.*

Incorporation's mortcloth, which was made available on hire for the funerals of deceased members or their relatives. A new mortcloth was ordered in June 1588, to be made 'of fit fassion'. The cost of this was £25 13s 4d, a fair sum, given that in September 1590 the entire funds of the Incorporation totalled £56 7s 6d.[6] The duties of the quartermasters were outlined at the election in 1589, when it was noted that they were to 'concur and assist with him (the Deacon) for the said year nixtocumin persewing arresting or poynding sic persones as transgress their privilege'.[7] The quartermasters were clearly elected in order to broaden the net of supervision, control and prevention of unauthorised practice – aims still recognisable today, albeit perhaps pursued with a little more subtlety.

The elections settled into an annual routine. The masters prepared a leet of six individuals proposed for Deacon; this list was submitted to the Town Council, which reduced this to a short-leet of three, from which the surgeons made their final choice. After the reform of the political sett of the burgh in 1583, when new guidelines for the composition of the Town Council were laid out (which remained largely unaltered until the major reforms of 1833), a surgeon was always elected as one of the six craft councillors, and invariably named first in Town Council sederunts. There was therefore considerable influence exercised by the Town Council over the Incorporation's choice of Deacon, though their constant representation on the Council ensured that the surgeons also had first-hand knowledge of events unfolding within the Council chamber. The Incorporation was not independent in its choice of Deacon, but co-operation ensured Council support in times of political difficulty, particularly in the second half of the seventeenth century during the often acrimonious triangular disputes among physicians, surgeons and apothecaries.

A pattern of office-holding gradually emerged, the Deacon normally serving for two years, unless prevented from doing so by illness, royal or military service, or death. The Deacon had often served in one or more of the other official capacities before his election to the highest office, but there does not appear to have been a strict or inflexible *cursus honorum* in operation. The quartermasters seem to have been discontinued from around the mid-1670s; examiners – known as examinators – were elected from 1698; and a librarian was added to the list of officials following the establishment of the library and collection of curiosities in 1699. Further changes took place according to contextual influences, so that a Deacon's council evolved to cope with day-to-day decision-making (though full executive power did not pass to the Council till 1971), together with a library committee, a museum committee, and a committee to run the Widows' Fund which was established in the second half of the eighteenth century. Separate groups to oversee finance and buildings were convened as the need arose. The Incorporation was nothing if not adaptable, within the constraints and limitations in force at any point in its history. The Town Council may have interfered in the choice of Deacon, but there is little evidence of wholesale interference by it or any other outside agency in internal organisation or surgical practice. It must be remembered that society and politics were rather different in this period, but despite these differences, the surgeons were apparently able to develop their organisation more or less along the lines which they desired. The Incorporation evolved against an ever-shifting backcloth of turbulence, war and general social and economic change, not to mention changes in the medical and surgical climate and the cosmological context within which everyone operated.

As noted, the Deacon and other office-bearers were elected annually, and this seems to have been a fairly straightforward system, though there were occasional disputes about the eligibility of some individuals to vote. Meetings generally consisted of the presentation of apprentices and new masters, notes about money, and disciplinary matters – seemly behaviour was considered to be of the greatest importance, a feature in society at large in this early-modern period. Whatever the level of society at which any individual found him or herself, correct codes of conduct had to be observed, to the extent of the oft-quoted example of the wife of a skinner, who, when her husband became a burgess of Edinburgh, was informed that she could no longer venture out onto the street wearing an apron.[8] A few examples will suffice to illustrate the concerns of the early Edinburgh master surgeons.

On 15 January 1588, the minutes contained the following items:

- 'Robt Lumsdell entered prentice to Henry Lumsden'
- 'William Watson servant to Henry Lumsden payet for his jewes to the craft xx schillings and ii schill. for the clerkis dewtie'
- 'Officer and common scribe payed 13/4d each'
- 'Input in the box mair nor [more than] was in it of befoir iii lib xv schillings and ivd'
- 'Act anent admission of simpill barbouris'. This stated that thenceforth barbers could only 'clip, cow, schaife and wesche allanerlie . . . under paine of penurie, defamation and tynsell [forfeit] of their friedom [of the Incorporation] for ever'

This was a fairly typical meeting, concerned with registration of apprentices, the available funds, payments to officers, and a decree concerning the barbers, who were from the start quickly and ruthlessly marginalised by the surgeons. Most regular meetings were of this nature, punctuated occasionally by adverse circumstances or events of wider historical significance. The elections in 1604 were cancelled and the serving officials obliged to continue in office for a further year because of 'the necessities of the present time and of the continowing of the plague of pestilence.[9]

The minutes for 25 August 1638 contain the following entry, which appears entirely without comment:

The qlk day in pns of the Deacon and brethren of the chyrurgians and barboris the covenant being put to them they have all subscryved the same and all ordains thar haill prentiessis and servandis to subscryve the samen als weile as thame selffis. And that there sall be in no tyme comming any freeman admitted ather chyrurgain or barbour nor yill any buikt prenteis or servand but sic as sall subscryve the covenant in witnes where-of this pnt act is maid and subscryved be me Alexr Henrysone thir clerk.

Though some six months had elapsed since the National Covenant was first read out and signed in the churchyard of Greyfriars Kirk, the surgeons clearly felt that it was necessary to sign on their own behalf and to make subscription a condition of membership or apprenticeship. In this and most other historically significant events, however, the minutes yield no information as to any debate which might have taken place at the meeting, or to any collective political thoughts or loyalties. It seems fairly clear, though, that the Incorporation was politically pragmatic; it took assistance from whatever source was most fruitful at the time, and it furnished surgeons to serve successive monarchs and their regiments as a matter of course. The only problem noted in the minutes during the Cromwellian occupation in the 1650s, for instance, was that the Incorporation's rented meeting rooms had been commandeered as a billet for English troops, and that the surgeons were experiencing difficulty in recovering their possessions from the building; there is no other comment.[10] It may be that caution in committing anything to paper that might generate trouble in the future was considered paramount – the result is, to say the least, frustrating for the historian.

Besides concerning themselves with registration of apprentices, admission of masters and maintaining Incorporation funds at as favourable a level as possible, the overriding concerns of the masters were to maintain discipline, instil correct behaviour, and prevent the unauthorised practice of surgery. It is important to remember that the Incorporation was emerging out of a completely unregulated medical market place, where individuals of all sorts offered opinions and advice. The respective designations of physician, surgeon or surgeon-apothecary all meant specific things to the practitioners in theory, but in practice the patients did not discriminate and the practitioners themselves were often happy to overstep their own self-imposed boundaries. The slightly paradoxical situation was that legitimate practitioners tried to impose demarcation, while ignoring the boundaries in their own practice, and at the same time many other individuals offered help 'out of motives of neighbourliness, paternalism, good housekeeping, Christian charity or simple self-help.'[11] The Incorporation regularly hauled before it recalcitrant individuals who persisted in performing unauthorised surgical procedures, however minor. These included barber Alexander Rattray, who appeared before the assembled brethren in 1585, admitted an unspecified offence, and was ordained to 'hummell himself to the deakin and ask thame forgivines on his knees and of his own consent binds and oblisses him that gif ever he fall in the lyk offence to tyn his freedom of the craft'.[12] The offence is not noted, but it would be safe to conclude that Rattray had been practising surgery. Incidents of this sort appear fairly regularly and it is clear that not only did the masters wish to prevent individuals with no affiliation to the Incorporation from carrying out surgical procedures, they were also equally determined to ensure that barbers did not venture beyond their area of certified competence, as noted above. In 1588 a general order was issued for an 'inquisition' of 'all unfriemen usurpand their privilges to be gevin in to the officer be thair names in quat poyntes they occupy and he to answer thairfor.'[13] This was very much in line with the defence of territory that came with corporate rights, though in this period, in which most people practised their own medicine, or consulted many 'irregulars' before restoring to an 'official' practitioner, demarcation was anything but easy to impose. It was not only the monopoly on surgery that was guarded. On 15 October 1595 the minutes note that the Incorporation chest contained, among other things, 'tua actis aganis unfriemen that makis aqua vita'.

All sorts of 'irregular' practitioners, variously designated quacks, mountebanks or empirics were a recurrent irritation. At this time the quacks were associated with public performances as well as selling potions or offering treatments and cures. One such individual who occupied the oppositional energies of the Incorporation was John Baptista Quarantine. He was given permission by the Town Council to set up a stage 'for the exercise of his airt and Calling in Public' in 1665. Ten years later he reappeared, and on this occasion the Incorporation took legal opinion and tried to persuade the Town Council to revoke Baptista's licence, but in the event he was able to stay until April 1667 before finally removing himself from Edinburgh.[14] The FPSG was also concerned with the problem of quacks and irregular practitioners, and it has been claimed that co-operation between physicians and surgeons was necessary in order to oppose those who indulged in unauthorised practice.[15]

The master surgeons, though, were not always blameless, and one of their number, Robert Auchmutie, who had entered as master in 1591,[16] was executed in April 1600 after killing his opponent in a duel at St Leonards Hill. Not without ingenuity, he had tried to escape his incarceration in the Tolbooth, and the anecdote amply repays rehearsing in full from a contemporary account.

> In the time of his being in Ward he hang ane cloke wtout the window of the irone-hous and another wtin the window yr, and saying yat he was seik, and might not see the light: he had aquafortis continually seething at the irone window, quhill at the last the irone window was eaten throw; sua, upon a morneing, he caused his prentis boy attend quhan the town gaird should have dissolvit, and quilk time the boy waited on and gaif hes Mr ane token yat ye said gaird were gone, be the show or waif of hes hand-curche. The said Rot hung oot ane tow, q'on he thocht to have comeit downe; the said gaird spyit the waiffe of the hand curche, and sua the said Rot was disappoyntit of hes intentione and devyse, and sua, on the 19 day he was beheidit at the cross upon ane scaffolt.[17]

Auchmutie seems to have been the only master of the Incorporation to pay the price for a capital offence, but many of his successors led less than wholly ethical surgical lives, and more modern volumes of the records contain fair numbers of cases involving Fellows or Licentiates who had been convicted of criminal offences.

In terms of organisational and disciplinary matters, there was relatively little change over the first century of the College's documented existence. As time went on more evidence began to appear about details rather than major changes to organisation. For example, although the kist was mentioned previously, it was not until 1595 that its current contents were listed. These were:

- 'Seill of caus'
- 'The chirurgeans exemption gevin be the queins ma[jes]tie under the previe seall' (Mary, Queen of Scots 1567)
- 'Ane confirmation given by King James the fift under the privie seal'
- 'Ane chart[er] or any annualrent of 32/- of Janet . . . hous'
- 'Tua acts aganis unfriemen that makis aqua vita given to Hendrie Lumsden to keep'
- 'In the said kist the silver box'
- 'John Naysmith dekin hes the mortclayt'[18]

These items, though few in number, illustrate the main areas of concern at the time – incorporating charter, money, demarcation, corporate possessions and service to their poorer members in terms of the mortcloth. References to the kist appear occasionally thereafter, including an order on 4 September 1628 for 'ane new kist of auk [oak], bandit with yrine wt ane fine lock' (orders were also given for a new fringe for the mortcloth and for it to be repaired 'qr it is faultie'), while a more disturbing note came in 1596 when John Naysmith had to repay over £40, the 'craftis kist and box being broken be som wicket persone'.[19]

## Correct behaviour

As part of the ongoing quest for recognition as a learned society, the Incorporation took great pains to ensure that the masters behaved correctly at meetings and elsewhere, and by the middle of the seventeenth century an Act of Ranking and an the Act of Civil Deportment had been instituted. The 'Act anent the ranking and placing of Deacons, masters and brethrane of the Incorporation', agreed on 15 October 1667, set out details about precedence and elections. It stated that in order to 'intertyne pece and unitie amongst thame selffis and finding that by reason thair hes not bene so clear rules hitherto for ranking the places and votes of Deacons, masters and boxmasters and other brethran their hes arisen some disensionis and annomosoties amongst the brethren', it was expedient to introduce rules and regulations 'according to the laudable example of all famous and weill governed Incorporations speciallie being numbrous as ours is now'. It was ordained that 'qhosoever sall be chosin deaken of qt standing soever he being in office sall have the prin[cip]all place in our meeting . . . and nixt him the old deakens are to tak yr places and to give yair votes in ye meetings and at other occasions to tak place lykewayes everie one according to ye priorite of tyme of his deakenship' (though any Deacon who had also served as Deacon Convener of the Magdalen Chapel took precedence over the other old Deacons). A further exception was made for Alexander Pennycuik of Newhall, who was allowed to sit next to the Deacon 'he being both the oldest master and oldest deaken of the haill Incorporation now of ane verie long tyme'. The Act went on to outline precedence for the rest of the company, the boxmaster following the old Deacons and the ordinary members taking the remaining places according to the date of their admission. Clearly such matters of protocol were designed both to maintain order and to give the semblance of an orderly society with a clear hierarchy – though were flexible enough to make exceptions for long-serving members or other particularly deserving individuals.

The order of precedence having been established, the next priority was to ensure a reasonable standard of behaviour at Incorporation meetings – again very much in line with the perceived orderliness of the learned society. Accordingly, on 18 February 1668, the Act of Civil Deportment was outlined. Its clauses included the instruction that no masters could speak 'till they be speared at be ye deakin or have leive askit or gevin be him'; speakers were not to be interrupted; no one was to 'profane the name of God by swearing, cursing and banning'; and no one was to take a place out of the agreed order of precedence. A further order was issued in 1677 prohibiting smoking or drinking during meetings.[20] Similar regulations were implemented by the FPSG from its foundation.[21]

It seems that the regulations were enforced as far as possible. In 1670, George Scott was censured for having 'foullie transgressit' by means of 'unchristian miscarriages (not worthie to re repeited named or again heard of)' against John Jossie, including a 'great oath that he would break his heid'. Scott was fined and ordered to 'crave the pardon of the masters'.[22] This was not an isolated incident. The Incorporation was also concerned with the morals of society at large as well as its own. At this time any disaster, natural, economic or otherwise, was considered to be punishment for sin, either individual or collective, and following the severe disasters of the ill-years of the 1690s and the ill-fated Darien Scheme, to which the Incorporation had subscribed (the Incorporation pledged £600 sterling – a considerable sum – while seventeen individual masters invested, as did sixteen physicians and two apothecaries), it was deemed to be a prudent move to issue a lengthy declaration against immorality, the colourful language of which needs no elaboration or explanation:

> Considering the many and dreadfull judgements and tokens of the wrath of an angry god which hath overtaken this sinful nation and city. Such as many years scarcity of victual and death qrby not only this nation and City has been mightily impoverished but many thousands of Christians perished with famine to the desolation of some corners of the land. The disappointing and blasting that great desire of advancing the Trade and wealth of the nation by the loss of the African and Indian Company and Colony of Caledonia and America qrby this nation and City have lost not only many brethren but a great part of this Treasure notwithstanding hopes of recovery.[23] Several dreadfull fires within these few years have consumed the

most glorious of our buildings and best part of our City whereby many families have been brought to ruine . . . The terrible blowing up of severall barrels of Gunpowder in our Suburbs of Leith qrby a great part of that place was reduced to a ruinous heap. The greit losses this City and nation have of late and dayly sustained in our trade by taking of many of our shyps by French pirates and that even in sight our our harbors so that trade and commerce even in our own parts is obstructed . . . the crying sins of atheism prophanity blasphemy vile hypocrysie Sabbath breaking and immoralitie of all sorts qlk flows thro City and nation like a flood. We doe therefore in the first place earnestly beg of the Eternal god to avert his deserved rods and for his own holy names sake yet preserve a remnant for himselfe and this poore afflicted nation and city. And in the next place we doe resolve in the Lords strength every one of us to be more watchful over our own habits and ways than formerly.[24]

Despite their claims to superior knowledge and organisation, members of the Incorporation still shared wider beliefs about the causes of natural disasters or other conflicts. This is one of the paradoxes of the seventeenth century. Scientific knowledge was advancing, but this process took place against a background of superstition and belief in divine retribution. This may be difficult for the modern psyche to comprehend, but was not at all contradictory in the seventeenth century.

### Money

As with any such institution, a reasonably sound financial basis was a prime concern. Most of the Incorporation's early income came from the fees charged to apprentices and entrant masters and their subsequent quarterly dues. Later on, borrowing money was common, and also lending out money in order gain income. Property transactions and legacies also helped, though rarely did the Incorporation have excess funds. The scale of fees charged to masters and those for apprentice and servant bookings were raised periodically, and the early records indicate that the booking fee for an apprentice was 40s, and for a servant 13s 4d. Entry fees for masters were around £6 6s for most of this period. By 1710 the entry fee for an apprentice had risen to six guineas and that for a servant £3 4s. In addition, small amounts were paid to the Incorporation Clerk and Officer. Quarterly dues of 40s were paid by each master and the payments and defaulters noted in the minute books. As in most crafts, the sons or sons-in-law of master surgeons could be admitted at a reduced fee, though it must have been somewhat difficult to enforce the precondition whereby 'in case any of the saidis friemans dochters beis deflorit and tynes hir virginitie sho nor he quah maryis his sall brouke no privilege nor ryt be hir father albeit he was and be freman of the said craft and burges alsua of the burght'.[25] The finances of the Incorporation also had to depend on the current state of the currency – in 1636, for example, the records note the King's proclamation in which the dollar (40s) had been 'callit down twa schillings', this to be taken into account by the boxmaster.[26] Once entered, masters were obliged to pay quarterly dues and defaulters were noted and pursued just as diligently as the masters pursued irregular practitioners. Then, as now, the Incorporation depended on its members for economic survival.

In an era without banks, the use of money was rather different and often more complex. The financial structure of society was based on the constant circulation of money, bonds and the rights to property. Borrowing and lending out money at interest was the core of the system, and even the smallest sum could be lent out, while at the same time the individual or group concerned may have been borrowing additional funds. Debts were not necessarily paid in cash or promissory notes, but could be paid in kind or by transfer of the rights to property rental or a debt owed to another person, so that an individual could receive payment in the form of rights to a debt which had been transferred to and from several intervening parties. The Incorporation in this regard was entirely typical of the early-modern financial situation, the records showing both borrowing and lending throughout this period, the borrowed money often coming from its own members. In 1680 it had been necessary to borrow 500 merks to cover the expenses of the Cunningham affair (see below);[27] In 1697, Walter Porterfield lent 2,000 merks and James Hamilton 3,000 merks towards the cost of building the new Hall, and on several occasions money had been borrowed from a Canongate tailor, Pierre Castile, who used the name 'La Pearle', and who seems to have been affluent enough to lend the Incorporation money whenever it was required.

**Table 3.1 Financial state of the Incorporation, 1665–1710.**
(Source: College Minutes)

| Date | Balance (£Scots) |
|------|------------------|
| 1665 | +351 |
| 1670 | +6 |
| 1675 | −106 |
| 1680 | +49 |
| 1685 | +249 |
| 1690 | +214 |
| 1695 | +858 |
| 1700 | −301 |
| 1705 | −113 |
| 1710 | −128 |

On the other hand, though, the Incorporation itself lent 3,000 merks to the Town Council in May 1692 – this was repaid with interest the following year.[28] There was a fairly consistent pattern of increased borrowing when legal advice was necessary or when the Incorporation was faced with unusual expenses. It was in the boxmaster's interest to try to balance the books, as he was liable to make up any shortfall from his own pocket. A brief survey of the Incorporation's accounts in Table 3.1 illustrates its fairly precarious financial state for much of the period.

## Clerks and Officers

In addition to the Deacon and his assistants, two other officials were necessary to ensure the smooth running of the Incorporation. The Clerk was important for record-keeping and maintaining the minutes of meetings and the registration of apprentices, servants and masters, and by 1723 it was ordained that he should keep an account book. The first recorded Clerk was writer (lawyer) Adam Gibson, appointed in 1587 at an annual salary of 40s, succeeded by three others in the next half-century. A curious step was taken in 1671 when, for reasons not detailed, it was decided to invite Sir Andrew Ramsay, current Lord Provost (and first Honorary Freeman of the Incorporation) to nominate a successor, he being 'an honest and abill man'.[29] Patrick Moubray was chosen, and he served the Incorporation till 1708, his physical decline over the years confirmed by the gradual deterioration in his signature at the end of each Incorporation minute.[30] (From the middle of the eighteenth century the office was, for a time, sold to the highest bidder, though this was amended to require a deposit paid by the incoming Clerk, and by 1825 the title was changed to Secretary, which was thought to be 'more consonant with their dignity as a Royal College'.)[31] Clerks occasionally left for higher office, such as Alexander Schaw, who resigned in 1774 because he had been 'appointed to an office abroad under the government'.[32]

The other appointment, that of Incorporation Officer, was more concerned with keeping order and with the more practical aspects of the running of the organisation, particularly in the early years when it had no permanent location or meeting place. At first these duties were devolved to the most junior entrant master, and included summoning masters to meetings, collecting dues and general supervision, but by 1614 it was agreed that such an arrangement was detrimental both to the junior master and to the image of the Incorporation, and Alexander Thomson was appointed as the first non-surgeon Officer in 1614, at an annual remuneration of £4, together with 6s 8d for each master admitted and 3s 4d per apprentice booking. Like the Clerks, the Officers tended to be long-serving, including George Cathcart, engaged in 1664 to care for the surgeon's medicinal garden as well as performing the Officer's duties. He served for over 30 years and might have remained longer, but when it was agreed in 1697 that the Officer should wear a uniform livery coat and silver badge, he refused to do so and left. In the same way that any uniform or badge of office is symbolic, it was entirely in line with the Incorporation's aspirations for recognition as a serious body that any of its servants should be recognisable and should be suitably – and formally – attired. Members of many organisations are distinguished by a livery of some sort, whether it be military uniform or academic gown, and in this period, when visual symbolism was of crucial importance in all aspects of society, it was quite natural that the Incorporation wished its Officer to

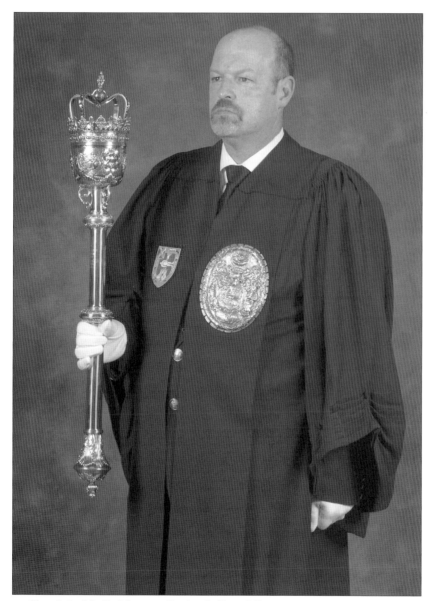

**FIG. 3.2**  *Mr D. Morcom, Senior College Officer, with the Officer's silver badge and the College mace.*

bear its badge – a badge which is still worn by the current incumbent of the office on formal occasions.[33]

### Charitable works

Most craft Incorporations were formed initially with social intent, in terms of caring for impoverished members and their dependants. This was no less the case with the Incorporation, despite its often less than solvent financial state. The surgeons did 'suffrage' for their own souls at the pre-Reformation altar in St Giles', and translated this into good works in terms of trying to care for the most indigent of their members. General appeals were responded to also – towards the end of the seventeenth century there were recurrent appeals for the sustenance of deposed Episcopal clergy. A few examples will suffice to demonstrate this aspect of the Incorporation's practices.

In 1635 it was decreed that if any surgeon received more then £10 Scots for a cure, 'considering the weill of the calling and supporting of the pure', he should pay 'ten schillings Scottis money' towards poor relief.[34] This would, of course, depend on the honesty of the surgeons concerned. Individual charity was apparent, as illustrated by surgeon James Brown, who in October 1643 gave £5 8s 'out of his own frie motive will to the use of the poore'. Charity was shown to William Temple, who had been 'by the good providence of God redacted to very great straits having little or no imployment for this long tyme bygane and a great chairge of a numer-ous family having very small means to maintaine himself and them, and for the present not being in a condition to go about his calling by reason of sickness'.[35] Temple was excused payment of his dues to the Incorporation and by November 1684 he had been granted a quarterly pension because of his 'low condition'. It was not just poverty that drew Incorporation benevolence, though. The minutes note on 2 February 1652 that £30 was lent to the wife of barber Hector McLay, 'for relies of hir husband from prissone out of Ingland and for his transportation homeward' – this at the end of the Civil Wars and beginning of the Cromwellian occupation.

Other recipients of Incorporation charity were Helen Beck, 'old and weak', paid 6s weekly; the widow of barber Adam Darling despite his being expelled from the Incorporation; Widow Burnett '28 years since it pleased God to remove her hus-band from her'; and, in 1700, 40s sterling was contributed towards the sustenance of 'upwards of ane hundred families' of the 'poor suffering clergy'.[36] Despite the fact that the Incorporation was often in parlous financial straits and forced to borrow money, this did not prevent it from attempting to care for the needy. This was also the case with surgery. The Town Council employed a surgeon to treat the poor, and these records show that it was possible to survive heroic surgery. The accounts for the surgeon to the poor in 1710 recount the case of Jean Beaton, who had a leg amputated in April that year, and survived to require the provision of a 'timber leg' in October.[37]

## ECLIPSE OF THE BARBERS

While the Seal of Cause was granted to the Surgeons and Barbers of Edinburgh, there was never anything approaching parity of status or influence within the Incorporation. The Surgeons saw themselves as the superior and dominant partner, and from the beginning attempts were made to marginalise the barbers. It would take until 1722 before there was final separation, but the evidence from the records is clear – the money accrued from barbers' quarterly dues and other fees was welcome, but they themselves were not. Of the sixty individuals who became master surgeons between 1581 and 1656, twenty-three had the dual qualification, including James Skaithmuire (1594), Bartilmo Aikman (1610), Archibald Hay (1621) and Walter Turnbull (1649). The last of these double entries seems to have been held by Peter Norrie, who became a master in 1656, having qualified as a barber in 1647. Thereafter there is no mention of any other surgeon taking this route. The process of eliminating the barbers can be seen almost as one of internal social construction, or indeed deconstruction – the construction of the elite society by means of the deconstruction of the original group. Whatever the case, the barbers were purposefully edged out of any influence in the Incorporation. In 1588 entrant barbers had been warned that in addition to barbering they could 'use the cureing of simpill wounds allanerlie and not use ony compount cureing', and early the following year it was ordained that entrants who did not meet the required standards would be allowed to 'clip, cow, schaife and wesche allanerlie'.[38] This is the closest that the Incorporation came to the regulations of the FPSG, which had a system of awarding lesser qualifications to entrant surgeons who did not fully meet the requirements of the examiners. From the mid-seventeenth century most of the barbers were forced to work in the suburbs, particularly Canongate and Leith, and were evidently not interested in adding a surgical qualification.

In terms of their potential role within the administration of the Incorporation, the barbers were again unlucky. The only offices which appear to have been held by barbers were those of boxmaster and keeper of the kist. The duties of boxmaster were undertaken by William Wood (1596), William Rattray (1597), William Lowson and John Flucker (1605) and John Davidson (1607). Flucker and Davidson became surgeons, and Flucker was a long-serving official, taking up the role of keeper of the kist in 1616, 1617, 1621, 1629 and 1631–4. The early seventeenth century was a time when the numbers of master surgeons were dangerously low, partly as a result of plague, and this may be one reason why a few barbers were allowed to become office-bearers. No barber achieved the office of Deacon, and the Incorporation sederunts note attending surgeons only.

Despite their lowly status within the Incorporation and their exile to the fringes of the burgh, the barbers were subjected to the same rigorous discipline that was applied to errant surgeons. Public humiliation was one of the measures taken, and one example was that of James Stevenson, who had been convicted of uttering 'odious and sclanderous words' against the Incorporation. He was paraded at the Mercat Cross 'with ane paper on his heid and thair to ask thame forgifness on his kneyis of the said falt'. This was, of course, very much in line with current punishment practices, and measures such as these would, in the view of adherents of the social control explanations of Foucault, be entirely predictable. They were public and visual and would serve as a deterrent to others and, therefore, help to maintain stability within society at large as well as within individual institutions.

There were other disputes. In 1651, Robert Priest, a barber who had taken the oath to practise only in Canongate, made friends in high places during the Cromwellian occupation, and felt able to break his oath and take a shop within the walls of the burgh. This, naturally, outraged those who had legitimate reasons for keeping shops in the town, and several complained that their trade was being adversely affected by Priest's activities. Priest was summoned to explain himself to the Incorporation, but refused to 'take in his basins', and produced a supporting letter signed by four of the English Commissioners for the Administration of Justice in Scotland. The high status of the signatories perhaps influenced the Incorporation which, surprisingly, did not try to enforce Priest's exclusion too aggressively. Further communications were received from Robert Lilburne, Commander of English forces in Scotland and matters rumbled on unresolved till 1654, when Lilburne had been succeeded by General Monck, and an investigation was held into the situation. Monck wrote to the Incorporation from his base at Dalkeith, giving his view that Priest should indeed remove himself from Edinburgh, within three weeks. This was an expensive process for the Incorporation and one which involved it in risky conflict with the political authorities of the day, but one which was ultimately successful.[39]

The surgeons were nothing if not even-handed, and mention should be made of the famous incident concerning David Pringle. Pringle had been appointed surgeon to Heriot's Hospital, and on Founders' Day in June 1670 he was requested to arrange for the hair of the sixty inmates to be trimmed. Unable to locate any of his own servants, Pringle took on the first barber he encountered to help with this formidable task. The problem was that this individual only had a licence to operate in the suburb of Portsburgh, which was very close to Heriot's Hospital (an institution for the sons of indigent burgesses) but still outwith the town boundaries, and therefore outwith his officially permitted area of operation. Both Pringle and his unfortunate subcontractor were incarcerated in the Tolbooth and Pringle began legal action, but in the end decided to back down and apologise to the Incorporation, which declared unctuously that it had 'never intended the said David his ruin nor ever had spleen or malice against him'.[40]

The forced removal of most of the barbers to the suburbs was also in line with trends. A number of other crafts had migrated from the centre of the town in this period, mainly textile workers. Skinners and tanners were socially unacceptable because of the noxious odours produced by their industrial processes, while by the end of the century the butchering of meat was prohibited in the inner burghs and Dalkeith emerged as the butchering centre for Edinburgh. This 'flight to the suburbs' took place partly for expediency and partly as a result of coercion.[41] Part of the reason for pushing out the barbers from the centre was that for the first half of the seventeenth century there was a fair number of surgeons with the barbering qualification, who wished to offer barbering services as well as surgical treatments, and eliminating the competition from the simple barbers would be a great help to them economically. From the start of the records in 1581 to the admission of the last doubly-qualified master in 1656, some twenty-nine entrant surgeons were also barbers. In February 1661 the Deacon and two masters were appointed to visit and inspect the shops of 'friemen in the town that uses trimming to sie that they have qualified and able servands for trimming togidder with fit instrumentis sic as cleane and neat dressing claythes combs, razors and pincers'.[42] However, the potential

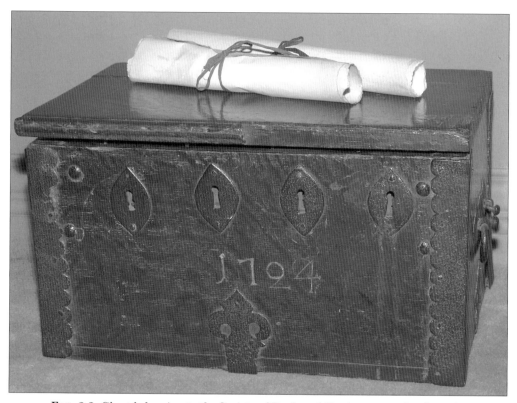

**FIG. 3.3** *Chest belonging to the Society of Barbers following separation from the Incorporation in 1722.*

clients and customers were not particularly gratified by these arrangements, as by 1682 complaints were made that they 'had to go to the suburbs to be barbarized'. The Incorporation responded to the 'clamour on that accompt' by allowing some entrant barbers to operate in the centre of the burgh, but at a raised entry fee of £333 (500 merks) as opposed to the average £40 charged to outlying barbers.[43] There was clearly a fine line to be drawn between putting the barbers in their rightful place and serving the needs of high-ranking clients, some of whom might be in a position to give political patronage to the Incorporation in times of difficulty. Some of the barbers, though, were not lacking in entrepreneurial skills themselves, and began to combine their barbering with the increasingly lucrative pursuit of wig-making. The needs of fashion and of the burgeoning legal profession meant that the wigmakers were one of the craft groups which was growing steadily by the turn of the eighteenth century, and the new breed of barber-periwigmaker gradually overtook the barber-surgeon group.[44] Final separation between the surgeons and barbers took place in 1722, and the Society of Barbers survived until the early part of the twentieth century. The Glasgow surgeons and barbers separated around the same time.

Relations between barbers and surgeons were rarely harmonious in any of the early-modern Incorporations, though in London and Paris it seems that closer links between the two were a feature, in contrast to the situation in Edinburgh, though in Paris by the middle of the seventeenth century the barbers and surgeons followed increasingly divergent paths.[45] Some London barbers were able to achieve high office in their organisation, but formal separation eventually occurred in the 1740s, shortly after that in Edinburgh, though it has been claimed that such 'unions' between surgeons and barbers were advantageous to both sides – the barbers gaining perceived social status and the surgeons achieving access to the guild or craft network.[46] The situation in Glasgow was a little more complex because of the unique nature of the FPSG. The Glasgow barbers had been adopted as a 'pendicle' of the FPSG as early as 1602, but in 1656 a separate Incorporation of Surgeons and Barbers was chartered by the Glasgow Town Council, in some ways similar to the Edinburgh Fraternity of Apothecaries and Surgeon-Apothecaries, founded a year later. Separation between the Glasgow barbers and surgeons came in 1719, shortly before the same process took place in Edinburgh.[47]

Relationships between barbers and surgeons in this period were complex. It may be that there was initial union and a degree of toleration because the procedures undertaken by the two groups were similar, and that once the surgeons became more knowledgeable and able to carry out more complex procedures, it was felt that to be associated with 'simple' barbering would be detrimental to their image and aspirations. Whatever the case there was, in most organisations, an eventual parting of the ways between two callings which had originally been relatively indistinguishable from each other.

## APPRENTICES AND APPRENTICESHIP

From the start apprentices were one of the central concerns of the Incorporation. Well-supervised training was deemed essential, and however unscientific that training might have been, the aims were there and steps taken to carry them out. As noted above, literacy was stipulated from the start, and since many of the available books were in Latin or French, insistence on literacy tests was important. The emphasis on Latin could be justified almost by a single book: Harvey's crucial work, usually cited by its short title *De Motu Cordis*, arguably the most important publication of the seventeenth century, which was not available in English before 1653.[48] Surgical books such as those of Lowe and Paré were also important. Some of the London apprentices would not have been able to benefit from these and other texts, in whatever language they were written, until the Latin requirement was reintroduced in the English capital in 1727.

During the course of the 'long seventeenth century' (a term used by historians to cover the period c. 1600–c. 1725), around 650 apprentices were indentured to members of the Incorporation, all of whom were literate (though of course the best of regulations can be flouted). Once literacy had been established and appropriate financial arrangements concluded between the parent or guardian of the aspirant apprentice and the surgeon to whom he wished to be bound, a formal indenture document was drawn up. These indentures were generally similar in content and

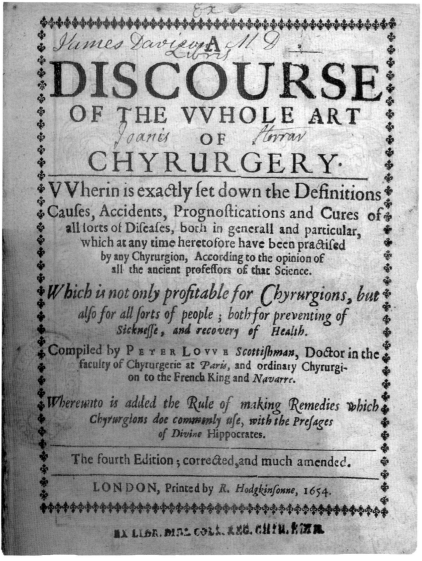

**FIG. 3.4** *(above and overleaf) Pages from Peter Lowe's* Discourse of the Whole Art of Chyrurgery *(1654 edition) and Ambroise Paré's* Opera Chirurgica *(1594).*

in intent to those issued by most of the other craft incorporations in terms of length and conditions of apprenticeship, although those of the surgeons did contain specific 'ethical' clauses. It was ordained that the apprentice would:

> serve his said master leitly & truely by Night and by day, holy day & work day in all things Godly and honest. And shall not hear of his said Masters skaith at any time by day or night, during the space foresaid but shall reveal the same to him, and hinder it to his power: and that he shall not reveal his masters secrets in his art nor the diseases of his patients to any

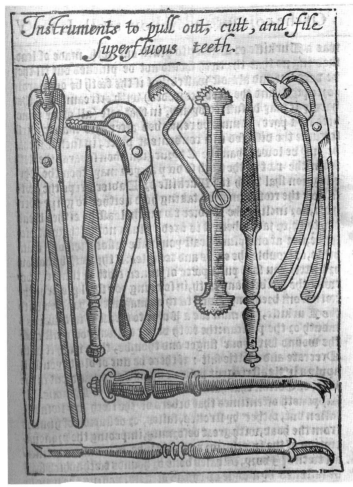

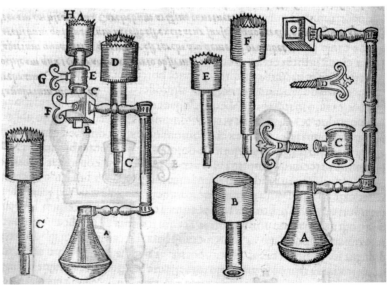

person whatsoever, Nor shall have any Patients or his own under cure upon any pretext whatsoever. Nor shall he absent himself from his said master's service at any time, during the space foresaid, without his Masters special licence, had and obtained of him for that effect. And that he shall not commit the filthy Crimes of Fornication or Adultery nor play at any games whatsoever; And that he shall not be drunk, nor Night-walker nor an haunter of Debaucht or Idle company, nor go to ale-houses, nor Taverns, to tiple or drink with any company whatsoever.[49]

The earliest indenture in the possession of the College is that of Patrick Cunningham, a somewhat notorious individual who never qualified as a surgeon but involved the Incorporation in expensive litigation over unauthorised surgery when he had allegedly performed bloodletting on two titled individuals. The outcome of this and other incidents was a decree issued by the Lords of Council in 1682 to the effect that surgery and pharmacy must be separated (Cunningham was by this time apparently practising as an apothecary). Before his notoriety revealed itself, however, Cunningham was apprenticed to James Borthwick, one of the leading surgeon-apothecaries of the day, in 1661. His indentures are fairly similar to those quoted above, but there were specific penalties for transgression of the rules, including the stipulation that for the 'fylthie crime of fornication or adulterie', the apprentice must serve a further three years before his indentures might be discharged.[50] It is tempting to conclude that such penalties might have been the reason why Cunningham did not qualify in surgery; he was by no means untypical, though, as less than a quarter of the indentured apprentices became members of the Incorporation.

Despite the Incorporation's strenuous efforts to inculcate seemly conduct, both master and apprentice resorted to violence on occasion. The masters voted to dissolve the indentures of James Harvey, apprentice to William Wood, in 1595, because he had allegedly 'put violent hands on his said master to the effusione of his bluid, as was sufficiently proven'.[51] Matters had apparently deteriorated to the extent that in 1612 it was decreed that apprentices were 'not to wair ony dager, quhinger or knyff (except ane knyff to cut thir meit wanting the point).[52] Half a century later, in 1666, a master's family was also involved. Francis Ogston was imprisoned in the burgh Tolbooth after he had 'beaten and strucken' Arthur Temple's wife and children and 'offered to put violent hands' on Temple himself.[53]

The fault was, however, not always with the apprentice. In November 1679 surgeon James Hopkirk was severely reprimanded by his colleagues for maltreatment of his apprentice John Tait. In addition to failing to instruct Tait in the art of surgery, Hopkirk was convicted of not feeding and clothing him adequately and also beating him several times 'not only to the effusion of his blood in great quantitie but to the hazard of his lyfe'.[54] Confirmation of the recurrent difficulties with apprentices is also to be found in the Dean of Guild Court minute books, and a further case involving Arthur Temple provides illustration. John Cuthbertson, the apprentice involved, sued Temple for breach of contract, but the Dean of Guild

Court took the view that Cuthbertson had 'absented himself wrongfully' and was ordered to return to Temple. Violence was also alleged, Cuthbertson claiming that he had been assaulted, but Temple stated righteously that he had merely 'moderatlie correctit him as he did his own children'.[55]

A further category of 'student' is also identified within the training pyramid. These individuals were designated 'servant' and were formally registered, but at a lower fee than the apprentices, being appointed either yearly or for a period of three years. Servants could transfer fairly freely among the masters and in many instances were registered servant 'in order to be prentice' to a master. It has been assumed hitherto that the servants had finished their apprenticeships and were about to become master surgeons or work as journeymen,[56] but it is clear from the records that this was not the case in Edinburgh, and from at least the mid-seventeenth century this type of pre-apprenticeship service was common. The duties undertaken by these individuals are never specified, but it may be assumed that their work was of a routine nature, perhaps assisting with dressings, carrying and cleaning equipment, and also brushing up their Latin in anticipation of full indenture as apprentices. Comparison may be made with the garçons-chirurgiens of Paris, where the garçon's status 'resembled that of a domestic servant',[57] though in the French capital the servants were not entitled to formal tuition, while the Edinburgh servants could attend sessions in the Physic Garden with their apprentice colleagues. There is no evidence from the London records of a similar category of trainee. Between 1581 and 1726, around 650 servants were booked – a similar number to the apprentices, the latter including a fair number who had already been enrolled as servants. This was one area also where, unusually, women were allowed to engage servants. In the case of deceased barbers, their wives were permitted occasionally to engage barbers and servants in order to keep the business going. On 4 November 1590, for example, William Wood was entered servant to Bessie Lundie (his mother-in-law) 'to remain in hir household and in ane buith during her lifetime'. The arrangement would be terminated should she 'deceise or marry'.

Though there was a formal apprentice structure and large numbers of indentures were concluded, the numbers eventually achieving the status of master surgeon were low. Between 1581 and 1726, some 160 master surgeons joined the Incorporation. They employed 650 apprentices, of whom only 108 (16.6 per cent) became master surgeons. The masters trained an average of five apprentices during their working lives (range 0–13). The Incorporation rules decreed that three years had to elapse between apprentice signings, with the expected exceptions for the death of an apprentice or other circumstances which deprived the master of his apprentice during that period. This would indicate an average 'operating life' for most master surgeons of between fifteen and twenty years, though, of course, the spectrum was broad. Each master employed an average of four servants during his career (range 0–27), of whom one-fifth became full apprentices.

An example of a master of the Incorporation at the more active end of the scale was John Baillie, who qualified as a master in 1681 and took a servant and an

50

apprentice the following year. He taught fourteen apprentices in all and employed a total of thirteen servants. Four of the servants became apprentices, and two of the combined number became master surgeons. One of these was David Fyfe, who began as Baillie's servant in 1686, was apprenticed in 1688 and entered the Incorporation in 1695. Fyfe, in his turn, took on eight apprentices and thirteen servants; five servants became apprentices but only one a master surgeon. These examples demonstrate fairly typical careers, and also the very narrow apex of the pyramid of training and qualification, this in spite of the universal literacy of the apprentices and masters and the increasing availability of teaching aids in the library and museum.[58]

The apprentices acted as their contemporaries in other crafts did – they followed their masters. Surgical apprentices observed procedures, cleaned equipment and generally absorbed the essence of surgery in the limited state that it was during this period. As they progressed, they were allowed to change dressings, initially under supervision and then by themselves, to the extent that daily visits to check on dressings and the state of wounds could be entrusted to the reliable senior apprentice. Following the establishment of the Physic Garden in the mid-seventeenth century, later supervised by James Sutherland[59] and then Charles Preston, lecture/demonstrations were given by the incumbent superintendent, at a cost to each student of one guinea, the lectures being delivered at the stimulating hour of 5 a.m. By 1711 the instructions to apprentices included orders that:

> no prentice or servant shall come to the garden any other time than what is above mentioned without acquainting their masters. And the intendant is to attend the garden for that purpose three days in the week, Monday, Wednesday and Friday betwixt the hours of three and five in the afternoon. All prentices and servants are herby discharged to pluck up any tree shrub or plant without leave asked and given by the intendant and as oft as any of the saids prentices or servants shall be found plucking or pulling any of the trees they shall be obleidged to pay six pence to the gardner every time and lose the benefits of being taught in the afternoon and of comeing to the garden at any time except betwixt the hours of five and seven in the morning.[60]

Though Alexander Monro *primus'* account of the foundation of the Medical School in 1726 may be less than objective, his autobiographical notes give some flavour of the life of an apprentice – albeit, perhaps, a highly privileged apprentice. He states that his duties comprised:

> assisting dissection, furnishing books and chemical vessels; putting the sick pensioners of the town under his care and obtaining of the Physicians and his brethren to let him attend their patients in uncommon cases gave him better opportunities of informing himself in medicine than the other students had. With several of these he attended the demonstrations of the pharmaceutical plants exhibited every summer by Mr George Preston; a

course of chemistry which Dr Crauford sometimes gave; and the dissection of the human body which was shewed once in two or three years by Mr Robert Elliot and after by Messiers Andrew Drummond and John M'Gill, surgeon-apothecaries who had the title of Professors of Anatomy.[61]

This gives indirect confirmation that dissection was performed relatively rarely by the Professors of Anatomy. Monro also states cryptically that he 'obtained the dismission' of Drummond and M'Gill when he obtained the Chair of Anatomy in 1720 (see below).[62]

## ANATOMY

The main academic focus of the Incorporation at this time was on the teaching and learning of anatomy, and it is a little surprising, perhaps, that no organised instruction seems to have been available until the mid-seventeenth century, and even then the evidence is flimsy. This may be explained in part by the fact that the Incorporation had no designated meeting house until 1647; prior to this meetings had been held in the current Deacon's residence, or occasionally in St Giles' kirk. Neither location lent itself easily to practical anatomical instruction or to storage of the body of the 'condampnit man efter he be deid' that had been promised annually to the Incorporation in the Seal of Cause. The individual credited with making the first moves towards anatomical teaching was James Borthwick, an apothecary admitted to the Incorporation in March 1645 as one of the first of a new genre of practitioner, the surgeon-apothecary. The minutes record that he had passed his examinations (but had not served a surgical apprenticeship), paid his dues and also given his oath *de fideli* to the Seal of Cause, 'especially that poynt therof anent descetting of anatome for the fardir instruction of prentisses and servants'.[63] No evidence has come to light to confirm whether Borthwick did any teaching, though the accounts for transporting goods to the Incorporation's rented rooms in Dickson's Close in 1647 included 6s as the cost of taking the skeleton to the new accommodation.[64] The Incorporation also passed an act in 1693 'discharging any member of the Calling from eviscerating any person within less space than sixteen hours after death'.[65]

The next hints at organised teaching came in 1694, when Alexander Monteith secured permission from the Town Council to obtain the bodies of prisoners who died in the Tolbooth or other places of incarceration. This stimulated a counter-petition from the Incorporation, which petitioned the Council to let it have:

the dead bodies of foundlings who die betwixt the time they are weaned and their being put to schools or trades, while they remain upon the charges of the Kirk, unless the friends of those concerned reimburse the Kirk Treasurer whatever they have cost the town. As also they allow the dead bodies of such as are *felo de se*, when it is found unquestionable self-murder and have none to own them . . . the petitioners always burying the dead bodies within ten free labouring days upon their own charges in what place that shall be appointed by the Council.[66]

Monteith's action appears to have been taken without the knowledge of the Incorporation. It was supported by Archibald Pitcairne, who reported acidly in a letter to a colleague in London that there was a 'vast opposition made to it by the chief-surgeons, who neither will eat hay nor suffer the oxen to eat it'.[67] Whatever the situation, it stung the Incorporation into action, and the Town Council granted its petition on condition that an anatomical theatre was built by Michaelmas 1697 for the purpose of carrying out annual public dissections.

Once the new Hall was completed in 1697 (to replace Curryhill House, bought in 1657 – see Chapter 7), arrangements could be made to carry out the Town Council's instructions, although the first public dissection did not take place until November 1702. Over the course of a week the various parts of the body were dissected, a different surgeon carrying out the work each day. An 'epilogue' was given by Archibald Pitcairne, who had by then left the College of Physicians and drawn his chair up to the surgeons' table. The schedule of dissection was as follows:

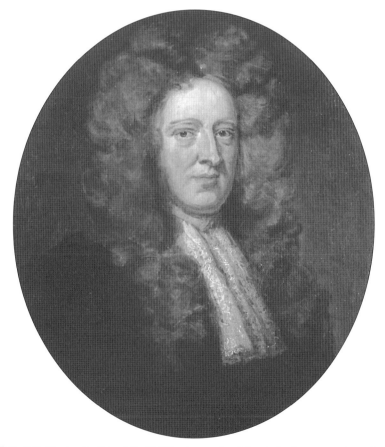

*FIG. 3.5* *Portrait of Archibald Pitcairne, who joined the Incorporation after quarrelling with the physicians.*

Day 1    A general discourse of anatomie, the common teguments and
         muscles of the abdomen (James Hamilton, current Deacon)
Day 2    The peritoneum, stomach, intestines, mesentery and pancreas
         (John Baillie)
Day 3    Liver, spleen, kidneys, ureters, bladder and parts of generation
         (Alexander Monteith)
Day 4    Brain and its nerves with a discourse of the animal spirits
         (Alexander Fyfe)
Day 5    Muscles of the extremeties (Hugh Paterson)
Day 6    Skeleton in general with the head (Robert Clerk)
Day 7    Articulations and the rest of the skeleton (James Auchinleck)
Day 8    Epilogue (Archibald Pitcairne)

The body dissected was that of David Myles, who had been convicted of incest with his sister; she was also hanged for killing the infant subsequently produced. A record of incidental expenses incurred by the Incorporation includes £18s 6d 'to ye officers & trone men for carrying David Mylle's corps', and 9s 6d for 'weights for weighing the body.'[68] Two years later the dissection comprised:

Day 1    Discourse in anatomie in generall with a dissection and
         demonstration of the common teguments and muscles of the
         abdomen (James Hamilton)
Day 2    Umbilicus, omentum, peritoneum, stomach, pancreas, intestines,
         vasa lactea, mesentery, receptaculum chyli, ductus thoracicus
         (John Mirrie)
Day 3    Liver, vesica sellis with their vessels, spleen, kidneys, glanduli
         renales, ureters and bladder (Alexander Nisbet)
Day 4    The organs of generation in a woman with a discourse of hernias
         (George Dundas)
Day 5    The containing and contained parts of the thorax with the
         circulation of the blood and respiration (Robert Swinton)
Day 6    Hair, teguments, dura and pia mater, cerebrum, cerebellum,
         medulla oblongata and nerves within the head (Henry Hamilton)
Day 7    The five external senses with a demonstration of the severall
         organs (Robert Elliot)
Day 8    The muscles of the neck and arme with a discourse of muscular
         motion (no name given)
Day 9    The epilogue or conclusion (Archibald Pitcairne)[69]

By 1704 an extra day was required, and there was no mention of animal spirits, which only two years previously had offered a curious juxtaposition of detailed anatomical dissection and ancient medical philosophy. The limbs were not dissected on the second occasion, and the convicted criminal was apparently female. Some of the leading surgeons of the day were involved in the dissections, and the Incorporation was clearly making every attempt to fulfil the provisions of the Seal of Cause and to prepare apprentices and fellow surgeons for further advances in anatomical and medical knowledge. Each day's dissection was subject to peer review by vote of the assembled members as to the sufficiency of the work.

In France around 1700 there were also problems obtaining bodies for dissection, and a religious dimension can be identified which would not have obtained in Scotland. It was claimed that Protestant inmates who had died within the Hôtel Dieu at Montpellier were especially suitable for autoptic study as 'they are more suitable for instruction than others since we can do what we like with these subjects'.[70]

The next logical step was to try to co-ordinate anatomical teaching, and in 1705 a significant appointment was made. Though there was not yet a formal medical school, the Town Council had appointed three physicians (James Halket, Archibald Pitcairne and Robert Sibbald) as Professors of Medicine in 1685. They received no salary or teaching accommodation, and there is no direct evidence that they carried out any teaching, but the title was created. In 1705 a similar anatomical appointment was made, when, stimulated by a report that 'a person now in the City' intended to approach the Incorporation for permission to carry out the annual dissection', Robert Elliot volunteered to perform these duties, so that the Incorporation would not lose out to an outsider (this kind of 'reactive action' was typical). Elliot was duly appointed by the Town Council at an annual salary of £15 sterling. Though not designated as such, Elliot can be seen as the first Professor of Anatomy in the University. He was joined by a colleague, Adam Drummond, in 1708,[71] and on Elliot's death in 1717, John M'Gill was appointed conjointly with Drummond.[72] The final anatomical link between the Incorporation and the University came in 1720, when political manoeuvring by John Monro and his acquaintances resulted in both Drummond and M'Gill demitting office in favour of Alexander Monro *primus*. The Chair of Anatomy was located within the University in 1725, as one of the last pieces in the jigsaw puzzle that was the foundation of the Medical School (see below). The Seal of Cause had urged the teaching of anatomy, and its transformation into an academic, university subject was a milestone, though perhaps not in the way that had been envisaged earlier, and one which would in time prove to be a millstone rather than a milestone for the College. The anatomy that was taught in 1725 was not significantly different from what it had been earlier, but in the following half-century progress would be made at a much faster rate and the structures and functions of the body elucidated much more clearly and reliably, though the domination of the Monros would turn sour by the middle of the eighteenth century as new knowledge clashed with classical anatomical rhetoric.

As well as dissection and general anatomical instruction, surgeons carried out post-mortem examinations. These were generally undertaken at the request of relatives in order to ascertain the cause of death, and were performed by surgeons, though a physician was usually in attendance, particularly if the deceased were of high social rank. There was a tradition in London (though no direct evidence for Edinburgh) of post-mortems being seen as an occasion for a social gathering – Samuel

Pepys recording just such an occasion in his diary[73] – but there is also evidence that 'guesstimates' of the cause of death were being superseded by more reasoned arguments. Two examples will illustrate this trend. Two surgeons were involved in opening the body of the Earl of Atholl, who had died in suspicious circumstances in 1579. Foul play was suspected and the report concluded that since no other cause was found, 'the said umquhile noble lord Athol was cuttit of be extraordinary means and his life shortnitt be the meanes of poysonn'.[74] The decision of the medical attendants was clearly influenced by outside factors, the conclusion being based not on physical evidence but on the lack of an alternative explanation. By the time of Lady Polwarth's death in 1701, though, the approach was very different. Patrick Telfer was the surgeon involved, and the report was much more detailed, the conclusion being that 'the substance of the lungs in both right left side was wholelie stuff'd with evident purulent mater in all the little cavities and cells thereof'.[75]

Long before the days of Burke and Hare, the question of the illicit acquisition of bodies arose. Ever mindful of its public image, the Incorporation set great store by correct behaviour (at least outwardly) and a serious threat to its standing came in the early 1720s, when accusations of grave-robbing were made. Various incidents were claimed and reported in the press, and in November 1725 the Incorporation felt it necessary to insert a lengthy disclaimer in the *Caledonian Mercury*:

> The Incorporation of Surgeons considering, that several malicious and evil-disposed persons, have industriously raised and spread calumnious Reports, importing, That the Bodies of the Dead have been by them or their apprentices, raised from their graves, to be dissected in their theatre in their Hall: Which reports have met with such great credit among credulous and unthinking people; in so much that they have created great uneasiness in their minds; and of late have been artfully improven by factious designing men, into Tumults and disturbances in this City. Therefore the Incorporation . . . Enact, that each apprentice who should be convicted of raising or attempting to raise the Dead from their Graves, should forfeit their freedom and all Privilege competent to them by their indentures, and be extruded their master's service.[76]

Rewards were offered to those who provided evidence that surgical apprentices were guilty of these offences, and it was stressed that only bodies authorised by the Town Council would be dissected. An unfortunate incident reported only five days later illustrates graphically why the surgeons had to take decisive action. It was reported in the same newspaper that:

> Richard Elliot, a centinel in Colonel Kirk's regiment, now in Canongate, came yesterday to the surgeons and offered (in presence of two Constables whom he supposed to be surgeons) to sell his wife, who is 8 months gone with child, in order to have her anatomised [the unfortunate woman being

alive]. The Magistrates, having been informed thereof caused seize the Centinel; and after a precognition, found the fact fully proven. But by the advice of their Assessors, finding the crime not capital, they gave him up to the officers of the regiment, by whome he is to be severely whipp'd and drumm'd out of the regiment.[77]

Matters did not end there, though, and in 1739 further accusations were made that 'there was a Corps taken out of the West Church Yard'. It was again denied that surgical apprentices were involved, and further rewards were offered for information.[78] Given the atmosphere of the age, when rumours spread rapidly, occurrences of this nature could not be allowed to continue.

## THE INCORPORATION'S LIBRARY AND MUSEUM

From the beginning the Incorporation enforced universal apprentice literacy. It also declared itself to be a learned society, and in keeping with that self-image, the acquisition of the appropriate intellectual accoutrements was a priority. It was not, however, until the Incorporation had existed for almost two centuries that these aims could be fulfilled. As described in detail in Chapter 7, the first fully purpose-built hall was completed in 1697. Very shortly thereafter moves were made to institute a library and a collection of 'curiosities', which formed the basis of the museum collection until the middle of the eighteenth century. Prior to this some books had been acquired by the Incorporation, including a 1661 edition of Hippocrates' *Aphorisms* presented by Alexander Monteith in 1696. By 1699, the foundation of a library collection was something of a natural progression, and orders were issued that 'a draught of laws and constitution for the Biblioteck' should be prepared, and the masters and apprentices made aware of the rules and regulations. Early donations included copies of Culpepper's *Herbal*, some of the works of Ambroise Paré and Wedely's *Phyiologia Medica* (one of a number of works donated by Archibald Pitcairne), while the curiosities included 'a case containing ten old German lancets'; 'a pair of tenailes incisive and a pair of tenailes for drawing of teeth'; 'a pair of Scots cocks spurs, clecked in Fife, prodigiously long'; 'a large eell skin stuff'd and taken in Cramond water'; and, most curious of all, 'an Italian padlock for women'. Alexander Monteith also gave 'some pictures with an glass cylinder by which they can only be discovered', and 'an American birds beak very curious'. The collection of books was by no means confined to surgical or anatomical treatises, with such works as *History of the Antiquities and Warres of the Jews*, published in London in 1576; 'a fine English Bible'; 'a French Bible with the Psalms'; and 'the Acts of Parliament from King James the second to King Charles the second'.

Shortly after this initial trawl for contributions from the masters, advertisements were placed in *Edinburgh Gazette* for donations of books and curiosities. The contributors and the books donated are listed in the minutes. Donors of items valued at £3 sterling or over were rewarded by having their names portrayed in gold lettering and payment was offered in any instance where the donor 'did not think fitt to bestow them gratis'. The request was for the donation of 'Physicall, Anatomicall, Chirurgical, Botanicall, Pharmaceuticall and other Curious books', as well as 'naturall and artificiall curiosities'. How many items were donated is difficult to assess, though merchant James Balfour gave 'a large African gourd with a silver stand', and fellow merchant Lawrence Oliphant offered sixteen books, including Culpepper and a copy of Harvey's *De Motu Cordis*. In any event a series of library rules was drawn up, which bear considerable resemblance to regulations in operation in most academic libraries nowadays. Borrowing of books would be allowed, but only to masters, though if the donor desired, he or she could provide the funds for a chain for their books; the library would be staffed for two hours each day, and no smoking or drinking would be allowed.[79]

From these relatively inauspicious beginnings the collection grew steadily and it was boosted considerably in 1708 when Thomas Kincaid's substantial collection was bequeathed to the Incorporation. Rather surprisingly, Creswell's history of the College makes no mention of this generous bequest, which was of considerable importance in widening the scope of the initial collection. Described as 'a great ornament to that stately fabrick which is erected of late to the honour and use of their society', Kincaid's books covered many subjects, including of course many medical, anatomical and surgical treatises. A recent account of this collection has concluded that the collection was compiled with care, in accordance with Kincaid's own views on medical and surgical matters, and indeed contained a wide range of medical as well as surgical books.[80] Perhaps as a result of this large influx of new material, a further set of library regulations was issued, ordaining that:

- books could be borrowed, but only by masters
- non-masters would have consultation rights only
- fines would be imposed for overdue books
- a catalogue would be drawn up and revised to include future donations
- 'a little table with chairs' was to be provided for reading purposes
- a collection of surgical instruments was to be available for borrowing
- a library committee would be established, with the requirement to carry out yearly inspections and stocktaking.[81]

Thus was founded one of the key elements of the academic 'package'. Unfortunately, though, only some 60 years later the parlous state of the Incorporation would see this valuable collection handed over to the library of the University of Edinburgh. The collection was re-started in the early years of the nineteenth century, but so far attempts by the College to retrieve the original books have been unsuccessful.

The establishment of library collections was a feature of most learned institutions. The FPSG library was started in 1698, shortly after the Faculty had acquired its Hall in the Trongate – there is a clear and obvious connection here between libraries and suitable institutional buildings. As in Edinburgh, Faculty members were invited to donate books and, unlike the Edinburgh situation, the

RCPSG still owns much of its original collection.[82] The RCPEd established a library very soon after its foundation in 1681, as witnessed by the appointment of the first librarian, Sir Archibald Stevenson, in 1683, with Archibald Pitcairne as his deputy.[83] In due course library committees were formed in most institutions to oversee their growing collections and to enforce the rules for borrowing and general behaviour. Though some books were bought by the Incorporation, the core of most of these collections was donations from individuals.

## EXAMINATIONS

Following the requisite period of apprenticeship training, the aspirant surgeon had to face the final hurdle of examinations. Once again, the Seal of Cause provided the impetus, stating that candidates must be 'diligently and avisitly examinit and previt', but the very early records offer little insight as to the content or conduct of these examinations. The first documented entry trial took place in June 1582, when William Bisset was examined and 'fund qualifiet'.[84]

The next entrant master was James Henryson, son of high-profile surgical parent Robert Henryson, who was examined in February 1584. He was followed in 1588 by John Naysmith. Naysmith's examination is not reported in detail other than that he was examined by the assembled Deacon and masters, found qualified, produced his burgess ticket and swore the oath of allegiance.[85] As customary, Naysmith also had to provide a banquet for the Deacon and masters. These dinners were obligatory but later discontinued; the revised regulations in 1723 ordained that:

> every Member pay at his admission, Five Pound Sterling whereof Two shall be given to the Library Keeper for the use of the Library, and the other Three to the Thesaurer for the use of the Society instead of the Treat formerly given, and that the intrant be advertised by the Clerk that the Calling are to meet with him and give him a Glass of Wyne, and that the Intrant be distinctly told that the Calling will take it amiss if he pay any thing on this Occasion, and that the Deacon have the naming of the Tavern.[86]

Though there is no evidence of examination content in the early period, concern with further study is revealed in the record of Andrew Scott. On his admission in 1593, the masters recorded their wish that he 'employ himself to the earnest studie in the said art as he hes begun'.[87] (Scott had been allowed to take his examinations early in view of his impending departure on royal service. This was not an isolated incident. On 20 May 1623, John Pringle was admitted early 'by the earnest request of ane potent lord the erle of Melross'. Patronage was the life-blood of the Incorporation, and the patrons clearly expected returns.) Immediately after qualification Scott left to serve as royal surgeon, and on his return held office as Deacon on eight occasions between 1598 and 1627.

The first information as to the content of examinations does not appear till

1647, when specific guidelines were set down, possibly at the instigation of James Borthwick, who had offered to teach anatomy at his admission in 1645. It was decided that a formal examination routine should be established in order that future tests could be applied 'without variance or discrepance', and it was agreed that:

> Every entrant on the day of his examination shall have one of the masters to be his examinator and this without prejudice to any of the rest of the brethren to question him upon that samyn days subject. The first day the intrant is to begin with the introduction to chirurgerie and to make ane generall discourse of the hole anatomie without any demonstration. Secondly he is to demonstrate be ocular inspection more particularly some pairtes of the anatomie qllk sall be aponyted to him by the Deacon and masters and to answer the demands of his examinators and masters thereupon. Thirdly he is to show some operations on the foresaid subjects as the Deacon and masters think fit and to answer the demands of his examinators and masters thereupon ... and accordynglie as the Deacon and masters fynds him qualified or unqualifiet they may remitt or repiett him or otherways continue his examination on the foresaid subjects by and quhyll they fund him qualifiet.[88]

These regulations clearly reflect the aims of the Seal of Cause and it is indeed possible to overlay present-day regulations and find a number of points of comparison. Though a specific examinator was to be nominated, the assembled brethren still had the right to participate in the examination, and this system remained unchanged till 1698, when it was decided that specific examinators, initially five in number, were to be elected each year. The examination would now stretch over five days and it was also decreed that the examinators themselves must offer a discourse on a topic of their choice – a further move towards increasing general knowledge.

The topics chosen by the examinators included:

- aneurysm
- animal oeconomy
- arteries and motion of the heart
- bite of a mad dog
- circulation of the blood
- dislocations and fractures
- empyema
- structure of kidneys
- wounds of nerves

Some of the topics were much more narrow and specific. In 1736 Thomas Gibson spoke on 'proving that there is no anastomosis betwixt the spermatick arteries and veins', while some five years later Walter Gibson offered the view that 'a derivation to the external parts of the head can be shown by opening the external jugulars'. Further evidence of the evolving state of anatomical knowledge comes from the examination of John Semple in 1719, when he was instructed to discuss the brain and its 'eleven pairs of nerves', not twelve, as now recognised.

In 1712 the examination was reduced to four days,[89] but the next major change came in 1723, when the syllabus was expanded to include tests on 'materia medica, bottany and the reading and explaining of receipts', and from the mid-1730s *methodus componendi* was added and candidates were obliged to offer samples of compounded medications or plasters. To assist the apprentices and masters in this new examination area, the librarian, Alexander Monro *primus*, was ordered to 'fill the chist in the library with Materia Medica'.[90] The background to this change was not simply one of broadening knowledge. It stemmed from attempts by the College of Physicians to participate in the teaching of pharmacy to surgical apprentices, the records indicating that 'the College of Phisitians were willing in ane amicable way to consort with the calling what method would be most proper for improving and regulating Pharmacy'.[91] The standard response by most corporate bodies of whatever sort to any perceived encroachment is to set up a committee to look into the matter, and this is just what was done. The inclusion of the extra examination topics came immediately thereafter. The questions posed to most of the entrants reflected the most common problems to be encountered, but occasionally there is confirmation that enduring belief systems must be remembered. On 31 August 1727, for example, William Wardrob sat his third examination and 'discoursed upon the Humane Body in a Religious and Anatomick way'.[92]

Among the topics allocated to candidates most frequently were: amputation; trepanning; bandages of head and face; contained parts of abdomen and thorax; operation for empyema; bloodletting; couching of cataract; fistula lachrymalis; and compound fracture of the leg. The examinations were normally undertaken over a period of several weeks, and occasionally entrants were delayed because the regulations stated that no trial could begin until the previous one had been completed. Most candidates were successful, with only three recorded instances of referral by 1737. Adam Darling embarked on his examinations in 1652, but after the third test was suspended until he 'had farder qualification and abilitie in the art',[93] while the records note on 2 November 1671 that Thomas Ker had failed to satisfy his examiners on the topic of the 'contained parts of the breast', and he was suspended from further examination 'till he be better qualifiet'. The third candidate was David Knox, who took his examinations in early 1718 but failed the third session on the Deacon's casting vote.[94] He was deferred for a year, but went to law, seeking an injunction against the Incorporation. The result of this litigation is not known, but Knox next appeared in the minutes when he passed his final test on 'bleeding of the jugular and bandages of the head and face' in January 1719. Once entered, the new masters could immediately take on servants and apprentices, and were also eligible for office-holding, as well as submitting themselves to the rules and regulations of the Incorporation.[95]

The examinations undertaken by entrant masters were probably comparable to those operated by similar Incorporations. The FPSG had a somewhat more complex examining system, some individuals being licensed to practise only those procedures in which they had been deemed competent. This, unusually, included permission given to perform bloodletting by individuals from other trades.[96] As far as the 'legitimate' surgical apprentices were concerned, regulation of apprenticeships seems to have been very much the same as in the Edinburgh Incorporation or, indeed, in any organised craft. There does, though, appear to have been a more rigorous system of formal examinations in Glasgow, the apprentices being examined three times during the course of their apprenticeship. Details are scarce – as they are for most Incorporations at this time – but it seems that by the end of the seventeenth century most of the Glasgow apprentices were tried in surgery and pharmacy in order to practise as 'general practitioners'.[97]

In the case of the London Barber-Surgeons there was the added complication that the Bishop of London had been authorised by Act of Parliament in 1511 to grant licences to surgeons. An agreement had apparently been reached that he would not grant any such licence unless the candidate had been approved by the Company of Barber-Surgeons, but this was not always adhered to, and the matter was not resolved finally till the early eighteenth century. The Barber-Surgeons had a Court of Examiners in 1555, four of whom were ordained to examine each candidate, though few details are available about the format or content of the tests.[98]

## WHAT DID THE SURGEONS DO?

It is all very well for any group to have a well-ordered organisation, good training and comprehensive examinations to ensure standards, but in early-modern Scotland the surgical lives of the masters of the Incorporation were limited, though they were, mostly, conscientious in their care of the patients. Whereas in more modern times a vast array of surgical procedures can be done on any part of the body, and while the surgical profile is still to some extent constructed by outside influences, such as state of war or peace, political unrest or natural disasters, the seventeenth-century surgeon's workload was determined to a much greater degree by violence and the environment. Unable to perform complex invasive procedures, what the Edinburgh surgeons could do was treat the wounds of conflict and the infections caused by wounds and the environment. They were expert in amputation, and also developed considerable skills in cataract removal and the treatment of fistulas. The care of patients with bladder stones, one of the most common afflictions of the day, was rather more controversial, and at times left to unqualified individuals who claimed specialist expertise in this area.[99] There is very little in the way of direct evidence about surgical procedures, though it is possible to gain a good general impression from records such as testaments and court books, as well as occasional mentions in the Town Council records. Fuller accounts of these have appeared elsewhere,[100] but it is necessary here to give some examples to illustrate the day-to-day work of the early-modern Incorporation master.

In 1617, James Henryson treated Mr Patrick Crawford, who had been 'deidlie hurt and woundit in Muscovia be an shott of ane muskett in the left thigh and the bullet being stuck and fixit in his thigh bane qrby he was unabill to gang bot only upone his teyes'.[101] After what must have been a difficult journey back to Edinburgh, the musket ball was removed and final cure took eleven weeks of treatment. Around 1670, John Forrest was involved in the treatment of a complex heel wound sustained by an apprentice, described as 'ane hollo ulser with ane flux of san[g]ui[nou]s humours upon the great tendon of his heill and towards his cuit [ankle] accompanied with inflammation and tumefaction which at first was occasioned with the stroak of ane ax, which wound forsaid was turned ulserus.'[102] Other cases included a head wound whereby the patient had been 'crewellie hurt and woundit', the surgeon having to extract 'seventeine brokin banes out of the said Walter's heid and face for preservation of his lyff and eye'; 'ane musket shott in the heil qrby the bones was brokin'; and 'thrie ulcers, ane qrof in his left shoulder, ane uther in his left thie and the other in his knie'.

There was also considerable blurring of the supposedly strict demarcations between what was deemed to come within the compass of medical as opposed to surgical work. A Town Council edict in 1643 confirmed that the surgeons were entitled to treat 'all kind of woundis impostumes ulceris fractures dislocatiouns, canceris, imbalming of dead corps, applying of sparadraps [waxed cloths]'.[103] Regulations were there to be contravened, though, and it is clear that many surgeons offered treatments for internal conditions. Alexander Pennycuik took the father of one of his patients to court for non-payment of fees concerning Pennycuik's treatment for scrofula (tuberculosis), with 'all kinds of inward and outward medicines'.[104]

Military surgery and service to royal houses and armies was an important part of the work of the Incorporation, and indeed of Scottish physicians and surgeons in general,[105] and the ubiquitous Pennycuik clearly had some difficulty in acquiring money and supplies for this purpose, as he had to issue a claim in 1644 for fees due to him during the bitter conflicts of the Civil War period:

> Forsameikill and be indentor of the dait at Edr the first of febr 1644 years betwix umqull colonell James Rae mert burges of ye said burt colonell to ye towne of Edr thair regiment on ye ane pairt and me on ye uyr part bering yat it was agriet betwixt us that I should undertake ye said regiment sould be sufficiently attendid and servit in maner specifiet for the qlk ye said umqul colonell obleist him to cause supplie me wt all necessarie medicaments in maner yrin mentionat and ye said pay as chirurgaine to ye said regiment that he sould procure payt yrof to me fra ye guid towne of Edr.[106]

The Colonel did not pay up and Pennycuik eventually went to court and obtained a decreet against him for £197 12s 3d sterling for the period 1 February 1644 to February 1647. He was eventually reimbursed by Rae's son.

What is clear from the scarce records is that the surgeons treated a limited range of conditions, determined to a great extent by violence and infections; they charged variable fees according to the means of the patients;[107] they did deal with medical conditions, though they were not supposed to; and often they treated the patients for lengthy periods. It is likely also that the surgical techniques involved were similar to, or derived from, those of Lowe and Paré.[108] By the time of the foundation of the Medical School in 1726, the spheres of anatomical knowledge and practical organisation were changing much more rapidly than the ability of the surgeons to carry out complex procedures. The situation seems to have been in most respects very similar to that elsewhere. Evidence from research on the work of London and English provincial surgeons confirms the general nature of surgical practice at this time.[109] The records of a seventeenth-century German barber-surgeon indicate that he was obliged to present difficult cases to a commission of inspection – these cases including instances where no improvement was seen after the fourth dressing, no change could be detected or there was 'danger to life, impending paralysis, or the possible amputation of a limb'.[110] As with the Scottish surgeons, the bulk of this particular surgeon's workload was dealing with wounds, together with ulcers, fractures, burns and gangrene. Unlike his Edinburgh counter-parts, though, this surgeon also carried out barbering duties, though similar demarcations existed about dealing with external and internal conditions.[111] At this time it must be remembered also that the balance of power between patient and practitioner was very different.

## THE BAGNIO

In addition to the well-proportioned meeting house and dissection theatre, the new Hall which was completed by 1697 (see Chapter 7) also incorporated a bagnio or Turkish bath within its complex, for both therapeutic and economic purposes – an extension of surgical treatment in its broadest sense. It was not the first one in Edinburgh, though, as barber and Incorporation member James Rae had erected one in 1686. The Town Council records note that he had 'erected baith stoves upon the north side of the head of the Cannongate with several conveniensyes thereto belonging', and had furnished it at great expense, with the intention that it would be 'verrie useful to the leidges as to their health'. His petition to prevent others setting up similar baths was granted, though it would not be long before the Incorporation built its own, apparently unopposed.[112]

By the end of the seventeenth century the medicinal use of baths was becoming more popular, probably influenced by Sir John Floyer's book on the topic.[113] In any event, a bagnio was constructed as part of the new building. From the start there were problems, though, not least because of poor water supply from the surgeons' own well, and it was not till 1701 that the Town Council allowed the Incorporation to make use of surplus water from other town wells. Eventually, though, the bath was made available to the public, and it was noted on 7 January 1704 that:

> there is now erected at the Chirurgeon-Apothecaries Hall Edr two fine Bagnios after the Turkish Fashion where all Noblemen Gentlemen Ladyes

and others may be conveniently sweated and Bathed. The men on Mondays, Wednesdays, Thursdays and Saturdays and the women on Tuesdays and Fridays (on which two days no man is allowed to come within the Garden). The price for each person is 3 pounds Scots. And if any person desires the use of a Bagnio alone they are to pay 6 pounds. The prices for the beds in the upper rooms of the Bagnio is to be two shillings ster. Per night for a single person and if two shall lay together they are to pay three shillings ster. Each night. There is nothing to be given to the Servants.

John Valentine and his daughter were employed to run the operation, being allowed to sell 'Coffee, Tea, Chocolate and other cordial liquors in the house'. The bagnio was, though, and quite naturally, open to misuse, and on 7 July 1707 the officer was disciplined and clear instructions issued that if any man came near the building on the days reserved for women, 'the doors leading to the bedrooms [should] be locked and neither master nor stranger enter these rooms at that time'. Despite attempts to improve the water supply, the bagnio proved to be expensive and difficult to maintain, and eventually fell into disrepair. It was put up for sale in 1740, with the 'marbles and piggs' to be sold off at best value. The Incorporation had experienced considerable financial difficulty since the separation with the barbers in 1722, which had resulted in a significant fall in income.

## HONORARY FREEDOMS AND VISUAL SYMBOLS

By the second half of the seventeenth century, the crisis of numbers had been averted, apprenticeships and examinations were well established, and the masters continued their driving aim to be viewed as an academic society. Although the Incorporation generally had the support of the Town Council in any dispute, it was considered expedient to try to broaden the network of potential political support – possibly motivated by the formation of the Fraternity of Apothecaries and Surgeon-Apothecaries (see below), and also the ongoing attempts being made by the physicians to gain a royal charter and set up a College. After discussion as to what could be done in this regard the masters agreed that it would be:

Highly expedient not only for the honour reputation and splendour of their art and Incorporation but also for the maintenance preservation and amplificatione of the liberties and priviledges thereof. That some select persons of eminence poure and place and of known good affection suld with societie be admitted honorary frieman of the Incorporation during thir lyftimes without any examination conforme to the laudable custom used by severall Incorporations and societies in foreign kingdoms who may countenance protest or otherways concurre to the preservation and maintenance of their just interests and concerns, albeit they are not to use nor exerce the practicall part and mannuall operations of the said profession of Chirurgerie and anatomie.[114]

Not surprisingly, the first individual to be accorded this honour was Sir Andrew Ramsay, Provost of Edinburgh, Privy Councillor and Lord of the Exchequer, who was admitted on 17 October 1671, in recognition of his 'very great affection and respects' for the Incorporation. Clearly this was someone who could give high-level political assistance. Not all of the presentations went strictly according to plan, though. On 20 August 1672 a deputation was sent to Holyrood to present the Duke of Lauderdale with his honorary freedom, but a second delegation had to be despatched later in the day, 'in respect he was not at home in the forenoon'.[115] Among the recipients of the honour later in the century were the Earl of Perth, the Duke of Queensberry and the Marquises of Atholl and Tweeddale. Though the political appointments have continued, the majority of recipients in recent times have been individuals deemed to have made a significant contribution to surgery and the wider medical field. The award of Honorary Freedoms can be seen perhaps as marking the beginning of the Incorporation's independent political activities, outwith the shelter of the Town Council chamber. The first Honorary Fellowship awarded by the RCPEd went to Patrick Hume, later the first Earl of Marchmont in 1696, together with four Lords of Session, confirming the political nature of honorary appointments in this period.[116]

Two years after the decision about honorary freedoms, the Incorporation's coat of arms was matriculated – yet another outward symbol,[117] while on completion of the new Hall in 1697, masters were ordered to have their portraits painted by Sir John Medina (see Chapter 7). All of these things had a common purpose – to emphasise and enhance the image of the Incorporation as a learned body.

## THE INCORPORATION AND PARLIAMENT

During the earlier years of the Incorporation's life, the Scottish parliament functioned very differently from its modern counterparts. It comprised a single chamber, and was only called at the king's desire, usually in order to acquire funds for wars or to finance the royal court (regular taxation in peacetime was not a feature until the early seventeenth century). The Privy Council was the main forum for politics between king and nobles. There was nothing equivalent to parliamentary debate on major issues in the modern sense. Politics had much more to do with patronage than parliament, though the latter had to ratify measures before they could be put into operation. An Act of Parliament of 1584 ordained that one of the commissioners to parliament representing Edinburgh should be a craftsman, and as the surgeons were the senior craft, this gave them direct access to parliament. Some of the measures recorded in parliamentary records relating to the Incorporation, though not necessarily Acts of Parliament in the modern sense, were:

- Confirmation of the Seal of Cause (1506)
- Letter of exemption granted by Mary, Queen of Scots (1567)
- Confirmation by King James VI of the Seal of Cause and Ratification, 6 June 1613

- Act of Parliament, 'dated at Edinburgh 17 November 1741, made and granted by his Majestie's umquhill deceased father, of eternal memory, with advice and consent of the Estates of Parliament, in favours of the said surgeons and barbers'
- Ratification in favours of the Surgeons, by the Parliament, of all their former Grants, 22 August 1670
- Grant by King William and Queen Mary, in favours of the College of Surgeons of Edinburgh and Ratification thereof in Parliament 17 July 1695

On a more individual level, parliament on occasion was asked to confirm payments to surgeons for services rendered. In 1641 it was noted that any surgeon appointed to armies travelling to England would be allowed £15 sterling to furnish his 'kist'; and £53 6s 8d was paid to a surgeon for 'curing the wounds of two prisoners in Edinburgh castle.' In October 1606 Andrew Scott was one of two delegates sent to attend the 'Seicrett Counsell at Lythgow [Privy Council at Linlithgow]'. Some years later he was sent as a commissioner to the Convention of the Royal Burghs and to the Scottish parliament.

Other Edinburgh surgeons who served parliament as well as royal houses and armies included James Borthwick, who attended on a number of occasions in the second half of the seventeenth century. He was a commissioner to parliament in 1649–50 and 1661, served on the Committee for Plantation of Kirks in 1649 and on the Committee of the Estates in the same year, as well as participating in pre-Restoration discussions with nobles and gentry in 1659–60. He was allowed to retire in 1662 because he was too busy 'attending persons of quality' in his professional capacity. Arthur Temple was a commissioner to parliament in 1669, but was 'called away by reason of his employment of Chyrurgion and his wife being valetudinarie'. George Stirling served as Commissioner to the Convention of Estates in 1689 and, following the accession of William and Mary, Commissioner to Parliament in 1689–93. Following the Union of Parliaments of 1707, the Incorporation had fewer opportunities to be directly influential, but there was ongoing contact with individual MPs and government ministers, which would intensify in the period leading up to the Medical Act of 1858. The nature of the Incorporation's political actions and contacts would change in the light of general political change, though it would be no less important.

## THE EDINBURGH MEDICAL TRIANGLE – PHYSICIANS, SURGEONS AND APOTHECARIES

In most towns large enough to have groups of medical practitioners there was some conflict and jostling for the limited space available. In Edinburgh the situation was no different, and the Incorporation was involved in bitter disputes with the apothecaries and the physicians in the latter decades of the seventeenth century, mainly over who should have supervisory rights over the apothecaries, who did not have a fully independent organisation of their own. In 1657 the Fraternity of Apothecaries and Surgeon-apothecaries was created by the Town Council.[118] This was a shadowy group – shadowy in terms of evidence – which seems to have survived for only a few decades, and whose relationship with the Incorporation is difficult to define. This group comprised simple apothecaries and apothecaries who had also qualified as surgeons, and seems to have originated with the admission to the Incorporation of Robert Borthwick and Thomas Kincaid in 1645. The general view is that they were admitted because of scarcity of numbers in the Incorporation, but a claim has also been made that they gained admission as a reward for assistance given to the surgeons during the military campaigns of the early 1640s.[119]

Whatever the case, the erection of the Fraternity was confirmed by Act of Parliament in 1670. It seems that from that point the surgical apprentices received training in dispensing of medicines, and the evidence confirms that the species of surgeon-apothecary dates from this time, though it was shortlived and there were few such admissions by the early 1690s. A Town Council act of 1643 had confirmed the demarcated duties of surgeons, so that 'the application of searcloths [wax cloths for preservation] to dead bodies, all manual operations and applications about dead of living bodies, and the curing of tumours, wounds, ulcers, luxations, fractures, and the curing of virolls, etc' were reserved to the surgeons.[120] The surgeon-apothecaries were one thing, but the simple apothecaries quite another, and the Incorporation maintained its pursuit of any infringement of privilege. The Cunningham affair, mentioned above, was fairly typical, though perhaps more high-profile than some, as it involved patients of high social rank. Following a tortuous legal path, the case was eventually put before the Lords of Council, and by the time it had reached the Court of Session, it had gone from the particular to the general, with the apothecaries in opposition to the combined forces of the surgeons, the surgeon-apothecaries and the Town Council. Legal argument centred on whether the pursuits of surgery and pharmacy should be separated, and in what would nowadays be termed a 'landmark judgement', the court found for the apothecaries (who would be backed by the physicians from 1681), and the subsequent Decreet of Separation in 1862 meant that for the next fourteen years the callings were officially separated and the problems centred on supervision of apothecaries and their shops.[121] The situation would be reversed with the William and Mary patent of 1694, which reconfirmed the surgeons' privileges, but for the moment the Incorporation appeared to have been adversely affected in terms of its areas of jurisdiction.[122] During the dispute the Incorporation engaged the legal might of Sir George Mackenzie, Sir John Lauder and Mr Colin Mackenzie, at considerable expense, as at least 1,000 merks (£666) was borrowed specifically for the purpose, and the minutes note on 15 July 1681 that there was a need 'to borrow more money'. In consequence of the judgement of 1682, the remaining surgeon-apothecaries were allowed to perform both functions, but were obliged to choose either to remain within the Incorporation, or join the surgeon-apothecaries' organisation. It appears that only one, John Jossie, took the latter option, and neither the species nor the Fraternity survived for much longer.

There is not enough space here to go into great detail about the many attempts which had been made by the physicians to gain a collegiate organisation from the early seventeenth century. At all stages, though, these moves were strongly opposed by the surgeons, particularly as some of the proposals, if successful, would have given the physicians sweeping powers over the surgeons as well as the apothecaries and appeared to be an unjustified encroachment on their historic territories and Town Council-backed responsibilities.[123] As the final attempt approached, the Incorporation appointed a committee to look into the matter and suggest ways of preserving its position, and meanwhile began attempts to gain a new charter for itself.[124] Again, money was borrowed for the purpose. In the event, as had happened with the foundation of the Incorporation, royal support was crucial for the physicians, though in this case rather different. James IV had ratified the Incorporation's Seal of Cause from a background of his own interest in medicine; in the case of the physicians, the support of the Duke of York was important, but it was particularly important for the duke himself, in the heat of the Exclusion Crisis and the need to canvass as much personal political support as he could.[125] He was clearly interested in patronage of the arts and learning, but this interest was more complex than a simple desire to support these areas of intellectual Scotland.[126]

The priority of the Incorporation during this period was quite simply to maintain its privileges against the perceived onslaught of the physicians. It might be assumed from the formation of the Fraternity that legal opinion would have been in favour of the Incorporation when it came to matters of jurisdiction over the apothecaries, but here again demarcation disputes continued and once the RCPEd came into being, the courts as well as the Town Council became embroiled in expensive legal argument. It may seem natural to assume that in any legal contest a ruling of the Court of Session would take precedence over an act of the Town Council. This was, though, a period during which Scots Law itself was in the process of being written down for the first time – Stair's *Institutions* saw its first edition in the Golden Year of 1681,[127] and indeed the Incorporation itself was older than the Court of Session, which was founded in 1532. So it was not necessarily the case that a Court decreet would be accepted immediately as the final word on any matter – in the case of the Incorporation, unlike the physicians, the weight of history and a succession of confirmations of privileges had considerable significance. The legal argument lay in the interpretation of history and precedence just as much as in any rule as to what should take place in the future.

This period was one of the most important for the Incorporation in terms of its attempts to maintain its jurisdiction and privileges against the backcloth of the new physicians' College and the temporary boost to the apothecaries given by the Decreet of Separation. Future disputes were played out in this complex triangle, each member of which justified its position from a different perspective – the surgeons from precedence and Town Council Acts, the physicians from their new Royal Charter, and the apothecaries from the Decreet of Separation. The contemporary context is clearly important here. A Town Council Act was seen by the Incorporation as fully equal to a Court of Session decreet. The hierarchy of the

Scots legal profession was no doubt just as keen as the Incorporation to make its mark in terms of the weight of Scots Law, and the whole background is one of jostling for position on the part of several groups in urban society – some well-established and others much newer. The emerging professions had a key role to play in the urbanisation process in general.

For the next two decades there was a rash of disputes as a result of the three entrenched positions. The terms of the Decreet of Separation meant that an apothecary should have been nominated by the Town Council to visit apothecaries' shops, but a surgeon-apothecary was appointed instead, and the Court was forced to intervene. This was only one of a number of similar disputes. The Incorporation made a strong plea to the Privy Council on this matter, part of the claim on its behalf being that whereas surgeon-apothecaries were 'for many years bred up in the skill of them [drugs], and it is a science that requires long and great experience, a Phisitian will be graduate upon a year's studie'.[128] A Privy Council Act of 1684 granted the physicians rights of visitation of the shops, and this was contested by the Incorporation, but in 1686 a simple apothecary was appointed by the Court of

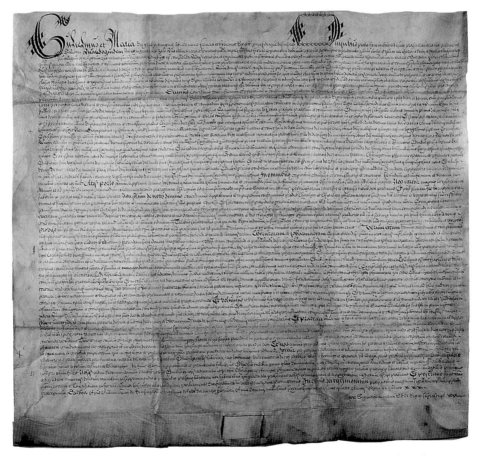

**FIG. 3.6** *Patent granted to the Incoporation by William and Mary (1694), reconfirming privileges.*

Session, adding still further to the confusion of the situation. This litigious and expensive three-cornered struggle continued till 1694, when the Incorporation managed to gain a patent or diploma from William and Mary, which reconstituted all of its previous rights and privileges, including control of pharmacy. This gained parliamentary ratification on 17 July 1695, and was, surprisingly, not opposed by the physicians, who had been making a few conciliatory gestures, including inviting the Incorporation in 1688 to comment on the draft of the first edition of the *Edinburgh Pharmacopoeia* (though this was not published until 1699).[129] An additional benefit gained from the new patent was the extension of the sphere of influence of the Incorporation to the Lothians, Fife, Peebles, Selkirk, Roxburgh and Berwickshire. Surgeons wishing to practise in these parts would thenceforth require certification by the Incorporation. When the Incorporation's diploma was introduced in the 1770s the opportunity was taken to require these surgeons to take the examination. In this way, then, the whole of the south of Scotland was under the control of either the Incorporation or the FPSG.

## THE INCORPORATION AND THE MEDICAL
## SCHOOL – WHY THEN?

A number of theories have been advanced about why the Edinburgh Medical School came into being in 1726. One view expressed by Cunningham, but since contested by others, is that the major stimulus was the need for Edinburgh to find new directions in the aftermath of 1707, a new identity with a calming or eirenic aspect to intellectual life, and that the system imported from the University of Leiden (which included clinical instruction and taught what was claimed to be a refined, classical medical philosophy) provided just that.[130] This is probably not the whole explanation. The strong Leiden connection was undoubtedly a factor, both in the actions of individuals and of the Town Council and University, but there were other influences. In most major events in history there seems to be a crucial combination – at the particular time – of background trends and the impetus of individuals and the pressure of immediate circumstance. In this case there were already in existence medical and surgical corporations in Edinburgh; the University was under the control of the Town Council and its current principal, William Carstares, was a devotee of Leiden; the most prominent politician of the time, the ubiquitous George Drummond, certainly had a wish to promote and develop the intellectual and cultural aspects of Edinburgh; the change from regenting to professorial teaching in the University was more appropriate to specialised subjects; and the Town Council had already appointed several individuals as Professors in the University. From the Incorporation's point of view the important factor here was the appointment of Elliot as Professor of Anatomy in 1705, and his successors. John Monro (who had studied at Leiden), master of the Incorporation (deacon 1712–14) and archetypal ambitious parent, saw his son, Alexander Monro *primus*, enter as master of the Incorporation in 1719, on a 'fast-track' examination, and very quickly manage to oust the incumbent Professors of Anatomy and install himself in that position.

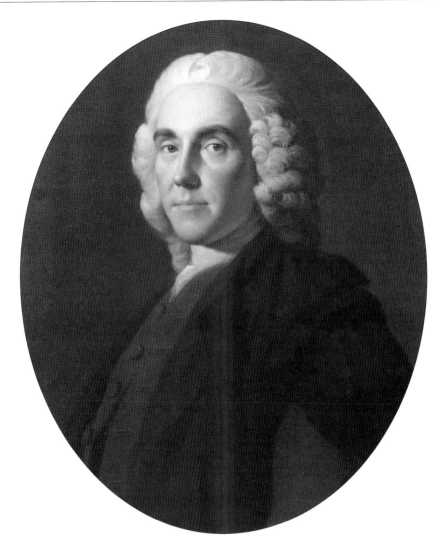

**FIG. 3.7** *Portrait of Alexander Monro* primus.

Monro operated extra-murally – and lectured regularly in the Incorporation's theatre, as well as donating dissected specimens – until 1725, when the grave-robbing scandal broke and he thought it prudent to try to move within the walls of the University.[131] A year later four physicians (Drs Innes, Plummer, Rutherford and Sinclair), all of whom had studied at Leiden,[132] were appointed Professors of Medicine, and so came into being the Edinburgh Medical School. A Professor of Midwifery was appointed in 1729 to complete the range of medical subjects. These individuals provided the teaching and examining.

But what of the role of the Incorporation in all of this? As mentioned, Monro senior was a master of the Incorporation, and so was his son, though subsequent Monros would give their allegiance to the 'other place' and become physicians, though maintaining a stranglehold on the teaching of anatomy and surgery for

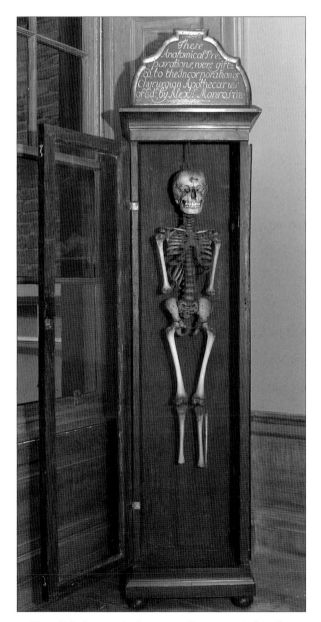

**FIG. 3.8** *Anatomical preparation presented to the Incorporation by Alexander Monro* primus *in 1718.*

most of the eighteenth century. The Incorporation clearly welcomed the initial appointment of Elliot in 1705, as this ensured that one of its own would take charge of anatomical instruction. It co-operated in the accelerated examination schedule applied to Monro *primus*, and approved his preference to the Chair of Anatomy, though the reasons given for the demission of the incumbents ring less than true.[133] The Incorporation itself may not have had direct influence on the process, but it was represented on the Town Council. Conflicts would arise later in terms of the teaching of surgery, and also with the moves to modernise anatomical teaching, but for the moment the Incorporation was involved with the Medical School indirectly, but involved none the less. Incorporation teaching and philosophy were still centred on the apprenticeship and the individual relationship between master and apprentice, but increasingly it would be the case that apprentices availed themselves of University courses, and in turn medical students would take the College diploma when it was instituted in the second half of the eighteenth century.

The College records are singularly uninformative about any corporate attitude towards the establishment of a medical school, but this does not necessarily indicate apathy or indeed opposition. In 1723 a general review of rules and regulations was undertaken. This volume of the minutes is less complete than others, with frequent gaps where information has not been inserted, but it was noted on 2 March 1723 that 'no Apprentice for five years shall for the first three years go to any of the Professors of Medicine, Chimie, Anatomy, Surgery or Materia Medica but with his Masters consent' – suggesting some degree of tension between the Incorporation and the University.[134] Though the foundation of the Medical School would prove to be both advantageous and problematic for the Incorporation, it caused few ripples in the records. By 1726, the Incorporation was soundly structured in terms of its organisation, rules and examinations. It had survived the challenges of the physicians, it had supplied the Professor of Anatomy, and had confirmed its status as the leading urban craft, despite its numerical disadvantage as compared with some of the other crafts. The potential political power of the crafts had been noted earlier by James VI in his book *Basilikon Doron*, in which he stated that 'if they [crafts] in anything be controlled . . . up goes the Blue Blanket [the banner of the Incorporated Trades]'.[135] This was all a little ambiguous for the Incorporation. University teaching of anatomy enhanced the veneer of learning, but at the same time it still required Town Council support as a craft.

Once the Medical School was a reality, though, it was one more influence on Edinburgh medicine with which the Incorporation had to deal. It must be remembered that throughout all of this period, the medical marketplace was teeming with practitioners of all sorts, claiming all sorts of powers and consulted by a public eager to cure its various ills by whatever means possible. The surgeons may have been awarded exclusive rights by the Town Council, but this did not mean that they were necessarily able to secure these rights. Whether threatened by physician, apothecary, mountebank, quack or other institution, this was a continual struggle for the maintenance of the Incorporation's position. It may have considered itself to be 'famous and flourishing', but, crucially, consultation was at the choice of the patient, who was not necessarily going to consult a qualified practitioner. The foundation of the RCPEd and Medical School were new difficulties towards the end of the early-modern period, and shortly thereafter would come the very early beginnings of hospital medicine, which would, in time, afford an entirely new aspect, to medicine and surgery, but also, importantly, to the nature of the relationship between practitioner and patient and the role of the Incorporation.

## CONCLUSION

For the first two centuries of its existence – or at least the period from 1581 when the written records commence – the Incorporation was shaped and influenced by a number of interacting and, at times, conflicting factors. The period saw the final secularisation of medical training and the emergence of an organised medical orthodoxy. This was a lowland, urban phenomenon, centred on claims made by emergent groups of trained practitioners for 'custody' of medical and surgical knowledge, which was then defined as the orthodoxy. The identity of Scottish medicine and surgery in this period was complex, and based on a multiplicity of traditions and influences, but in terms of the role and status of the Incorporation, the key factors were the secularisation and, importantly, the early institutionalisation of the orthodoxy. If from that point 'legitimate' medical or surgical practice must be linked to professional institutions, then the Incorporation had had a very good start indeed. In terms of the nation itself, Scotland had been transformed from a feudal to a mercantile society, the urban network was strengthening, there were rather more marked contrasts between highlands and lowlands, and European connections were still strong. What must be remembered, though, is that the Incorporation was part of a world in which the orthodox and unorthodox were comfortable partners. 'Professional' medicine and surgery operated in a complex cosmological context, and masters of the Incorporation were no different. By the time that the Incorporation had to consider its links with the newly formed Medical School in 1726, the nation had experienced two unions with England, and from that point it functioned within the context of Great Britain. It had also gone some way towards general recognition as a profession – indeed from the 1690s members of the Incorporation had been taxed individually at the same level as physicians, lawyers and ministers, unlike the other crafts which were taxed corporately rather than individually (for nationally imposed taxes such as the Poll Tax of 1694).[136] On the other hand, it had not been possible for the Incorporation to eradicate unauthorised practice. Though it was less easy for amateurs to perform heroic surgery such as amputation, as opposed to the concoction of potions and remedies or the dressing of wounds, there was still more than enough to keep the Incorporation's officials active. The next period in its history would reflect this, together with the rapid increase in knowledge, the considerable effects of the Enlightenment, the role of 'big government' and the push towards medical reform.

## NOTES

1. College prayer, attributed to John Knox.
2. Brown, K. M., *Kingdom or Province? Scotland and the Regal Union 1603–1707* (Basingstoke, 1992), covers the politics of the period. For a more anglocentric view of James VI's reign from 1603, see Lockyer, R., *James VI and I* (London, 1998).
3. For a recent account of the historiographical controversies surrounding the union, see Whatley, C. A., *Bought and Sold for English Gold? Explaining the Union of 1707* (East Linton, 2001).
4. College Minutes, 4 February 1583.

5. Primrose occupied the office of Deacon in 1581–2 and 1602. The College Museum contains a replica of his mortar and pestle, presented by the Rosebery family.
6. College Minutes, 30 June 1588 and 15 September 1590. It was ordained on 18 April 1614 that if any master failed to contribute towards the buying of a mortcloth, 'thay, thir wyff and bairnis sall nowayes have the use of the said mortclaith at thair buriall'. This is understandable as the new cloth cost £175 Scots.
7. Ibid., 16 September 1589.
8. Quoted in Lynch, M., 'Whatever happened to the medieval burgh?', *Scottish Economic and Social History*, 4 (1984), p. 13.
9. College Minutes, 21 September 1604. Deputies were also elected should the Deacon or other officials be called away on royal or military service, or if any should die while in office.
10. After a gap in the minutes from September 1650, the records restart in March 1651, with the comment that a meeting had been held in the home of the Deacon, James Borthwick, and that Thomas Carter, one of the four assistant masters, had been despatched to visit the rented rooms in Robert Hay's tenement in Kirkheugh, to ascertain the state of their goods.
11. Porter, R., *Disease, Medicine and Society in England 1550–1860* (Cambridge, 1993), p. 14; Hamilton, *Healers*, pp. 34–7.
12. College Minutes, 30 May 1585.
13. Ibid., January 1588 (exact date illegible). This is similar to the actions taken by other bodies. The RCPEng indulged in pursuit of 'irregulars' in the same period. See Pelling, M., *Medical Conflicts in Early Modern London. Patronage, Physicians and Irregular Practitioners 1550–1640* (Oxford, 2003).
14. Thin, R., 'Medical quacks in Edinburgh in the seventeenth and eighteenth centuries', *BOEC* 22 (1938), pp. 135–7. See also Porter, R., *Quacks, Fakers and Charlatans in English Medicine* (Stroud, 2000), which is relevant to the situation in Scotland in general terms.
15. Geyer-Kordesch and Macdonald, *Physicians and Surgeons in Glasgow*, pp. 22, 34–5.
16. At his entry examination in 1591, the Incorporation had 'dewlie usit ane exercise in mony of the poyntis of chirurgerie'. College Minutes, 30 September 1591.
17. Dalyell, J., *Fragments of Scottish History* (Edinburgh, 1798), pp. 48–9.
18. College Minutes, 15 October 1595.
19. Ibid., 11 October 1596.
20. Ibid., 18 December 1677; Dingwall, *Physicians, Surgeons and Apothecaries*, pp. 49–50.
21. Geyer-Kordesch and Macdonald, *Physicians and Surgeons in Glasgow*, pp. 101–3.
22. College Minutes, 13 December 1670.
23. It was estimated that Scotland lost a quarter of its financial assets in the Darien Scheme alone. See Prebble, J., *The Darien Disaster* (Edinburgh, 1968).
24. College Minutes, 25 May 1702.
25. Ibid., 26 September 1591.
26. Ibid., 1 March 1636.
27. Ibid., 10 November 1680. Further sums were borrowed in January, July and September 1681, partly to cover the expenses incurred in opposing the foundation of the RCPEd.
28. Ibid., 12 May 1692 and 9 May 1693. The following year money was borrowed from Porterfield to finance the attempts to gain a new Royal patent.
29. Creswell, *Royal College of Surgeons*, p. 306.
30. In 1699, when the library and museum collections were instituted, Moubray donated 'a pair of cocks spurs, prodigiously long'.
31. Creswell, *Royal College of Surgeons*, p. 307.
32. College Business Papers, 23 May 1774. The title of Clerk to the College reappeared in the twentieth century, but has once again been eclipsed and lost within the modern administrative organisation of the College. There was, therefore, an early and strong link with the legal profession in practical as well as political matters.

33. Unlike the Clerks, who appeared relatively comfortably-off, at least two of the Officers died in poverty, and when the new Hall was opened in 1831, the Officer, John Dodds, complained that he could no longer keep animals behind the Hall. Nowadays the College Officers are assisted by a team of Officers who are often ex-servicemen. Their duties are much more complex, but they still carry out tasks which would have been done by their predecessors in very different social and historical circumstances.

34. College Minutes, 25 August 1635.

35. Ibid., 10 April 1680.

36. A large number of Episcopal clergy had left their charges in 1690 when the Presbyterian settlement was reached, as they felt unable to comply with the requirement to pray for William and Mary in their churches every Sunday. (The link between Episcopalianism and Jacobitism is not straightforward, but inferences were certainly made at the time.)

37. ECA, Moses Bundle 135/5321, 'Accompt of Medicaments and Drugs furnished to the Poor of Edinburgh by Thomas Gibson, from January 1710 to January 1711'.

38. College Minutes, 30 June 1588 and 15 January 1589.

39. For a fuller account of the case see Creswell, *Royal College of Surgeons*, pp. 37–42. Incorporation master Christopher Irvine was surgeon to General George Monck, Commander-in-Chief in Scotland, an appointment he maintained till 1660. A confirmed Royalist none the less, Irvine wrote *Medicina Magnetica*, published in Edinburgh in 1656 and dedicated to Monck. Irvine was just as politically pragmatic as his fellow masters of the Incorporation. There is a general account of the Cromwellian period in Dow, F. D., *Cromwellian Scotland, 1651–60* (Edinburgh, 1979).

40. Dingwall, *Physicians, Surgeons and Apothecaries*, p. 58. See also Creswell, *Royal College of Surgeons*, pp. 42–5. Pringle had been engaged by Heriots as the nearest living relation to the founder, and his duties included 'cutting and polling the heads of the scholars, external applications to surgical diseases and operations'.

41. Lynch, M., 'Continuity and change in urban society 1500–1700', in R. A. Houston and I. D. Whyte (eds), *Scottish Society 1500–1800* (Cambridge, 1989), p. 109.

42. A second such visitation took place in June 1670.

43. See Dingwall, *Physicians, Surgeons and Apothecaries*, pp. 56–7. Two of those allowed to practise within the walls were French Huguenots who had been 'educat and brought up fra yr infancy in the protestant religion'.

44. By the end of the seventeenth century periwigmakers employed the largest numbers of apprentices. Dingwall, H. M., *Late Seventeenth Century Edinburgh. A Demographic Study* (Aldershot, 1994), pp. 137–8.

45. Gelfand, *Professionalising Modern Medicine, Paris Surgeons and Medical Science Institutions in the Eighteenth Century* (London, 1980), p. 36.

46. Geyer-Kordesch and Macdonald, *Physicians and Surgeons in Glasgow*, p. 80.

47. Duncan, *Memorials of the Faculty of Physicians and Surgeons of Glasgow, 1599–1850* (Glasgow, 1896), pp. 88–9.

48. Harvey, W., *Exercitatio Anatomica de Motu Cordis et Sanguinis in Animalibus* (Frankfurt, 1628).

49. College Minutes, 4 February 1595.

50. Ibid., 4 May 1661.

51. Ibid., 4 February 1595.

52. Ibid., 7 May 1612.

53. Ibid., 20 July 1666.

54. Ibid., 18 November 1679.

55. ECA, Dean of Guild Court Books, 28 November 1688. Other incidents referred to in Dingwall, *Physicians, Surgeons and Apothecaries*, pp. 147–64.

56. Creswell, for instance, claims that 'at the expiry of his apprenticeship he became an assistant or "servand"'. Creswell, *Royal College of Surgeons*, p. 17.

57. Gelfand, *Professionalising Modern Medicine*, p. 46.

58. This high drop-out rate was common to most crafts in the period. See discussion in Ben-Amos, I. K., 'Failure to become freemen. Urban apprentices in early-modern England', *Social History*, 16 (1991), pp. 155–72.
59. Sutherland petitioned the Incorporation on 11 June 1695 for teaching rights, as he had 'brought the Botanick garden in order and furnished it with a great number of plants as could hardly be expected in any garden of this Country'.
60. Creswell, *Royal College of Surgeons*, p. 153.
61. Erlan. H., 'Alexander Monro primus', *University of Edinburgh Journal*, 17 (1953–5), pp. 80–1.
62. Ibid., p. 82.
63. College Minutes, 20 March 1645.
64. Ibid., 20 August 1647.
65. Ibid., 7 November 1693.
66. *Burgh Recs*, 2 November 1694.
67. Letter to Robert Gray in London. Quoted in Johnston, W. T., *The Best of Oure Owne: Letters of Archibald Pitcairne 1652–1713* (Edinburgh, 1979), p. 19.
68. College Business Papers 4 February, 1703, Account of incidental charges disbursed for the Chururgions of Edr by David Fyffe.
69. College Minutes, 8 March 1703 (recording dissection in November/December 1702); 18 May 1704 (procedure undertaken in April of that year).
70. Brockliss and Jones, *The Medical World of Early Modern France* (Oxford, 1997), p. 713.
71. College Minutes, 5 August 1708. Robert Elliot requested that Adam Drummond be conjoined in office with him as Professor of Anatomy, having already obtained an act from the Town Council to that effect. It was agreed that he could have 'use of the publick dissection theatre for publick and private courses'.
72. Ibid., 1 February 1705; 5 August 1708; Creswell, *Royal College of Surgeons*, pp. 195–7; Dingwall, *Physicians, Surgeons and Apothecaries*, p. 77.
73. Wheatley, H. B. (ed.), *Diary of Samuel Pepys* (London, 1893), pp. 53–4, describes a visit made by Pepys to the Barber-Surgeons' Hall, where he attended lectures and viewed the body of a recently hanged criminal, following which Dr Scarborough showed 'very clearly the manner of the disease of the stone and the cutting'.
74. NLS, ms 3157, later copy of Depositions of the Chirurgeons and Apothecarys upon the Earl of Atholls death, 1579. The report was dated 12 June 1579. For a general account of the history of the period, see Lynch, M., *Scotland. A New History* (London, 1991), pp. 222–33.
75. NAS, GD158/926, account of post-mortem on Lady Polwarth undertaken by Patrick Telfer, chirurgeon, 12 December 1701.
76. *Caledonian Mercury*, 20 November 1725.
77. *Caledonian Mercury*, 22 April 1725.
78. College Minutes, 31 March 1739; further instances in 1742.
79. Ibid., 19 October 1699.
80. Stott, R., 'The library of Thomas Kincaid, a seventeenth-century Scottish surgeon', *Canadian Bulletin of Medical History*, 12 (2) (1995), pp. 351–67. The selective nature of the collection is confirmed, according to Stott, by, for example, the absence of any work by Harvey but the presence of works on the circulation of blood by a number of authors who had disagreed with Harvey's views.
81. College Minutes, 26 May 1709.
82. Duncan, *Memorials*, p. 211.
83. Craig, *Royal College of Physicians*, p. 120.
84. College Minutes, 4 June 1582.
85. Ibid., 30 June 1588.
86. Ibid., 23 May 1723.
87. Ibid., 15 May 1593.

88. Ibid., 15 July 1647. See also Dingwall, H. M., 'Original fellowship examination', *J. Roy. Coll. Surg. Edinb.*, 36 (1991), pp. 357–61 for a full discussion of the examinations.

89. College Minutes, 7 February 1712. It was ordered that the 'Intrants first lesson to be a speech by him on any chirurgicall case operation or surgery in general as he pleases, and to answer all practicall questions that shall be enquired in any case or operation in chirurgery by the examinators or any other member of the calling. That the intrants second lesson be anatomicall and that the said lesson be appointed by the calling and the time when the intrant is to make the same. That the other two subsequent lessons be operations of chirurgery and that these also be appointed by the calling'.

90. Ibid., 24 November 1724.

91. Ibid., 23 May 1723.

92. His final examination was more conventional, consisting of 'the operation of the trepan with its proper apparel and bandages with the bandages of the head and face, the composition of Electuarium Diacathholicon and the trochisi alberhasis'.

93. College Minutes, 14 October 1652. Darling was not successful until 1656.

94. Ibid., 2 January 1719.

95. Further assessment of examinations in Dingwall, 'Original Fellowship Examination'; Dingwall, *Physicians, Surgeons and Apothecaries*, pp. 83–91.

96. See Geyer-Kordesch and Macdonald, *Physicians and Surgeons in Glasgow*, pp. 116–25. These included the case of a weaver who was authorised to 'draw blood with a horn and such things as pertain thereto alone'.

97. Ibid., pp. 96–101. See also Duncan, *Memorials*, p. 50.

98. Dobson, J. and Milnes Walker, R., *Barbers and Barber-Surgeons of London* (London, 1979), pp. 46–7.

99. A stone-cutter (William Souter) had been appointed in Glasgow in 1655, and in 1656 the FPSG examined Iver McNeill, 'who has been in use these ten years or thereby bygone in cutting of the stone'. Geyer-Kordesch and Macdonald, *Physicians and Surgeons in Glasgow*, p. 123. For an account of operating technique, see Geyer-Kordesch and Macdonald, pp. 122–3. There is a history of the treatment of urinary calculi in Ellis, H., *A History of Bladder Stone* (Oxford, 1969).

100. Dingwall, H. M., '"General practice" in seventeenth-century Edinburgh: evidence from the Burgh Court', *Social History of Medicine*, 6 (1993), pp. 125–42; Dingwall, *Physicians, Surgeons and Apothecaries*, pp. 149–64.

101. Dingwall, 'General practice', p. 131.

102. ECA, Burgh Court Acts and Decreets, 17 June 1657; 10 December 1611; 25 November 1623.

103. *Burgh Recs*, 8 December 1643.

104. ECA, Burgh Court Books, 2 April 1659.

105. See Blair, J. S. G., 'The Scots and military medicine', in D. Dow (ed.), *The Influence of Scottish Medicine* (Carnforth, 1988), pp. 17–30.

106. ECA, Moses Bundle 32/1321, petition by Alexander Pennycuik.

107. The fees were often paid in kind rather than cash. Salmon, poultry and cloth were among the means of payment, and in 1640 James Rig claimed that he had been promised 'ane pair of new schoone guid and sufficient'. ECA, Burgh Court Acts and Decreets, 17 March 1640.

108. Lowe, P., *Discourse of the Whole Art of Chirurgerie* (London, 1597); Geyer-Kordesch and Macdonald, *Physicians and Surgeons in Glasgow*, pp. 53–78.

109. Beier, L. M., *Sufferers and Healers: The Experience of Illness in Seventeenth-Century England* (London, 1987), gives a detailed account of the work of individual physicians and surgeons in this period; also Beier, L. M., 'Seventeenth-century English surgery: the casebook of Joseph Binns', in C. Lawrence (ed.), *Medical Theory, Surgical Practice. Studies in the History of Surgery* (London, 1982), pp. 48–84; Pelling, M., *The Common Lot: Sickness, Medical Occupations and the Urban Poor in Early-Modern England* (London, 1998).

110. Jütte, R., 'A seventeenth-century German barber-surgeon and his patients', *Med. Hist.*, 33 (1989), pp. 185–6. The evidence indicates that this surgeon, Gerhard Eichhorn, was one of the most popular and frequently consulted practitioners at the time in Cologne.

111. Ibid., p. 189.

112. Boog Watson, W. N., 'Early baths and bagnios in Edinburgh', *BOEC*, 24 (2) (1979), p. 58.

113. Floyer, J., *An Enquiry into the Right Use and Abuses of the Hot, Cold and Temperate Baths in England* (London, 1697).

114. College Minutes, 13 June 1671. The honorary members could not practise surgery or be elected Deacon, though they could attend and vote at meetings.

115. There is an entry in the minutes dated 3 April 1663, which orders twelve masters to 'provide themselves with horses and wait upon the Deacon' in order to attend Lauderdale's funeral.

116. Craig, *Royal College of Physicians*, p. 1072.

117. College Minutes, 12 August 1673, note that the boxmaster was authorised to 'cause matriculat yr armes in the Lord Lyon his books'.

118. *Burgh Recs*, 5 February 1657.

119. Worling, P. M., 'The Edinburgh Apothecaries', *Pharmaceutical Historian*, 33 (3) (2003), p. 39. An alternative view is that the Incorporation was keen to resist current attempts being made by the physicians to gain their own organisation, in which they proposed to have sweeping supervisory powers over the apothecaries. NLS, Adv. Ms. 33.5.20, 'Memoirs for compiling the history of the Royal Coledge of Physitians at Edinburgh done from the Records by Sir Robert Sibbald', p. 7.

120. One apothecary was prosecuted for draining fluid from a corpse so that it could be fitted into its coffin. Eccles, M., *An Historical Account of the Rights and Privileges of the Royal College of Physicians and of the Incorporation of Chirurgians of Edinburgh* (Edinburgh, 1707), p. 15.

121. A complicating factor was that the surgeons were still permitted to 'buy and sell simples as any Drugist or Merchant may do'. See fuller accounts of the 'battle for pharmacy' in Creswell, *Royal College of Surgeons*; Craig, *Royal College of Physicians*; Dingwall, *Physicians, Surgeons and Apothecaries*, pp. 187–9.

122. There is a fuller account of legal proceedings in Creswell, *Royal College of Surgeons*, pp. 114–16.

123. Craig, *Royal College of Physicians*, pp. 39–57; see also Dingwall, *Physicians, Surgeons and Apothecaries*, pp. 109–13; McHarg, J. F., *In Search of Dr John Makluire, Pioneer Edinburgh Physician Forgotten for Over 300 Years* (Glasgow, 1997).

124. College Minutes, 5 January 1682, indicate that the committee had managed to procure a royal signature ratifying all former rights and privileges, but that this had to be shown to the physicians, so that there was 'nothing to be expected but a greate deale of trouble'.

125. James' succession to the English throne was in considerable doubt because of his Roman Catholicism.

126. See Ouston, H., 'York in Edinburgh: James VII and the patronage of learning in Scotland 1673–1688', in J. Dwyer, R. A. Mason and A. Murdoch (eds), *New Perspectives on the Politics and Culture of early Modern Scotland* (Edinburgh, 1982), pp. 133–55.

127. Dalrymple, J. (Viscount Stair), *The Institutions of the Laws of Scotland* (Edinburgh, 1681).

128. For the full text of the petition see Creswell, *Royal College of Surgeons*, p. 120.

129. College Minutes, 19 January 1688. The physicians had petitioned the Privy Council for an order to publish the work, and had asked that it be reviewed by 'such phisitians as are not of the number of the College and such Chirurgeon-Apothecaries as the Privy Council should think fitt'.

130. Cunningham, A., 'Medicine to calm the mind: Boerhaave's Medical System and why it was adopted in Edinburgh', in A. Cunningham and R. French (eds), *The Medical Enlightenment of the Eighteenth Century* (Cambridge, 1990), pp. 40–66.

131. Creswell, *Royal College of Surgeons*, pp. 197–9. Monro joined the College of Physicians in 1756 and was, therefore, obliged to leave the Incorporation.
132. For an account of Scots who had studied at Leiden, see Innes-Smith, R. W., *English-Speaking Students of Medicine at the University of Leyden* (Edinburgh, 1926).
133. Monro's four examination sessions comprised questions on 'chirurgerie and anatomy in general', 'containing and contained parts of the thorax with circulation of the blood', 'fistulas in general with the operation of the fistula lachrimalis', and 'bandages of the head and face'.
134. For the final two years there would be no restrictions and apprentices could attend without the consent of their master. All apprentices were allowed to attend the Physic Garden without restriction.
135. Quoted in Croft Dickinson, W., *Scotland from Earliest Times to 1603* (London, 1961), p. 288.
136. Dingwall, *Late Seventeenth Century Edinburgh*, pp. 62, 229.

# 4

# Enlightenment to Reform,
# Incorporation to College, 1726–c. 1830

The Petitioners humbly hoped they had been no less deserving of royal patronage than their predecessors, and their numerous pupils serving with reputation in His Majesty's Army and Navy might be mentioned as evidence of the attention bestowed by the present members of the said College to improve the art of Surgery.[1]

## INTRODUCTION

By the time of the foundation of the Edinburgh Medical School in 1726, the nation had changed just as much as had Edinburgh or any of its institutions. The Union of Parliaments of 1707 meant that Scotland was more firmly attached to her southern neighbour than ever, though it can be claimed with some justification that full incorporating union did not really take place, as Scotland retained separate and distinctive legal, religious and educational arrangements. There is no doubt, though, that the outlook and focus of Scotland had changed a great deal from the heady days of the Renaissance, when Scots looked towards Europe for culture, trade, education and travel. By the start of the equally heady days of the Enlightenment, the direction of overseas trade, now dominated by Glasgow, was firmly westwards, to America and the West Indies. Glasgow was rapidly overtaking Edinburgh in terms of population numbers and mercantile activity, but equally Edinburgh was consolidating as the intellectual and cultural capital of Scotland. While a timely case has been made in recent times for the recognition of the contribution of Glasgow to the Enlightenment,[2] Edinburgh was very much the focus of debate, in which College Fellows participated.[3] This is one area where the European influences remained strong, in terms of philosophical discussion on the human race and its relationships with the universe in a secular context. There is a view that a combination of Presbyterian ethics and European science combined to make the background for a 'Protestant scientific exchange', which was at the root of sceptical thought about medicine and about the long-standing humoral, Boerhaavian tradition.[4] It may be that this was more of a factor in the development of medicine rather than surgery, but the surgeons were part of

Enlightenment Edinburgh, they attended many of the philosophical and other societies which flourished at the time,[5] and their library contained a wide range of books, not just writings on surgery. It was also the period in which plans for the New Town were taking shape,[6] and the influence of Provost Drummond had been a fairly constant background to events. The surgeons were, therefore, aware of the directions in which intellectual debate was proceeding.

There is some historiographical debate as to whether the Enlightenment process in Scotland was distinctively Scottish. The main argument for this is that debate took place in, and was channelled through, the major institutions of the church and the universities, unlike the situation in other parts of Europe, where such ideas were generally mooted outside these bodies. The moderate Church of Scotland minister or university professor embraced new ideas and helped to maintain the debate in a climate of 'moderation' – the great exception, of course, being David Hume, who did not have a university chair, was not a minister or lawyer, but was keeper of the Advocates Library. The other distinctive feature attributed to the Scottish Enlightenment was its dissemination through most levels of society in terms of practical application, such as agricultural improvement or developments in industrial chemicals. This sort of climate was very favourable to the surgeons, who were ideally placed to take advantage of both the intellectual debate and the application of scientific progress. This was also the perfect background for the encouragement of anatomical exploration and reassessment of the detail of the structure and functions of the body without fear of religious recrimination.

The first half of the nineteenth century brought new problems and challenges, most particularly in relation to the rapid expansion of the cities and the public health problems this created. There were economic problems during the period of depression following the close of the Napoleonic Wars in 1815, and this helped to intensify the political debate about reform of parliamentary and local government. The Reform Act of 1832 brought the franchise within the grasp of more Scots men – though not significantly more – but it would take until 1867 for political reform to have significant effects on the composition of the electorate. Scotland was at the forefront of empire-building and led the world in industrialisation, but the cost was high in terms of disease and urban squalor. Though entering the Victorian period in a confident frame of mind, a number of factors would serve to destabilise the nation. Not least of these was the fragmentation and ultimate split in the national church, with the Disruption of 1843, and the end of kirk responsibility for education and poor relief by the 1870s, which marked the end of the historic 'parish state'. Industrialisation meant that by 1850 a quarter of all Scots lived in Edinburgh, Glasgow, Dundee or Aberdeen, and by the turn of the twentieth century this had risen to over half – with obvious practical, social and health problems.[7] By the 1850s the clamour for medical reform was loud; that for general political reform was even louder. So this was a period of contrasts – urbanisation and highland clearance, which resulted in realignment of the demographic map of Scotland; industrial progress and urban poverty; a rise in the influence of national and local government; and increasing health problems, not to mention the changing and complex nature of the Scottish identity in the context of North Britain.[8] This latter is significant here in terms of the question of whether by 1858 it can be claimed that there was anything distinctive or Scottish about medicine or surgery in Scotland.

The age of the 'great doctors' was one of progress and problems in almost equal measure for the Incorporation. By the turn of the nineteenth century it had gone through serious financial problems, had been forced to give over its library and museum collections to Edinburgh University, and was struggling to survive – this survival eventually enabled by the introduction of the diploma examination, much more than by the acquisition of a Royal Charter in 1778. The Charter, though, was symbolic of the final achievement of a key aim – recognition as a learned and academic society. The surgeons were still severely hampered in their abilities to cure patients or to advance surgical techniques, so this period in the College's history is one of contrasts and paradoxes rather than unfettered travel along the road to improvement and elevation of status. The bitter conflicts with the physicians were, largely, over, if grudgingly; what the future held would be enforced, and occasionally willing, co-operation rather than internecine warfare. The medical and surgical colleges in Britain as a whole were faced with growing opposition from the universities and the increasing influence of central and local government.

The general social background was of some significance here. The milieu of the Enlightenment did not only affect surgeons and other professionals. The climate of reasoned argument and wider availability of knowledge in the public sphere in general, thanks in some measure to the burgeoning culture of print and increasing levels of general literacy and educational availability, meant that knowledge previously restricted in its dissemination could now be acquired by many more interested individuals. This phenomenon is at the basis of Habermas's view on the functions of changing spheres of knowledge as a factor in stimulating change. The increasingly public discourse of this time meant that any group which sought exclusive possession of a body of knowledge had to defend its claim more forcefully than in the past.

This period also saw the emergence of a complex set of relationships – between the College and the University; between the College and the Royal Infirmary; between the College and the physicians; and, eventually, among the British and Irish surgical colleges as a group. While the FPSG was rather more complicated, in that it contained both physicians and surgeons, it was no less easy for the Edinburgh College to maintain its status in the light of fairly rapid social, economic and political change. Always politically pragmatic, the College saw fit to award an Honorary Fellowship to the Duke of Cumberland in the wake of the 1745 Jacobite uprising, and would go on to make very good use of Henry Dundas and the other Scottish political managers later in the eighteenth century.

During the late-eighteenth century the future of the College was in considerable doubt at times, mainly because of severe financial problems, which prompted the surgeons at one stage to put their Hall on the market in an attempt to lessen their financial burdens. Membership of the Incorporation at that point was not expanding rapidly enough to sustain the organisation financially. Between 1758 and 1768, for example, only two new masters were admitted. Though overall numbers were never reduced to the crisis levels of the early part of the seventeenth century, and indeed ninety-six surgeons entered between 1730 and 1800, the mid-century saw a net reduction in active membership from the forty-seven individuals recorded in November 1727, to a mere twenty-nine in January 1747. There was a slight improvement by 1756, when thirty-seven names were noted, but by 1762 numbers were back to twenty-nine. In 1723, the complement had been as high as fifty-nine, so the Incorporation was clearly in a little difficulty by the mid-eighteenth century. This was, however, the last period of real threat to the viability of the organisation, at least until the late twentieth century, and the situation did improve, as between 1800 and 1860 some 190 masters (by now termed Fellows) entered the College, and the average number of resident Fellows (and income) rose in consequence. By the 1830s the numbers had risen to around 250, but not all of these were resident or practising in Edinburgh, and this large number belies difficulties with finance and attracting Fellows. The situation in France at this time seems to have been rather different, with an apparent proliferation of surgeons from an estimated 5,250 in 1700 to around 15,000 on the eve of the revolution in 1789.[9]

It has been claimed that in the eighteenth century the Incorporation's 'principles of value were largely economic and utilitarian'.[10] Evidence for this was that in most of the surviving documentation relating to litigation and maintenance of rights, the language was of 'legal rights and social utility' rather than 'learning and rank'.[11] This is true in some ways, but does not adequately reflect the much broader spectrum of 'aims and objectives' held by the Incorporation. Events which helped to draw the Incorporation out into a more public forum, in spite of the difficulties, included the foundation of the Medical School at the University in 1726; the small beginnings of hospital medicine following the opening of the first Infirmary building in 1729; the institution of a diploma examination in the later decades of the century; and, of course, the achievement of Royal College status in 1778. All of these factors ensured that the surgeons became more prominent in Edinburgh medicine and medical politics. This chapter will consider all of these factors in terms of the combination of continuing and new influences within the sphere of Scottish medicine and the much larger one of Britain.

## GENERAL INCORPORATION MATTERS

The day-to-day organisation of the Incorporation changed relatively little over the period covered in this chapter. Officials were elected as usual and meetings continued to take place in Surgeons' Hall. One of the main administrative changes was the consolidation of the Deacon's council, which gave general assistance to the Deacon in matters such as the pursuit of unauthorised practitioners, and also formed or headed sub-committees to deal with specific problems. *Ad hoc* committees were set up to deal with various difficulties as they arose, usually matters concerning the University or the RIE. These committees would be of considerable importance in the first half of the nineteenth century during the lengthy period of debate, argument and consultation with the other British corporations, lawyers and members of parliament about proposals for national legislation to standardise medical education in Britain.

Day-to-day business was concerned mainly with what it always had been – discipline, money, apprentices, entrant masters, behaviour and buildings, though new status required some minor practical moves. One guinea was paid to Alison Cockburn on 16 June 1778 for a 'white iron charter chest', no doubt to house the new Royal Charter, while David Deuchar charged ten shillings for 'repairing and graving a new motto on their seal'. The symbolism of the new status had to be clearly displayed.

A further case of alleged grave-robbing on behalf of one Incorporation member occurred in 1742, and was dealt with by the burgh court. Martin Eccles was accused of acquiring a recently buried corpse and it was claimed that he had 'most indecently exposed, cut and mangled the same.' Although it was found proven that Eccles had the body in his premises, the uniquely Scottish verdict of not proven was delivered, as it could not be proved that he had dissected the body, despite its being in his possession.[12]

Administrative changes in the first half of the nineteenth century were relatively few, and concerned mainly the re-establishment of the library and museum, with appropriate committees and curators to oversee these developments. Major change to administrative structures would not come until the second half of the twentieth century, stimulated by the needs of a modern business, and for the moment the energies of the College were channelled towards development of teaching and examinations, and with the complex issue of national medical politics.

### The Widows' Fund and the Royal Charter

When a Widows' Fund was established in 1778, with the purpose of providing some financial support for the widows and children of surgeons, a standing committee was elected to oversee its workings and calculate potential numbers of widows and sums of money which would be accrued by means of the scheme. The main instigator of this scheme was Thomas Hay, who joined the Incorporation in March 1773 (Hay's examinations had comprised a discourse on hydrocele; an examination on the anatomy of the bones of the face; a session on botany and *Materia Medica* together with the production of samples of *syrapus balsamicus* and *unguentum citrinum* (a mercury-based ointment frequently allocated to examination candidates); and tests on the operation for hare lip with appropriate bandages and dressings).[13] Hay served as Deacon in 1784–5 and 1794–5, and was also chosen as Deacon Convener of the fourteen Edinburgh Trades, whose meeting place was the historic Magdalen Chapel in the Cowgate (despite Collegiate status, the surgeons still maintained a foot in both camps, though it would not be long before they began to try to separate themselves from their links with the Town Council as a means of ridding themselves of any possible accusations of being mere craftsmen rather than members of a learned profession).[14]

As with several features of the College's development, one decision or process prompted the surgeons to consider something perhaps more significant for the longer term. In this case, the desire to provide for the dependants of members stimulated the surgeons to take action to achieve something considerably more prestigious – a Royal Charter. It is evident throughout the College's history that chance, or immediate fortuitous circumstance, could bring about important developments. As discussed below, outside influences played a significant part in the changes made in the College's examinations; and it seems to be the case that sometimes the incidental, or secondary, action produced a more significant result. On this occasion, a proposal was made that a fund should be set up, into which each member would pay £5 each year, and on the death of a contributor his widow would receive benefits of £25 *per annum* from the funds accrued by these means, provided that the individual's contributions were not in arrears. This measure required the sanction of a Royal Charter, and, almost as a second thought, the Incorporation decided that this would also be an opportune moment to apply for the title and charter of a Royal College. Given the historic jealousies and rivalries between surgeons and physicians, it is perhaps surprising that it took almost a century after the foundation of the RCPEd for the surgeons to seek equivalent status (though, of course, in the postmodernist view this would not be at all surprising).[15]

Some investigations had taken place as early as the 1690s on the question of whether the Incorporation was entitled to designate itself College, because in a number of documents issued by the Crown, the Incorporation had been referred to as *'societati et Collegio chirurgorum'*. Legal opinion was obtained, and the advice was that in strictly legal terms the surgeons were an Incorporation, and it would not be appropriate to use the term *Royal* College, but there could be no objections to the assumption of the designation of *College* to describe the group.

Eventually both charters were applied for, and a petition submitted to George III in January 1778, stating that:

> The Petitioners hope that they have been no less deserving of Royal Patronage than their predecessors, Their numerous Pupils serving in Your Majesty's Army and Navy may be mentioned as an evidence of the attention bestowed by the present members of the said College [note that the surgeons refer to themselves as College in the petition] to improve the art of Surgery. That they may maintain an equality with similar institutions in several neighbouring Kingdoms they are solicitous that your Majesty may be graciously pleased to confer upon them the Title of Royal College of Surgeons – When they reflect on the liberal patronage and support your Majesty has been uniformly pleased to bestow on literature and useful Arts They are encouraged to hope this their request will not be refused.[16]

Even the practicalities of acquiring the charter were not straightforward. A letter was received from Mr Chalmers, the Incorporation's legal agent, about the

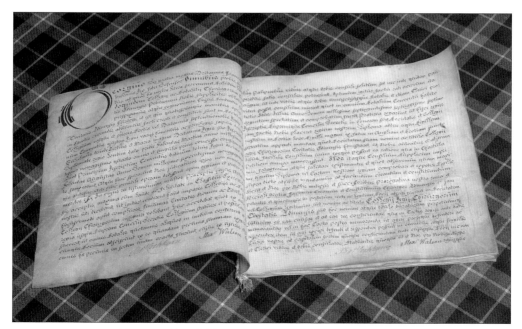

*FIG. 4.1 Royal Charter granted to the College in 1778.*

warrant for the charter, stating that he would not send it by post in view of its bulk, but would wait till 'some private hand casts up'.[17] It appears that no suitable hand did cast up, though, as the Incorporation accounts, under the hand of George Balderstone, contained the cost of 'postages from Mr Chalmers with the King's warrant', some two months later.[18]

The petition was successful and Royal status was achieved on 22 May 1778. Almost immediately, discussions began about breaking the links with the Town Council, in an effort to further elevate the status of the new Royal College, as it 'was found from experience that their connection with City Politicks had been a source of much dissention in the Society, and as it had long been the earnest wish of most of the members to be entirely disengaged from the Town Council, there could not be a more proper time than the present to effect a separation'.[19] Once higher status had been achieved, the surgeons seem to have conveniently forgotten the almost three centuries of support which they had enjoyed from the Town Council, support which had been vital in the protracted conflicts with the physicians for much of the seventeenth century.

Coupled with this desire to distance the College from its trade associations, the question arose as to whether a separate Deacon might be elected in addition to the President; the Deacon would continue to represent the interests of the College on the Town Council. The elected head of the College was referred to as President from 1778, and so the proposed appointment of a Deacon as a subordinate officer was an attempt to reduce the status of the link with the Town Council. Legal opinion was, though, that this move could not be supported by law and no further action was taken at that point – final separation did not come until a new Charter was granted in 1851.

Whether or not the application for a Royal Charter and its attendant confirmation of learned status had come of primary intent, an instance some nine years prior to the achievement of collegiate status neatly illustrates the view that, despite the unavoidably practical nature of surgery, it was not thought seemly for surgeons to indulge in such activities as keeping shops or selling. The relevant minute repays full quotation, as it eloquently portrays the image of surgeons as being set apart from such inferior pursuits as these.

> And further considering that there are at present a number of keepers of laboratories, who are a sort of whole sale dealers in drugs and at the same time retailers and compounders, who may perhaps apply to be admitted into this corporation. And as it is certain that no person of this profession however well qualified in fact he may be, will ever be considered by the public as an adept fit to be a member of this corporation, which has hitherto been considered as one of the first societies of the kind in Europe. That consequently a slur will be thrown upon it by the admission of such people who will prove not only a disgrace to the corporation but a general loss to the whole Kingdom. Therefore the Corporation hereby resolve and declare, that for the future no person shall be admitted a member of this Corporation till he obliges himself not to sell drugs as a merchant or shop keeper, that it to say by whole sale or retail to every person who comes to purchase in the stile the keepers of laboratories do and that for this purpose he shall subscribe a formal bond to the Corporation whenever required to comply with the above resolution under such penalty as the Corporation shall order to be inserted in the Bond in case of contravention over and above performance.[20]

Though entirely in keeping with the sentiments of the Incorporation, this seems just a little ironic, given the fierce struggles of the previous century, when the Incorporation had fought long and hard to retain the right of its members to practise pharmacy. The composition and preparation of prescriptions remained a constant examination topic for many decades thereafter, and though knowledge of these things was necessary in order to cater for the requirements of individual patients, trading commercially would not reflect well on the 'literary' nature of the Incorporation.

Once the Charter had been received and the scheme activated, the Widows' Fund soon accrued a large sum of money in excess of the mathematical predictions which had been calculated, and by 1782 it was already in credit by some £120, but fairly quickly began to be something of a millstone around the neck of the College. Many widows outlived their husbands by several decades and proved to be a considerable drain on the Fund, though it was never particularly short of money. In addition, the cost of becoming a Fellow with access to the Fund was thought to be deterring many individuals from coming forward for examination. The burden of administration of the Fund was also troublesome, and it was not long before some regrets began to be expressed. Further legislation was required in 1787 to regulate the Fund, in terms of possible shortfalls and the rules for contributions.[21] An Auxiliary Widows' Fund was established with the aim of catering for deficiencies in the main Fund, particularly in circumstances where a Fellow died before making his fourth annual contribution to the Fund – the threshold for widows to benefit. Various attempts were made in the early nineteenth century to transfer it to the care of one of the fledgling private insurance companies, but they were equally reluctant to take on the task. Attempts were made in 1812 and 1813 to achieve an Act of Parliament to alter the terms of the Fund, with financial penalties to be imposed on Fellows who married over the age of 50.[22] Late marriage might mean that a widow could benefit for many years on a relatively low cumulative contribution from the 'elderly' Fellow. This legislation was brought in despite the fact that the Fund was generally in a very healthy state, even with several widows who displayed a very determined longevity.

From the start the Incorporation had demonstrated its charitable intent (see Chapter 3 for examples), but the Widows' Fund was a very different manifestation of collegiate altruism. The burden of duties associated with administration of the Fund was recognised when in 1817 William Balderstone, who had collected the contributions for over forty years, was awarded an honorarium of £105 and remuneration of £20 *per annum* thereafter to compensate for his efforts. The Fund eventually ended by natural wastage, and Fellows thereafter made their own arrangements with one of the commercial insurance companies (though the College was quick to take out fire insurance once that became available). The FPSG had a comparable scheme, which produced very similar problems.[23]

### Loss of library and museum

Despite their determined efforts to increase academic standing and gain acceptance as a learned society, practical problems resulted in the loss of one of the main symbols of a learned organisation, the library. As will be discussed in Chapter 7, the first half of the eighteenth century saw the surgeons in deep financial difficulty, which necessitated renting out various parts of their buildings, including on occasion the Hall itself. Consequently the library collection needed to be rehoused, and in 1762 a proposal was put forward to offer the books to the managers of the RIE, so that students could consult them on payment of a subscription, which would then be used to purchase new books as recommended by the Professor of Anatomy or the RIE managers.

For reasons not entirely clear, this plan was not implemented, and the following year a new solution was found, when it was agreed to transfer both the library and museum collections to the care of the University. Thereafter the College would pay £5 to the University each year to secure the privilege of consultation rights for the surgeons.[24] Some 478 books and a number of pamphlets were transferred.[25] The records of the University Senatus indicate that 'all members of the Corporation shall be free cives of the University Library and Museum and have access to the use of them as the Professors of the University'.[26] The move had also been approved by the Town Council. This arrangement, which took effect during the long tenure of Principal William Robertson, caused much friction between the two organisations, with frequent complaints by the University about the growing numbers of surgeons consulting books and the inadequacy of the annual fee paid to the University. A dispute arose in 1825, when the University, apparently seeking a way out of the 'contract', took legal opinion from the Law Faculty as to whether it had ever had the right to admit 'outsiders' to the library. This dispute was partly brought about by the removal of the University library to the new buildings in 'Old College', when free admission tickets had been issued to professors, but not to College Fellows (who were also seeking access to new periodical publications).[27] These disputes rumbled on until 1860, when it was eventually agreed, after lengthy legal arguments about the nature of the original agreement, that resident Fellows could continue borrowing on payment of one guinea each year. By that time the College's own library had been re-established and the problem was not quite so pressing.[28]

Though these arrangements, however unsatisfactory, did allow continued access to academic books, it does seem a little unfortunate that practical and financial problems had brought about the loss of an important collection, which could not be recovered, as it was eventually dispersed within the main holdings of the University library. Efforts have been made by the College in recent times to identify and retrieve these books, though without success as yet. Similarly, the museum collection, which had begun with the library in 1699 as a small number of exotic curiosities, does not appear to have been re-established on any scale until the early years of the nineteenth century. In 1807, nine Fellows were appointed as curators, and £30 voted to cover the expenses of preserving and displaying pathological specimens donated to the museum, demonstrating the intention of providing adequate funding to support the collection.

## College laws

By the closing years of the eighteenth century the College found it necessary to undertake a major review of its laws, given the new considerations of hospitals and diploma examinations. A comprehensive recasting of the laws appeared in September 1793, the first occasion on which these were printed, and further amendments were added at regular intervals thereafter.[29] The preamble to the printed version of the laws states:

> The Royal College and Incorporation of Surgeons of the City of Edinburgh, having taken into consideration, That the Laws and Regulations have not been revised and arranged for a great number of years, and have fallen into confusion, in consequence of the numerous alterations and new enactments which have taken place since the last revisal, so that it has become difficult to ascertain what is the existing law, as applicable to many cases that

frequently occur: Therefore, to prevent such inconvenience in future, and that no one may plead ignorance in excuse for transgression or omission, the Royal College and Incorporation has ordered the several Laws and regulations as they at present stand in the Sederunt Book, to be revised and digested by a committee appointed for that purpose; and the same having been laid before the College, together with such alterations and additions as were proposed by the Committee of Revision, and by other Members, and having considered the whole with all due deliberation – It is Enacted and Declared, that the following shall be the Laws and Regulations in all time coming; subject to such alterations and additions as may hereafter by judged expedient, according to the forms provided by the particular Laws therein contained for regulating the same.[30]

The review of the laws had been several years in the making. On 11 January 1788, the minutes note, without explanatory comment, that 'the meeting appointed the Deacon, Dr Walker, Mr Hay and Mr Benjamin Bell as a committee to go through and arrange under proper heads the whole laws of the Society and to report thereof at Whitsunday next'. No further mention of this appears till 15 September 1791, when a brief reference in the minutes indicated that the committee was continuing its deliberations, and a further note to the same effect, in August 1792.

The committee finally reported in August 1793, and the new version of the laws appeared in full in the minute of the meeting on 12 September 1793. The revised laws outlined the regulations and procedures for calling ordinary and extraordinary meetings, including fines to be imposed for absence (though the new version of the laws allowed unpunished absence if the absentee were on duty at the RIE, a provision which had not been necessary in seventeenth-century regulations – by 1793 the second Infirmary was well established, and involved many of the College Fellows in its operations and management); the composition of the Deacon's council, which was to be 'six ordinary members' who should meet monthly; the duties and responsibilities of the librarian, including the instruction to 'purchase such books as he may judge proper for the University Library'; and regulations for the appointment of examiners, who were to be elected by ballot, each member giving in a list of twelve names, the top twelve being appointed for the forthcoming year. From that point the College administration consisted of the President, treasurer, council, auditors, librarian, library council (three members), twelve examiners, a four-man feuing committee, the Clerk and the College Officer. At that point the entry fee for a Fellow's son was £8 6s 8d sterling, a son-in-law £16 13s 4d and a time-served apprentice £43 6s 8d. Those who had not served an apprenticeship would be charged the much larger sum of £166 13s 4d.

Rules were set out for contributions to the Widows' Fund, and for the appointment of future Clerks, who would be obliged to pay to the College 'a moderate adequate sum' before being allowed to take up the post, the salary for which would be £20 sterling *per annum*, together with the usual fees for admissions, indentures and examinations, including, of course, the duties concerning the diploma examination and the certificates issued to military candidates and surgeons for slave ships.

Amendments and additions to the examination rules were a major concern in the revised laws, indeed examinations had been in large part the stimulus for the review. Examinations for entrant Fellows would in future consist of four sessions: firstly a discourse by the candidate 'of his own composition in English' on a surgical or anatomical topic; secondly an examination on the anatomy and diseases of a particular part of the body 'with the Surgical Operations necessary for their relief and the requisite Bandages with the method of applying them'; thirdly a session on botany, *Materia Medica*, Chemistry, Pharmacy and the uses and doses of medicines; and fourthly 'the candidate shall perform, if so required, some Surgical operation in presence of the College, and shall produce specimens of some compounds in the *Edinburgh Pharmacopoeia* prepared by himself, and shall answer such questions on both subjects as the Examinators may judge proper'. It is not quite clear how this last session would be organised. The specific operation to be tested was allocated to the candidate at the end of the third session, so that 'he may have a proper Subject and Instruments provided at his own expense', though it may have proved a little problematic to find a patient with the required condition at relatively short notice, and, indeed, one who would be willing to undergo surgery. Conveniently convicted cadavers were also hard to come by.

The changes in methods of training (see below) are reflected in the clause stating that a failed candidate could not present himself for trials for a year, 'or after having attended one Winter Session at the University'. When the Seal of Cause was drawn up in 1505, it could hardly have been envisaged that Edinburgh would have a university at all, far less that apprentices might be allowed to study there. This coming together of surgical and medical training, which resulted in surgical apprentices studying academic subjects and medical students taking surgical diplomas, was important to the construction of professional medicine, both in terms of the immediate context and in the longer term.

Though detailed regulations for the various diploma and certificate examinations were included in the new laws, no specific details were given as to what the content of these examinations should be. It seems to have been anticipated, though, that many of the resident surgical apprentices would wish to obtain this preliminary qualification, for which they would be allowed to sit the examination no earlier than the end of the fourth year of their period of indentured apprenticeship. As with most trades, there was a high and difficult-to-explain drop-out rate amongst apprentices (too high to be accounted for by the prevalent high death-rate).[31] By the early years of the nineteenth century it is likely that a number of apprentices who did not become masters had settled for the diploma.

Although the College needed the subscriptions of its Fellows, some controversy arose when it decided to alter the laws regarding non-resident Fellows, who paid a lower fee, debarring them from partaking in the decision-making processes of the College. The debate became public, as many such controversies did at this time.

One aggrieved country Licentiate, Dr Strachan of Dollar, wrote bitterly that the attitude of the College seemed to be 'Gentlemen, we shall be happy to receive your money, but on no account can we suffer the infliction of your company'.[32] An anonymous response from a College Fellow claims that the institution of the non-resident Fellowship was the result of a positive desire from country Fellows to pay a reduced subscription, and that they could have full voting rights by paying the difference.[33] During the first half of the nineteenth century, most of the subsequent amendments to the laws concerned required curricula and examinations with, of course, the retrograde step of discontinuing a separate examination for the Fellowship from 1850 to 1885 (see below).

## THE INFIRMARY

Apart from the usual day-to-day business and financial difficulties facing the surgeons, during this period they were closely involved with the Infirmary and also with the University, both of which relationships caused not inconsiderable problems and frustrations. The general background in the eighteenth century, in addition to the perceived needs of a medical school, was the continuing efforts on the part of practitioners to separate themselves from the unqualified. As the century progressed there was also a close relationship between the rise of academic anatomy and the development of surgery, which required a hospital setting. At this time the designation of physician, surgeon or apothecary was not clear-cut, and indeed then and for some considerable time to come, the 'general practitioner' formed the dominant force, at least in numerical terms (a situation not lost on the College when it came to the introduction of diploma examinations).[34] The notion of the hospital consultant, practising exclusively hospital medicine, was also far in the future, but whatever the case, the small beginnings of the Edinburgh Infirmary were significant. The Infirmary was founded for reasons which were shaped by the immediate context, and was, in the view of Drummond and Monro senior at least, the final key element in a comprehensive medical school. Clinical instruction had been a central feature in Leiden, although the influence of Boerhaave on European medicine has been brought into question recently.[35]

The Infirmary was established in 1729,[36] containing only six beds, in a house in Robertson's Close. However small-scale, this was the start of a new phase in medicine and surgery.[37] Firstly, no matter how few were the patients, they could now be closely observed; this would lead eventually to the important standardisation of case-history taking and close observation of signs and symptoms. Humoral medicine gradually gave way (perhaps somewhat later in Scotland than in England) during the eighteenth century to new theories of disease and their classification,[38] and, importantly, to more extensive use of physical examination. Here, then, was the beginning of clinical teaching, however rudimentary.[39]

Secondly, an important change occurred gradually in the relationship between patient and practitioner. Despite the fact that for most of the period home-based treatment was still predominant, particularly for those higher up the social scale (who would not find it socially acceptable to go into a hospital even if one were available), the hospital was a place were the patient was removed from the influence of family, had less control over the acceptance or rejection of treatments, and had (perhaps) less opportunity to indulge in amateur medicine. Multiple consultation was still possible, indeed widespread, but the low-key beginnings of hospitals in the early eighteenth century marked the start of the eventual demarcation between hospital doctor and general practitioner as well as alteration of the socio-medical interface between patient and practitioner.[40] The following case history is a graphic example of the consequences of multiple consultation:

> Ane old man of about 63 years of age of a sedentary life thin habit and phlegmatic ... was seized in the middle of winter with a stoppage of urin, pain in the os pubis and from the perineum reaching to the extremity of the yard. He had felt a constant pain there after making of water for some days before when at length the urin was wholly obstructed. He was ordered first to use baths of warm water in a sow's bladder applied to the os pubis then was sounded with a catheter by Mr Robinson who at the first said he felt a stone but afterwards found it no more and in trying to get entrance into the bladder found the catheter stopp'd ... He was afterwards bath'd in the outer room of the bagnio (probably the one at Surgeons' Hall), got several diureticks of pariera brava and sal. succini with some kinds of liniments on the os pubis and perineum. Dr Clerk order'd him to be bled upon which there came on again a small drilling of water that relieved a little for a day or two afterwards. Mr McGill in trying to sound him judg'd he felt the catheter stopp'd by some tumour in the perineum and ordered emollient cataplasms of cow's dung or bread and milk to be applied ... he was again bled by order of Dr Clerk upon which ensued a pretty plentiful drilling of a very red and foetid frothy urine which did not much relieve. He soon after this slept calmly as if well at night but had great tremors and startings of the nerves in the daytime with a vast uneasiness at last fell wholly insensible with a comatous stupor and dy'd. Some few hours before his death it was resolv'd to make an incision in the perineum but this was laid aside upon the appearance of mortal signs. Upon opening the dead body there was found in the curvature of the urethra a small hard stone about the bigness of a pea.[41]

This is a classic example of the problems of multiple consultation, one which involved a senior surgeon such as John McGill, who had succeeded Robert Elliot to the Chair of Anatomy in 1717 – the observational opportunities afforded by hospitals perhaps helped to obviate some of these problems. Bladder stones were one of the most common and distressing conditions of the day, often affecting children, and not sparing the most prominent individuals in Scottish society. In 1725 the Lord Chief Justice had succumbed to the stone, it being reported in the press that at post-mortem 'there were found in his bladder four stones, the largest whereof weighed seven ounces and an half'.[42] It appears also from the few surviving accounts that catheters were used as diagnostic aids, not as a means of relieving the problem. In 1741 consideration was given by the Incorporation to the appointment of a Professor of Lithotomy, 'whereby not only many poor people afflicted with the dreadful distemper of the stone may be relieved, but students in surgery instructed in that difficult and usefull operation'.[43] It was suggested that Thomas Glen, a member of the Incorporation, who had 'for several years past successfully practised the said operation of lithotomy or cutting for the stone', should be recommended. Objections were raised by other surgeons, who felt that this would be a slur on their own abilities, and nothing further was done in this regard.

The Incorporation wished to become involved in the Infirmary from the outset, and in May 1729 the minutes record the first attempt to participate:

> The Deacon presented to the Calling a Minute of the Infirmary which being read and considered by them, the Calling adhered to their former proposal of furnishing the sick and wounded in the Infirmary with medicines and operations in a society way for two years gratis. And agreed to the list of Medicines given in by the Committee. And in consequence thereof to ordain the Deacon and William Mitchell to attend in the termes foresaid for the first moneth and the Treasurer and John Douglas the second moneth. And for the remainder of the two years the Eldest and Youngest Members of the Corporation successive each moneth. And in case any member shall omit or be necessarily absent by sickness or otherways then the next in order shall supply their place.[44]

This was entirely in keeping with charitable sentiments expressed routinely by the surgeons, and also an instance of proposed co-operation with the physicians. It seems that this was not the only one. In August 1732 the surgeons were consulted by the physicians about amendments to the forthcoming edition of the *Edinburgh Pharmacopoeia*. A sub-committee considered the draft edition, and it was agreed that members of this committee would 'wait on the presces of the Colledge of Physitians . . . to lay their remarks on the said pharmacopoeia before them'.[45] It was around this time that the *Pharmacopoeia* began to be divested of some of its more outlandish contents and appeared in rather more streamlined form than the early editions had been. Despite co-operation in various matters, though, any surgeon who wished to become a Fellow of the RCPEd was obliged to resign from the Incorporation immediately.

The Incorporation's offer to assist in the hospital was not acceptable to the management, and a rival bid, submitted by Monro *primus* and five colleagues, who offered to attend the Infirmary on a rota basis to care for the surgical patients, was accepted. Provision was made for second opinions to be given on difficult cases, and medicines were to be offered *gratis*. Medical politics clearly played a part here. In accepting the Monro bid, the Infirmary managers were able to prevent the Incorporation from participating as a corporate body in the running of the Infirmary, though all members of the RCPEd had the right to offer their services, a situation which was less than pleasing to the surgeons, and one which would cause problems in the future.

The provision of hospital beds, or perhaps the public image of those who provided them, continued to exercise the mind of the Incorporation, and in 1736 it was felt that it would be prudent to set up a separate surgical hospital, ostensibly because of 'the deplorable condition of the many indigent and diseased poor who languish under various diseases and are ready to perish for want of that timely assistance which they might find in an Hospital erected for their entertainment'.[46] It was decided to urge members to contribute to the project, and, as always in this age, the scheme was justified in religious terms, so that the proposed hospital would assist in 'carrying out the pious and laudable work that it may become more usefull and extensive to the Honour of Almighty God and unspeakable relief and comfort of the diseased and indigent poor'. These were indeed laudable sentiments, and no doubt expressed sincerely, though the more cynical observer might justifiably see an element of getting even with the physicians under the gloss of noble charity.

The surgical hospital was set up in 1736, probably in College Wynd, though this is uncertain.[47] The same year, the contributors to the Infirmary achieved a Royal Charter, forming them into a legal corporation. This charter allowed for a new, much larger hospital, in which the patients would be 'entertained and taken care of by the Royal College of Physicians of Edinburgh and some of the most skilful surgeons'.[48] This, needless to say, was the nub of the surgeons' complaints and a major factor in the decision to set up their own hospital.

Further overtures were made by the Incorporation to the Infirmary managers, making the reasonable point that it would be to the advantage of all if the two hospitals and their staffs were combined. Generous terms were offered, including the provision of free medicines and the transfer to the Infirmary of funds which had been donated to the surgeons' institution. The offer was rejected on the grounds that the current building was too small, but it was stated that the matter would be reviewed and 'so soon as a large house can be got that inconveniency will be removed, and no time is to be lost in providing one'. It is difficult at times to assess fully the complex nature of the relationships between surgeons and physicians and between surgeons and Infirmary. The old hostilities remained, but excuses were occasionally of a plausible nature.

The Incorporation made a further offer two years later, and this time the Board of Managers agreed that as soon as the first phase of the new hospital building was completed, all Incorporation masters would be admitted as attending surgeons in rotation. By July 1738 the arrangements were complete and the financial stock of the surgeons' hospital had been transferred to the RIE. The agreement was recorded as follows:

Agree that William Mitchell, Adam Drummond, John Kennedy, William Wood, George Young, Francis Russell, William Wardrob, George Langlands, George Murray, Thomas Glen, Gilbert Laurie, Joseph Gibson, Robert Smith,

John Kirkwood, Charles Ramsay, John Wallace, Harie Osburn, George Lauder and Martin Eccles, with the six surgeons now serving in the Infirmary and such other members of the Corporation of Surgeons of Edinburgh shall oblige themselves to serve the Royal Infirmary in terms of the said Act of the Ordinary Managers, or who shall hereafter subscribe such an obligation within three months after being received into the corporation of Surgeons of Edinburgh shall be Surgeons to the Royal Infirmary. So soon as that part of the house now about to be built shall be fit to take in Patients under such Regulations as shall be appointed by the Managers of the Royal Infirmary, and the General Court of Managers hereby appoint the above named surgeons to be surgeons to the Royal Infirmary in the aforesaid terms . . . The house now called the Surgeons Hospital shall be called and esteemed a part of the Royal Infirmary, to be continued and keept up under the Government of the managers of the Royal Infirmary until the new house is finished and recommend to the Ordinary Managers to cause the names of the several donors to the Surgeons Hospital with the sums to be paid in by each of them to be enrolled in the List of Donors to the Royal Infirmary. So as they may be entitled to the same privileges which other Donors to the Royal Infirmary have or enjoy . . . And they also recommend to the Ordinary Managers to Regulate and sett the attendance of the six present surgeons of the Infirmary and of the Surgeons formerly attending in the Surgeons Hospital with the expence of both Houses and every thing else relating to them in such manner as may lend most to unity and harmony and the welfare of the whole.[49]

The new Infirmary opened its doors in 1741, but, needless to say, this was far from being the end of the story. Practical arrangements for the hospital staff were in the hands of the hospital managers, who decreed that four surgeons should attend *per vices* monthly, two for each ward, and that the members of the Incorporation should be divided into seven groups of four 'classes', in order to facilitate these arrangements.

The system was modified in November 1742, when the managers' records noted that:

Every new Intrant who hereafter becomes one of the surgeons of the Infirmary when every other Surgeon has a companion, and after that every surgeon in the above list who becomes single by the death of demission of the Companion he is now classed with, shall each of them when it is their turn to attend, have the care of a whole floor or ward until such time as they can get a Companion either by the death of demission of one of the former surgeons or by the entry of a new one.[50]

Though animosities remained, a more settled atmosphere began slowly to prevail. By December 1751 it was noted that 'in cases wholly internal the physicians

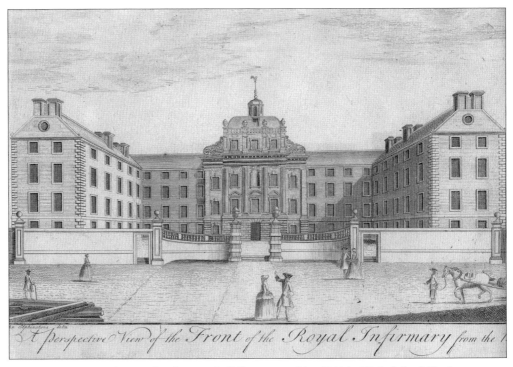

**FIG. 4.2** *The Royal Infirmary building, opened in 1741 in High School Yards.*
*(John Elphinstone.)*

are to be the judges of the patients . . . And in like manner the surgeons in cases wholly external', while 'they are to consult together' in cases 'of a mixed or complicated nature'.[51] Some indication of the continuing predilection for using mercury as a major tool of treatment comes in the note that in 1749 two wards were to be 'fitted up in a warmer manner for such patients as are to undergo sallivation'.[52] More 'modern' thinking was, though, apparent in the regulations for the surgeons' clerks in 1792, which contained the instruction that 'he is to electrify at state house the patients to whom electricity is ordered'.[53]

Relations with the Infirmary managers may have been thawing a little, but those with medical students still left room for improvement, particularly when students claimed to have been excluded from clinical instruction. A particularly strong complaint was lodged in January 1758, when 'a letter signed by sundry students of physick was laid before the meeting representing that the surgeons of the house had determined to perform ane operation for a strangulated hernia in a private manner and to seclude every student . . .'.[54] Permission to operate in private was given but without specifying the reasons for the decision. One area of surgery where privacy was enforced, though, was gynaecology, as it was ordained in 1758 that 'no operation whereby the private parts of women are exposed shall be performed by any surgeon of the Infirmary in the public theatre or in presence of the students, unless the allowance of the ordinary managers is previously obtained'.[55]

An even more explicit instruction was issued in 1769, when it was stated that 'as some chirurgical operations on women cannot be performed in the presence of many male spectators, or in a public theatre, without doing greater violence to female modesty than conflicts with decency, a discretionary power is delegated to the surgeons to conduct these operations in private rooms, and with no more assistants than shall be found necessary.'[56] 'Everything that he werkes' was subject to some constraints in the interests of the female patients.

Despite heated protests that the surgeons were being used 'more like hired servants than useful members and benefactors',[57] the arrangements continued relatively unaltered until 1766, when the first step towards surgical 'residencies' was imposed, by the RIE managers, though not without protest on the part of the surgeons. Though the four individuals to be appointed as 'ordinaries' would not be obliged to live in the hospital, they would attend in addition to the rota surgeon, and 'in his absence advise the chirurgical cases and perform the operations that shall occur'.[58] An annual salary of £10 sterling would be payable to these surgeons.

Meanwhile the day-to-day life and organisation of the hospital had to continue, and here again the surgeons faced some irritating rules and restrictions. It had been decreed in 1742, for example, that 'no operation of surgery by which the life of a patient is endangered shall be performed unless by the joynt opinion of three Surgeons and of the physicians under whose care the patient is'.[59] The latter part of this rule was the real cause of resentment. Regulations for the conduct of post-mortem examinations were also laid out, to the effect that 'when the Physicians shall require a body to be opened the surgeon in attendance or one of the ordinary surgeons in his place do attend the same and either make the dissection himself or employ a single hand under his direction to perform the same, that the dissection being finished he see the body decently sewed up and dressed before being delivered to the dead persons friends.'[60] Trouble was caused some time later, and indeed seems to prefigure modern organ-removal controversies, when John Bell was accused of 'carrying off certain parts of the dead bodies of patients on whom he had performed operations contrary to the standing regulations of the house'.[61] Some signs that post-mortems were intended for instruction as well as revealing the cause of death come from the minute of 9 November 1818, which ordered that any surgeon undertaking a post-mortem examination should 'point out to the students the morbid appearances that are discovered, and shall draw up with as little delay as possible a particular account of them, which shall be inserted in the journals of the house after the history of the case'. The didactic concerns of the post-mortem examinations were in keeping with the context of careful observation in all scientific areas at this time. James Syme became embroiled in a lengthy and bitter dispute with the Infirmary managers about his failure to fulfil the regulations relating to signing the journals compiled by the clerks.

Despite Incorporation grumbles, this rota arrangement continued, but after a further protest two years later, the managers decided that one of the four 'ordinaries' should be substituted each year, in order of seniority of those surgeons who had intimated their willingness to act in this capacity. This may be seen as the beginnings of the eventual distinction between hospital doctors and general practitioners, and indeed in 1786 the post of House Surgeon was created, the appointee to serve in that capacity for five years.[62]

After much delay and negotiation, a tentative framework for surgical arrangements was drafted in November 1800. Several College Fellows, including John Thomson and John Bell, had submitted lengthy opinions as to the best solution, the main basis of their argument being that the system should have enough flexibility to allow for surgeons to have adequate time to develop their surgical skills in the RIE, but that opportunities should be available for younger surgeons to gain experience.[63]

This plan was rejected by the RIE managers, who instead put forward a scheme whereby the surgical departments would be attended by six surgeons elected by the managers, and, crucially, excluding all of the other College Fellows. Six Fellows were duly elected and the College became embroiled in costly legal proceedings. The court initially found for the RIE, and after further consultations on the possibility of appeal, it was decided not to pursue the matter further.[64] One consequence of this was that disagreement arose in the College about the rectitude of the decision, roughly between the senior and the more junior members, one of whom, John Bell, was said 'never to have quite recovered from his exclusion from the Infirmary.'[65] In 1819 a further stormy meeting discussed proposed changes to the organisation of the RIE at length, during which the Deacon tried unsuccessfully to vacate the chair, and proposals put forward by Dr Gairdner for reform of the surgical arrangements were rejected.[66] In April 1822, the College received a strongly worded letter from one of its most famous Fellows, Robert Liston, complaining that he had been prevented from attending the RIE, which he accused of 'interfering improperly with the surgical department of the house'.[67] Liston had enjoyed persistently strained relationships with the RIE (see below) and it is clear that however carefully the regulations were worked out, the force of individual personality or the perceived slight, however minor, was enough to destabilise the situation. This would continue to be the case for much of the nineteenth century. Not only did the surgeons have to contend with the physicians, but also major decisions on surgical staffing were taken by the Board of Managers.

Though clinical instruction had been carried out by physicians since 1748, there had been problems with arrangements for surgical teaching, and, again controversially, the managers decided in 1852 to allow the University Professor of Surgery (at the time James Miller) to receive a permanent appointment to the RIE. This was opposed by the College as a whole, and by James Syme in particular, who saw it as intrusion in his own area of jurisdiction. The objections to the allocation of beds to Miller were based on the contentions that: it was a departure from agreed practice; it would result in the loss of three wards from the ordinary surgeons; and 'Mr Miller had founded his claim upon untenable grounds'. Backing the College stance were some of the noted surgeons of the time, including Syme, Gairdner and Andrew Wood. The managers replied in considerable detail in justification of their position, and the matter seems not to have been pursued by the

College thereafter. This was somewhat typical of the actions of the College in several areas. It always opposed any perceived slight or detriment in the loudest possible terms, but did not always continue the fight beyond these initial protestations. Part of the reason of course may have been the high cost of legal action and the production of lengthy memorials, but political posturing was a core element of the psyche of the College.

## THE COLLEGE, THE UNIVERSITY AND THE PROFESSORS OF SURGERY

As well as problems with the library, there were more serious difficulties with the University, when efforts were made to establish a chair of surgery separate from that of anatomy. In 1776, James Rae, who had joined the Incorporation in 1747, asked the Incorporation to submit a petition to the Town Council on his behalf, requesting that a Professorship of Surgery be established in the Town's College. It was noted that opposition had already been voiced by Alexander Monro *secundus*, who considered himself to be the rightful and best-qualified teacher of surgery as well as anatomy. The Incorporation agreed to submit a petition to the King, and the backing of the Lord Advocate was sought. Unfortunately, however, the latter was forced to admit that he had already been approached by the University, at the instigation of Monro, inviting him to oppose any such petition and that he would, therefore, be unable to act on behalf of the Incorporation.[68]

Meanwhile, Monro *secundus* petitioned the Town Council to have himself declared Professor of Surgery as well as Anatomy, a move opposed strongly by the Incorporation. It was declared that 'no man can teach both branches completely within the usual time employed in a Course, nor can this Professor do more by this additional nomination than has been done already by him'. However skilled the Professor of Anatomy might be, 'he can only give the rudiments of the Art, the surgeons must be formed by witnessing the practice on the living body.'[69] What rankled greatly also was that Monro was a physician, not a surgeon. There followed a series of heated exchanges with the Town Council, but to no avail, as Monro achieved his wish, and Rae's campaign failed. This was the start of a series of difficulties with the University, and was in large part responsible for the growth of extra-mural teaching in Edinburgh. A problem for all sides, though, was the open and unregulated student market place in which economic success depended on attracting students and their fees. Meanwhile Rae continued to deliver a course of lectures, supported by the College, covering surgery and also dentistry, which would become his speciality and account for his lasting reputation.

Rae's son, who followed in his footsteps (and was the first Fellow of the College in 1778), was not at all embarrassed to advertise his services as a dentist as well as his academic lectures:

Mr James Rae, Surgeon and Dentist, Member of the College of Surgeons, takes this opportunity of rectifying his gratitude for the patronage of the public. He begs leave to inform them, that he continues to Transplant Teeth, and to perform every other operation, relative to Natural Teeth. For that branch of his business which regards artificial teeth, he has lately procured a valuable collection of the best materials. Mr Rae attends families or individuals by the year. NB Mr Rae continues to give his assistance to servants and poor people gratis every morning at his house, Lady Stairs Close, Lawn Market where at the shop of Mr Johnston, Front of the Exchange, may be had his powder and tincture for the teeth and gums.[70]

In 1802, College Fellow James Russell was appointed by the Town Council to a Chair of Clinical Surgery in the University. This move was made without reference to the College, which protested its rights as 'a public body vested with the sole and exclusive privilege of teaching as well as practising surgery within the City', rights which should have necessitated at least the courtesy of consultation as to the best candidate. Legal advice was again taken, but the response was guarded. In its own turn, the University, while approving the appointment of Russell, recognised the need to impose limitations 'for the security of the professors of medicine, anatomy and surgery', who were not to be deprived of any of their rights. It was stipulated particularly that Russell's courses would not 'upon any pretence whatsoever, be converted into a general course of lectures on Anatomy, or on the Practice of Surgery, but shall consist of remarks falling immediately under his own observation, and that the appellation of the office be the Professor of Clinical Surgery only.'[71] The RIE managers emphasised that they could not guarantee similar accommodation for any successors to Russell. The College eventually agreed to Russell's appointment, but took the strong view that it would require to have strict limitations imposed.

By 1804, in a move similar to the foundation of the surgeons' own hospital in 1736, the College resolved to appoint its own lecturer in surgery, and in spite of questions concerning the legality of the move, John Thomson was appointed to the post, which carried the title of Professor of Surgery of the Royal College of Surgeons.[72] The duties of the post included the delivery of a course of lectures comparable in duration to those offered by the University professors (though anatomy would not be taught), and the formation of a collection of morbid anatomy, plaster casts and illustrations. (Thomson was probably spared such incidents as that which took place in the University in November 1811, when an 'outrage' was reported 'which had taken place in the Anatomy Theatre previous to the lecture, when a Pistol was produced by one of the students and a considerable confusion ensued'.)[73]

Not surprisingly, loud protests emanated from the University, and the Town Council was, of course, appealed to by both sides. Thomson was endorsed publicly by the College, and, as with many aspects of their activities, intimation was placed in the press, in terms which reveal between the lines much of the hostility towards the University and those felt to be less well equipped to teach surgery:

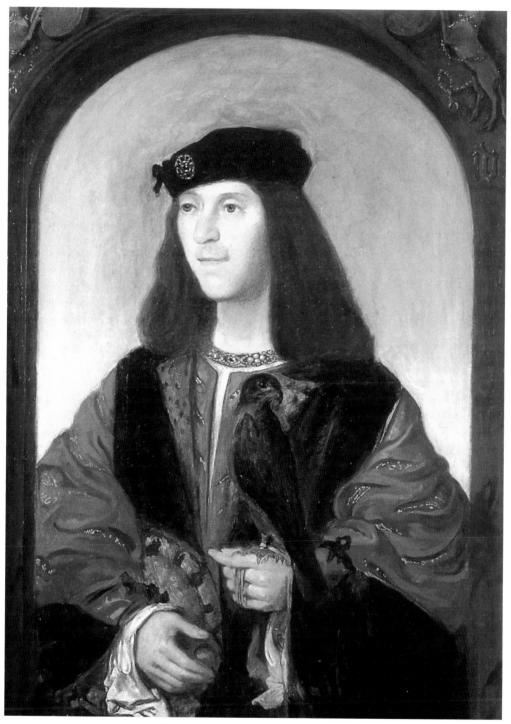

**PLATE 1** *Portrait of King James IV.*
*(H. H. R. Woolford, copy of original by Daniel Mytens.)*

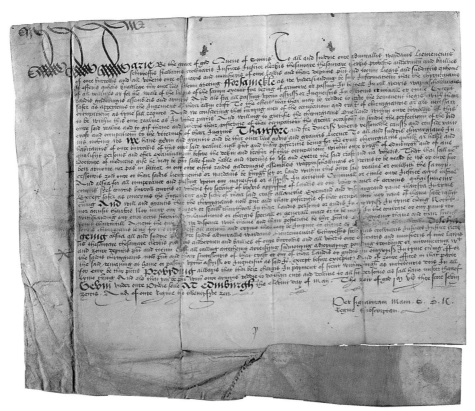

PLATE 2 *Letter of exemption granted by Mary, Queen of Scots (1567).*

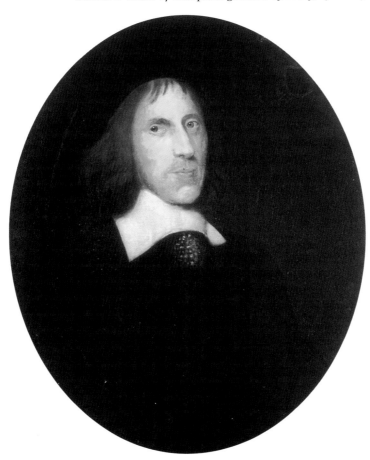

PLATE 3
*Portrait of James
Borthwick of Stow, first
surgeon-apothecary.
(Painter unknown.)*

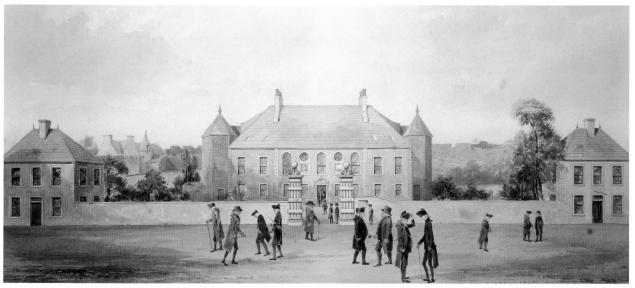

**PLATE 4** *Watercolour painting of Old Surgeons' Hall, High School Yards. (After Sandby.)*

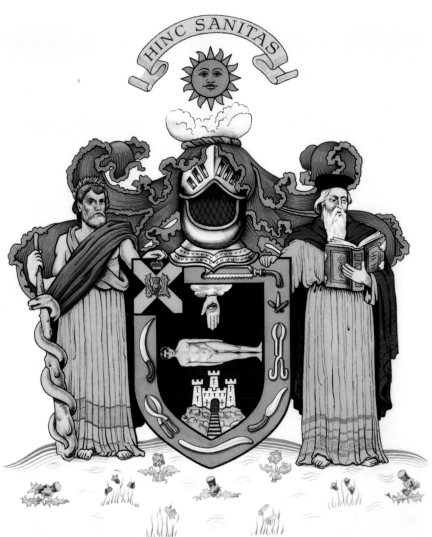

HINC SANITAS

**PLATE 5** *Armorial bearings of the College. The Honourable Colledge of Chirurgeons of Edinburgh Gives for Ensignes Armoriall:*

Azur a humaine Body fess wayes Betwixt a dexter hand having ane eye on the Palme issuing out of ane cloud downward and a Castle Situate on a rock all proper within a bordur Or Charged with severall Instruments peculiar to the Art On a Canton as the first A St Andrews cross argent surmounted of a thistle vert Crowned as the third: Above the shield ane helmet befitting their degree mantled azure doubled Or And for their crest on a wreath Or and Azur The sun dissipating a cloud proper Supported by Aesculapius vested argent mantled azure crowned with a Laurell Holding in his hand a baston nue reaching down to his foot wreathed about a Serpent proper armed gules and Hypocrates vested as the other with a mantle gules And on his head a Bonnet sable holding in his left hand a book expanded both standing on a Compartment And for their motto in ane escroll above all Hinc Sanitas. (From Volume 1, Part 3 of the Register of Arms in the Lyon Office, New Register House, Edinburgh, c. 1672)

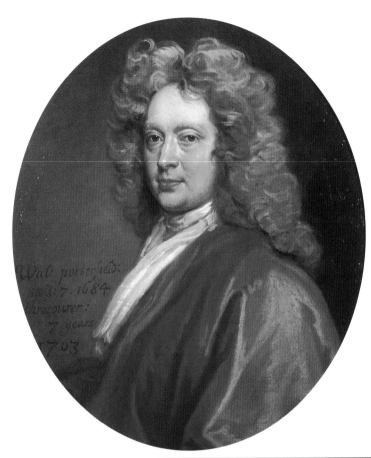

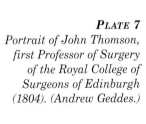

**PLATE 6**
*Portrait of*
*Walter Porterfield by*
*Sir John Medina,*
*1703.*

**PLATE 7**
*Portrait of John Thomson,*
*first Professor of Surgery*
*of the Royal College of*
*Surgeons of Edinburgh*
*(1804). (Andrew Geddes.)*

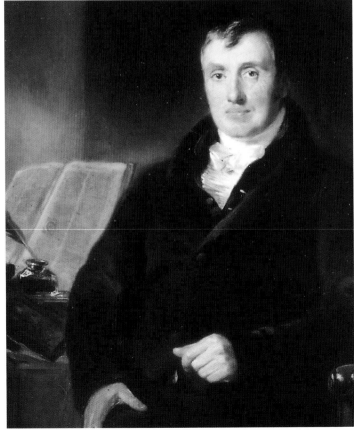

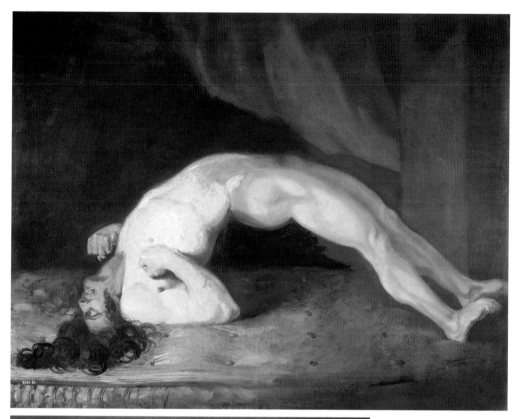

**PLATE 8** Opisthotonus, oil painting by Sir Charles Bell (c. 1809), who recorded injuries sustained by troops at the Battle of Corunna.

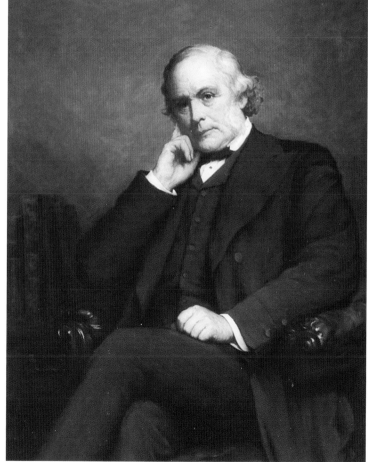

**PLATE 9** Portrait of Joseph Lister, first surgeon to be elevated to the peerage, and only holder of the Fellowship and Honorary Fellowship of the RCSEd. (Dorofield Hardy.)

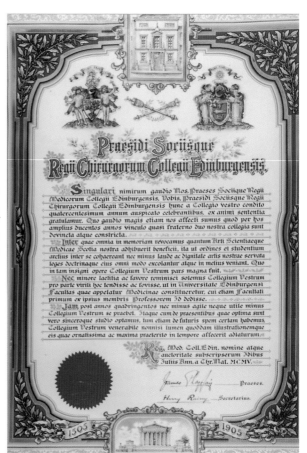

**PLATE 10**

*Congratulatory greetings from the Royal College of Physicians of Edinburgh on the occasion of the 400th anniversary of the College in 1905.*

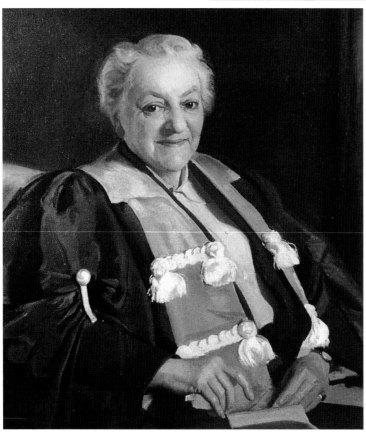

**PLATE 11**

*Portrait of Gertrude Herzfeld, second female Fellow of the College and first practising female surgeon in Scotland. (Sir William Hutchison.)*

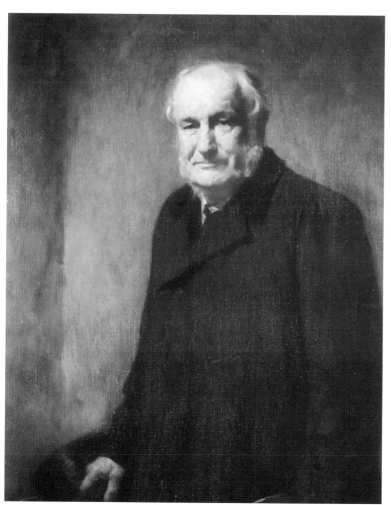

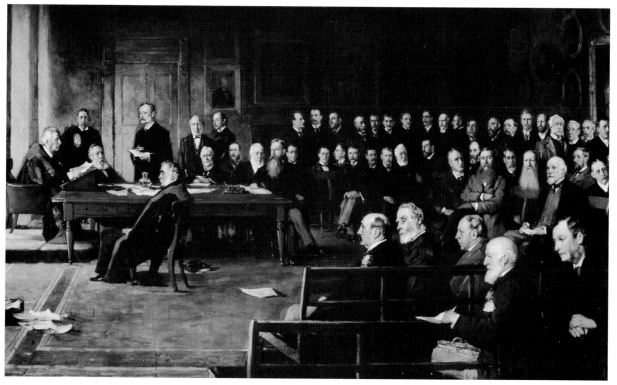

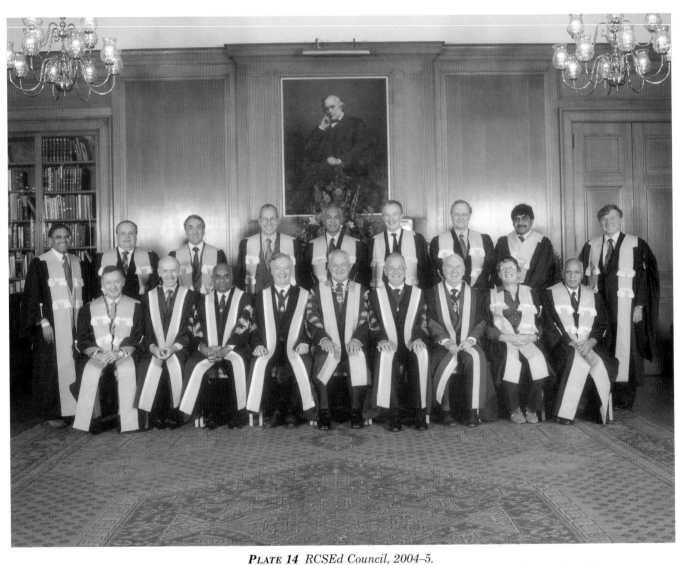

**PLATE 14** *RCSEd Council, 2004–5.*
*Back row: A. Bakran, D. I. Rowley, S. Nixon, C. J. K. Bustrode, U. Chetty, D. Lee, O. Eeremin, S. Kumar, D. A. Tolley*
*Front row: W. S. Hendry, J. R. C. Logie (Treasurer), P. K. Datta (Secretary), I. M. C. Macintyre (Vice-President), J. A. R. Smith (President),*
*J. D. Orr (Vice-President), J. P. McDonald (Dean and Convener of Dental Council), C. Evans, M. Khan*
*Absent: C. W. Oliver, I. K. Ritchie.*

The Royal College of Surgeons at their quarterly meeting held this day ordered notice to be given, that their Professor, Mr John Thomson, has by their appointment, commenced his course of lectures on the principles and practice of surgery. The Royal College, impressed with the conviction that these lectures will supply a most material deficit in the system of medical education in this place, feel it to be their duty to give them all the countenance and support in their power. The College are at the same time extremely desirous that these gentlemen who may be engaged in qualifying themselves for the profession of surgery should be fully aware of what importance to a chirurgical education an institution must be, which has for its object to afford them an opportunity of acquiring a knowledge of surgery, by studying it under the guidance of a practical surgeon. It is with much satisfaction that the College announce, that this institution has met with the fullest approbation of the Army Medical Board and of the Board for Sick and Wounded Seamen. Officers of the Medical Staff, Surgeons and Assistant Surgeons of the Navy, on producing proper vouches of their commissions, will be intitled to attend these lectures gratis.[74]

This advertisement speaks eloquently about the surgeons' views both on their growing status with the military and on who should teach surgery in Edinburgh, as well as their well-practised use of the available media. It also illustrates the continuing problems experienced by the College, and also the difficulties faced by the Town Council, which had close relationships with both College and University. Once again, long-term consequences were important, particularly for the future of extra-mural teaching. If it were not possible to teach surgery within the walls of the University, the College was determined to take other measures to ensure that the subject would be taught adequately. A note of controversy appeared, though, when John Thomson admitted to his colleagues that he had been in the habit of admitting military personnel to his lecture courses without taking a fee, so as to gain the favour of the Army Board. The College was careful to state that this should not be taken as a precedent.[75]

A further twist in the Thomson narrative came only two years later, when he was appointed to the Chair of Military Surgery in the University (see below), and carried out the duties of both appointments. This appointment once again was not without controversy, on this occasion the University complaining to the Town Council about perceived interference with the rights of the University. Legal advice was taken as usual, but the University was informed that it did not have a strong case, as a precedent had been set with a similar appointment in Conveyancing by the Society of Writers to the Signet.[76] University chairs at this time were overtly politicised and political appointments.[77] By 1819 Thomson was clearly becoming rather less able to carry out his heavy teaching load, as he successfully petitioned the College to be allowed to appoint an assistant to help him with 'the operative part of his lecture course'.[78]

Following Thomson's resignation, John Turner was appointed to the College chair. However, in 1831 the University instituted a Chair of Surgery separate from the Chair of Anatomy – something which the College had long desired – and Turner was nominated for and appointed to this post, the second time that the College Professor had accepted a University Chair. According to College regulations, any Fellow accepting a University Chair was obliged to resign from his College post, and Turner duly demitted office. James Syme immediately put his name forward to succeed Thomson, but the view was expressed in some quarters of the College that the post was effectively obsolete, since many College Fellows by that time gave lecture courses on surgery, and also because, importantly, a Fellow had now been appointed to the new University Chair. This opposition of views engendered a debate in which 'considerable warmth was displayed',[79] but after consulting legal opinion yet again it was decided to reappoint to the post, at which point Robert Lizars declared himself to be a candidate, and proceeded to outvote Syme. The post would be short-lived, though, and it came to a somewhat ignominious end in 1839 following a quarrel between Lizars and Syme over an alleged libel in one of Lizars' publications. Though the offending material was deleted, Lizars resigned and it was agreed without controversy this time that the post should not be filled again.

### Military surgery

Surgeons had been involved in military surgery for centuries, and by the early decades of the nineteenth century, against a background of increasingly academic aspects to surgical training and also of the immediate context of the Napoleonic War, it was quite logical that this important facet of surgery should be given academic status. As with most things, though, the road to academic military surgery was not straightforward. At Edinburgh University during the days of the Monro empire, any sort of modernisation or extension of anatomical or surgical teaching was faced with stiff reactionary opposition from the Monro camp and its heavyweight legal backing. A recent history of the Regius Chair of Military Surgery at the University of Edinburgh makes the claim that a major stimulus came from the wartime experiences of College Fellow John Bell, who had been apprenticed to the famous Lang Sandy Wood[80] and who had treated casualties of the Battle of Camperdown in October 1797. It was here that he had witnessed what he considered to be serious deficiencies in the surgical competence of the naval surgeons and their assistants.[81] Following this experience Bell made public his opinion that there should be a school of military surgery set up in Scotland, along the lines of some of the well-established centres in Europe, such as the Academy of Surgery in France, the Military College of Surgery in Germany and the Surgical School of Prussia.[82] No such school was founded in Edinburgh, but for a brief period military surgery would be taught at the University. The first incumbent of this chair in 1806 was John Thomson, who, as mentioned, had very recently been elected as Professor of Surgery of the Royal College of Surgeons. The Town Council may have been stimulated to set up the chair in the light of the renewed hostilities between Britain and France, and Thomson was the obvious candidate as he was already

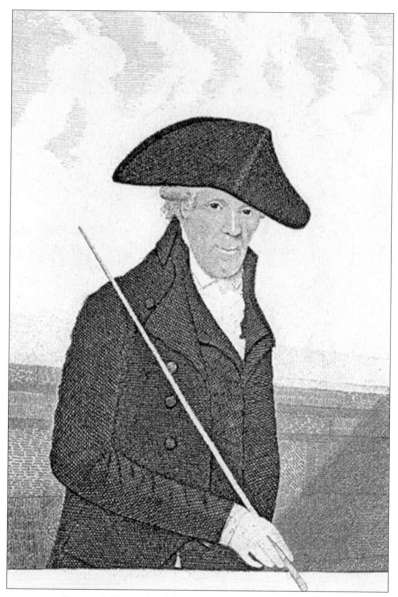

**FIG. 4.3** *Portrait of Alexander ('Lang Sandy') Wood.*
(Kay's Edinburgh Portraits.)

delivering a course of lectures on military injuries. He was confirmed to the new chair in May 1806, and continued to deliver lectures (which still considered the works of Paré), as well as offering clinical instruction at the military hospital in Edinburgh castle.[83] Thomson resigned from his College post in 1821, as he was a candidate for the vacant Chair of Physic – he was unsuccessful in this application, though he was eventually appointed to the first Regius Chair of Pathology in 1831. This is a good illustration of individual ambition perhaps overshadowing institutional loyalty. Surgeons were free agents, just as much as medical students.

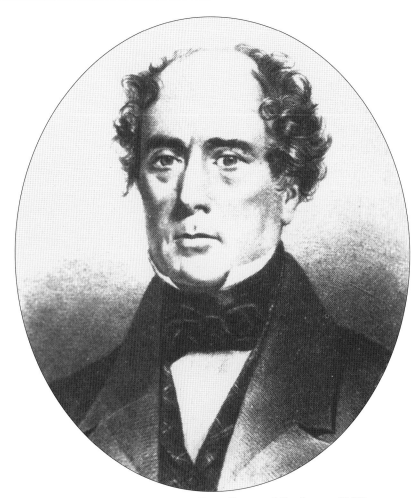

***FIG. 4.4*** *Portrait of George Ballingall, second Professor of Military Surgery at Edinburgh University.*

Thomson resigned the Chair of Military Surgery in 1822 and was succeeded, within the space of a few days, by George Ballingall, another prominent College Fellow, who served as President from 1836 to 1838 and who was one of those chosen by Robert Knox to investigate his involvement in the Burke and Hare episode.[84] He continued the teaching of military surgery, and during this time students were allowed to count Military Surgery as an alternative to lectures on Clinical Surgery. Ballingall was the last incumbent of the chair, as crown funds were withdrawn in 1855. It has been claimed that this was at least partly due to Ballingall's quarrels with Syme, who was apparently influential in convincing the government that a separate chair of military surgery was no longer necessary.

In line with the culture of print that engulfed Enlightenment Scotland, many College Fellows published, and the Professors of Military Surgery were no exception. Thomson published *Report of Observations Made in the British Military Hospitals in Belgium after the Battle of Waterloo*,[85] while among Ballingall's many publications was his *Outlines of Military Surgery*.[86] Evidence from lecture notes, museum specimens and other sources confirms that both Thomson and Ballingall dealt with all sorts of wounds inflicted by contemporary military hardware, particularly musket balls, and that they considered new treatments as well as continuing more long-standing methods of treatment. Penetrating wounds of the thorax and abdomen were particularly difficult to treat.[87]

The College professorships and the Chair of Military Surgery were short-lived posts. They quite quickly rendered themselves obsolete, in part because of the rapid development of surgical teaching in general, and the final separation of Anatomy and Surgery within the University. Their short lifespan, though, is not to suggest that the posts and their incumbents had not made valuable contributions to their surgical fields. They were constructed and deconstructed by immediate contextual influences and the changing relationships between the College and the University, as well as the roles played by enterprising individuals.

## TRAINING

For most of the period covered in this chapter, the apprenticeship was still the main entry to a full surgical career, though by the 1820s the servant category was disappearing rapidly. Table 4.1 gives the numbers of masters, apprentices and servants who entered the service of the College between 1730 and 1820.

**Table 4.1 Numbers of entrant masters/Fellows, apprentices and servants, 1730–1820.** (Source: College Minutes)

| Date | Masters | Apprentices | Servants |
|---|---|---|---|
| 1730–9 | 9 | 51 | 77 |
| 1740–9 | 14 | 50 | 72 |
| 1750–9 | 17 | 35 | 40 |
| 1760–9 | 6 | 29 | 37 |
| 1770–9 | 15 | 83 | 67 |
| 1780–9 | 16 | 49 | 54 |
| 1790–0 | 18 | 77 | 63 |
| 1800–9 | 18 | 62 | 25 |
| 1810–19 | 34 | 127 | – |
| Total | 147 | 563 | 435 |

The demise of the servants was relatively sudden, and probably reflects the impact of the diploma examination and the increasing popularity of University and extra-mural courses. The apprenticeship was fairly common for most of the nineteenth century, though by this time this was not necessarily with a single surgeon, but could be with a group or partnership.

The major new teaching feature from the later eighteenth century was the growth of extra-mural classes, and a number of factors combined to encourage this.

The financial situation of the College was becoming a little more secure, helped by the increasing popularity of the diploma (see below). The College had been in dispute with the University about the teaching of surgery, and though a solution was achieved eventually, tensions and restrictions remained. Importantly also, there was a growing trend towards the imposition of a required curriculum for examination candidates. Perhaps less directly influential, but none the less important, was the fact that the anatomy being taught by the Monros was classical, and consequently becoming less relevant to the needs of practical surgeons. This stimulated the growth in extra-mural teaching outwith the walls of the University, as anatomists who took a different approach to their subject were growing in popularity with students, in, it must be remembered, a free and rapidly expanding student market.

One of the earlier contributions to corporate teaching had come from James Rae, who offered a course of lectures in surgery, 'chiefly founded on the practice of the Society of Surgeons in Edinburgh'. This was publicised in the *Edinburgh Advertiser*:

- The different operations will be shown and made plain, by demonstrating the parts concerned in the disease, the parts that necessarily suffer in the operations and those which should be shunned for the safety of the patient.
- A discourse on the several instruments used in surgery, their mechanisms explained, and some new instruments of his own invention, which have been used with advantage in the Royal Infirmary, will be also exhibited.
- A lecture on each case of any consequence that may occur during the above course in the Royal Infirmary will be given occasionally, and the practice and observations on it.
- A course of lecture on the diseases of the body depending on those of the teeth, thro' all the stages of life, will be introduced in their proper place, such particularly as affect the head, eye, glands, and neighbouring parts.
- A method has for some years been followed by him, of preserving the real appearance of the different tumours, ulcers etc by taking their external forms in moulds of Paris plaister, and casts from these in the same material, or wax; these are coloured from the life, and kept among other preparations he has of diseased parts. In order to throw light on such parts of the above lectures as require anatomical illustration, recourse will be had to the human skeleton, to several drawings, to the figures by authors of established character, to preparations etc.[88]

This course contained a number of elements still central to surgical training: clinical demonstration, pathological anatomy and surgical pathology.

The background to the relative demise of the reputation of University anatomy is interesting and illustrates a number of key factors which influenced this period – the culture of enquiry, the practical application of scientific 'improvement' and the rise in power of the surgeons within the medical sphere. It was not surprising that the College wished to see the establishment of a separate Chair of Surgery; this was entirely in keeping with the prevailing atmosphere and the need to provide anatomical and surgical teaching that was appropriate to the needs of the medical and surgical practitioners of the early nineteenth century. Lawrence has identified the surgeons as 'the new power in medicine', and this power was wielded at a corporate as well as individual level.[89] This power was partly due to the carefully cultivated political contacts which the College had made in the past and would continue to use in the future. The combination also of anatomists outwith the University in opposition to the Medical Faculty, which claimed that it still offered comprehensive teaching, and the open student market was powerful and encouraged the growth of extra-mural teaching, involving many College Fellows. More and more students began to take the College diploma in preference to – as well as in addition to – the MD degree. Part of the reason for this upsurge in the College's profile in the town was that new subjects were offered by the extra-mural teachers, particularly in the area of pathology and physiology, which was important, as by this time the surgeons were claiming increasingly that internal disorders caused by local pathology rather than systemic abnormality came within their remit. It would be several decades before anaesthesia allowed them to cure many of these conditions surgically, but surgical pathology and physiology, together with comparative anatomy, were key components of 'everything that he werkes'.

Many more College Fellows would become involved in extra-mural teaching when the School of Medicine of the Royal Colleges was founded in 1895, but in the earlier period many surgeons offered classes, including John and Charles Bell, both of whom were eventually forced out by the Edinburgh anatomical establishment and moved to London, and John Barclay, who advertised his course in the following terms:

> Besides demonstrating as usual every Organ of the human body in regular order and illustrating their functions by Comparative Anatomy, he will among other improvements of his course, attend particularly to the simple and compound motions of the Animal System; which are not only calculated to throw much light on their form and structure, but an accurate knowledge of the organs which produce them is of much more importance than is generally imagined both in the Practice of Surgery and Physic.[90]

There is always a human aspect to any situation, and amusing insight into the physical attributes of one of the more notorious extra-mural lecturers, Robert Knox, comes from the diary of College Fellow Benjamin Bell, which states that 'although he had a bald vigorous, intellectual head, he was a very ugly man with one eye completely gone, and coarse rather repulsive features. The other eye was very keen and seemed to monopolise the sight which ought to have belonged to its comrade'. Bell conceded that 'he was listened to with invariable attention and

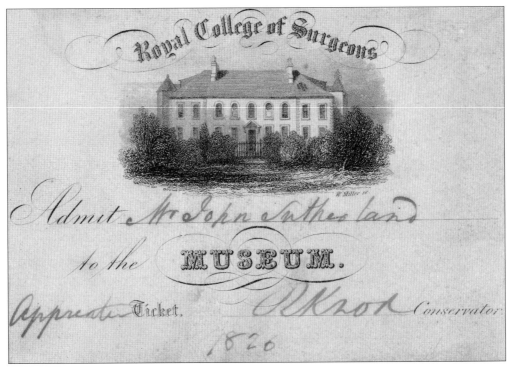

**FIG. 4.5** *Class card for the anatomy class of Robert Knox, 1826.*

respect', and noted that he 'indulged in elegant sarcasm against the Professors in the University'.[91] Barclay may have been a little more subtle in his criticism of the University, but it is apparent, none the less.

The teaching of anatomy would be placed on more sound footing once formal regulations had been put in place. The minutes of November 1831 note the College's approval of the terms of the proposed Anatomy Act, and the decision to submit petitions to both houses of parliament in support of the measure. The College was particularly sensitive about the Burke and Hare scandal, involving as it did one of its own, Robert Knox. Knox had claimed that he did not know that the bodies brought to him for dissection were murder victims, and that there was no evidence of foul play on examination. The pamphlet and newspaper press was active on this, of course, and the claim was made by 'Echo of Surgeon Square' that if Knox really was not aware of the provenance of his subjects, he was 'equally as ignorant as his students'.[92] Another anonymous letter to the same recipient (Sir William Rae) claimed that it was impossible that Knox had not known the circumstances. The Anatomy Act had been proposed partly in order to allay the fears of the people following such scandals, but 'Aristedes' claimed that 'no method of disanimation [was] more easily detected than that which Burke and Hare adopted', and that 'it was never imagined that any member of an enlightened College of Surgeons, honoured by their sanction as a teacher of anatomy could be either so unskilful or so iniquitous as to purchase slaughtered human beings, and, by so doing, hold out a premium for the commission of murder'.[93] Rae had, in Aristides' view, called into question the integrity of the entire medical profession, and claimed that no Anatomy Act would be effective 'when it is claimed that medical knowledge [of the surgeons] is so poor'. Despite these misgivings, though, the Anatomy Act of 1832 did provide a structure and guidelines for the acquisition of bodies for dissection in the anatomical schools which were proliferating at this time. This Act remained in force until 1984, when it was replaced by a new Act, and subsequent legislation has had to be constructed to deal with retention of human tissue and transplantation procedures.

The earlier decades of the nineteenth century were characterised by tensions between extra- and intra-mural teaching rather than between the College and the University itself. Following the report of the Royal Commission on the State of the Universities in Scotland of 1828, efforts had been made to revitalise the reputation and standards of these institutions, and by the middle of the century, the universities were in a better position to stake a stronger claim once again. The flourishing of extra-mural teaching served to provide an alternative to university anatomy as well as building the reputation and income of the teachers. The situation would be reversed, though, once the universities began to succeed in their aim to dominate the field of basic medical and surgical qualification.

## EXAMINATIONS

From the start, entry examinations had been clearly focused on the tenets of the Seal of Cause, and the Deacon and brethren seem to have acted from 'professional' motives. It is, of course, impossible to make any kind of judgement as to the conduct of the examinations, or the scope of the questions, or indeed the professionalism of the examiners. Life as an examinator was not without problems, though. In December 1818 John Gairdner was attacked by a disgruntled candidate who had arrived at his house, 'produced a whip and told him that he had been rejected by him as an Examinator at Surgeons' Hall and that he was come to give him a little chastisement on that account and that he immediately began to attack him with the whip'.[94] The culprit was sentenced to seven years' transportation (a fairly standard punishment for crimes deemed to be of a moderate degree of severity). The College, however, having achieved the conviction, magnanimously resolved to submit a petition to the Prince Regent for clemency, since 'the dignity of the College had been so sufficiently vindicated by the trial'.

Further threats to the examiners appeared in 1826, when a campaign was waged against one of their number. One of the letters contained the following threat:

> This is to inform you that a determined band of medical students, exasperated at the frequent rejections at Surgeons' Hall which they say you have invariably been the occasion of, have agreed to punish you most severely, in what manner I do not as yet know; yet this I know, that should you be found

off your guard, any advantage will be taken. They, it seems, lay the death of the unfortunate young man who, after rejection a few days ago, put a period to his existence on Arthur's Seat to your charge. This has roused their angry feelings, and they have sworn to have revenge. You will not despise this caution from – A FRIEND.[95]

It was decided to counter these threats by drawing up an address to be read out by professors at their lectures, 'in which way it would be made known to the students without being made so public in the town'.[96] This was one occasion on which the surgeons were reluctant to use the press to put their side of the case. The newspaper press had consolidated considerably during the eighteenth century and had been used to good effect by the College as a means of publicising and emphasising their exclusivity and worth, to students and to the general public.[97] Some things, though, were better dealt with in-house if possible.

Some amendments were made to the entry examinations in the mid-eighteenth century. As mentioned in the previous chapter, botany and *Materia Medica* were added in 1723 consequent on a perceived threat from the physicians. Examples of the examinations taken by pre- and post-1723 apprentices illustrate the expanding scope of the tests at this time. Colin Mackenzie petitioned for examination in June 1719 and passed his final test on 10 September. His four examination sessions were as follows:

- General surgery
- Demonstration of the skeleton except for the cranium
- Fistula *in ano*
- Compound fracture of the leg and appropriate bandages

Some fourteen years later, George Lauder underwent rather more searching tests:

- General anatomy and surgery with a speech on scrofulous humors
- Demonstration of the chylopoetic viscera of the abdomen, with their functions and uses
- *Materia medica*, botany, reading and explanation of prescriptions
- Preparation of *unguentum basilicum* and *emplastrum diapalma*, together with the operation of trepanning with the relevant bandaging techniques[98]

This is good example of outside pressures enforcing, or at least stimulating, development. Knowledge of these extra subjects was doubtless useful and their inclusion in the examination syllabus (together with the boosting of the library stock) is a clear indication of immediate response to an external challenge. The changes may not always have been made from the best of motives, but the results were probably beneficial.

During the next three decades examination regulations remained relatively intact, though it was decreed that when the new Royal Infirmary building was completed in the early 1740s, 'all the young gentlemen attending the Study of Physick or Surgery in Edinburgh either as apprentices or students shall be privileged to attend the patients in the infirmary...'.[99] One minor relief for the examinators was that their discourses were discontinued in 1742. It was also stipulated in 1755 that no surgeon could act as an examinator until one year after admission, a sensible precaution against very inexperienced examinators, though the rota examinators tended to comprise the most senior and most junior members of the Incorporation.

Unlike the FPSG, which acquired extensive powers for examining and licensing midwives in the eighteenth century,[100] there is only a single example of this in the College records, and it appears that in Edinburgh midwives were authorised by the Town Council on the basis of testimonials rather than examination. The individual concerned was Mrs Ann Ker, who in 1751 sought 'a license to practice Midwifery in any Town or Shire to which the Corporation their priviledges do extend'.[101] She apparently satisfied the examiners appointed to test her knowledge, as it was reported on 19 February 1752 that:

> having accordingly examined her upon all the different sorts of births, Natural, Laborious and Preter Natural and on the Methods of treating women after delivery and new born Children. Find that the answers she gives to the severall Questions We put to her are Judicious and satisfying and that she is in every respect Extremely well Qualified to discharge the Office of a Midwife and well deserves the favour of a Licence from the Corporation to practise the same.

### The diploma

In March 1757 a letter was delivered to the Incorporation from the War Office in London, asking the Incorporation to 'try the qualifications' of John McLean, who had applied for a post as surgeon to Lt. Col. Fraser's battalion of highlanders.[102] Four examinators were nominated, and the candidate appeared for examination. Nothing is recorded as to the content or standard of the examination in comparison to the entry tests for master surgeons, but the qualification awarded to McLean was the first of many. The diploma evolved from this inauspicious beginning to become a widely sought after subordinate qualification, the revenue from which would also prove vital to an institution whose financial basis was precarious, to say the least.

Stimulated by the McLean diploma, and probably also with an eye to monetary rewards as much as altruism, the Incorporation decided in the late 1760s to reassert its supervisory rights over surgeons in Fife, Lothian and the borders. An advertisement was inserted in various newspapers to the effect that the country surgeons must come in and submit themselves to an examination in order to obtain a diploma of competence and permission to continue in practice.[103] The first of these diplomas were awarded to John Stewart and Alexander Bruce, both surgeons in Musselburgh, on 7 February 1770. They were followed by around twenty others in the next few years, contributing both to the surgeons' supervisory conscience and territorial ambitions and to the usually empty Incorporation money-box.

A link with the Medical School came a few years later, when, in 1777, two medical students took the examination and were awarded diplomas on payment of a fee of two guineas.[104] This stimulated a further trend, whereby medical students began to acquire surgical diplomas. The potential market was large, as at this time Edinburgh was the mecca for medical students from most corners of the globe,[105] and would prove financially beneficial to the College as well as increasing the profile and acceptability of its diploma, and, importantly, attracting students to extra-mural lecture courses.

By 1778 it was becoming apparent that the diploma rules would have to be recast. The two main groups of applicants were country surgeons and members of the armed forces (together with a small number of individuals licensed to act as surgeons in ships involved in the African slave trade),[106] but it was increasingly the case that medical students were applying for surgical diplomas to add to their medical qualifications. The question was now whether 'it would not be proper to have two forms of diplomas', and after the usual discussion this was agreed, the cost of a full diploma being 100 merks and a military or naval diploma two guineas (there is no mention of scope or content of either examination, but it may be inferred that the 100-merk diploma was a little more detailed and searching than the less expensive military equivalent).

Within a few years, a threat to the College's licensing of surgeons for slave trade ships appeared in the form of an Act of parliament passed in 1787, by which surgeons could thenceforth only be licensed by the London surgeons. This, naturally, greatly offended the College, and a memorial was quickly dispatched to Henry Dundas requesting him to 'do his endeavour to get the above privilege extended to the College when this subject is again brought under the consideration of Parliament'.[107] Dundas's intervention was successful, as by 10 September 1789, the President was able to report that the College had achieved its aims and that intimation would be placed in the press to the effect that examinations for this category of candidate would take place on the first Monday of each month. This was just one instance of the many services rendered to the College by Henry Dundas, at that time the key figure in Scottish politics. The next few decades would witness recurrent disputes over the jurisdiction of the RCSEng, and although the trade in human degradation stirred the consciences of the surgeons, nevertheless it was thought essential to have equal examining and licensing rights to those of the London surgeons. The examinators were ordained to 'test the knowledge of the diseases most prevalent on board the ships employed therein'.[108] In the event, only around twenty diplomas were issued to slave ship surgeons, and while the College may be criticised for participating in such a venture, it is also possible to argue that perhaps the surgeons were able in some small way to alleviate the distress of some of those transported. A few years later a letter from the Society for Abolition

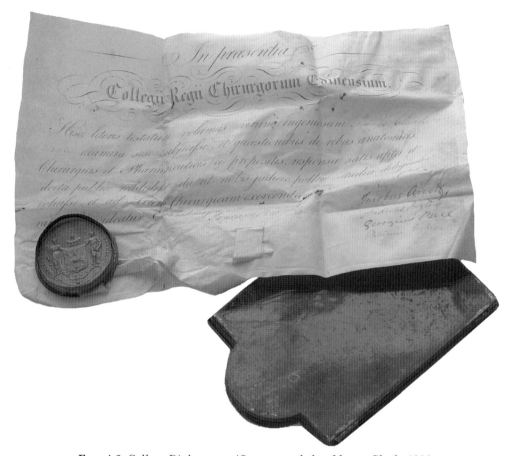

***FIG. 4.6*** *College Diploma certificate awarded to Mungo Clark, 1806.*

of the Slave trade was discussed, but it was decided that however much the members disapproved of slavery as individuals, they 'cannot take it upon them as a corporate body to interfere in the business'.[109] Shades of fence-sitting perhaps, but political pragmatism had long been a hallmark of survival for the College, and it must be remembered that this was the eighteenth century.

New diploma regulations were introduced in 1809, producing an examination which included most of the subjects taken by university medical students, as well as specified periods of hospital practice. Though the regulations were by now set out formally, there was still some opportunity for deserving cases to be allowed some flexibility. A candidate from Nova Scotia was allowed to take his diploma without having fulfilled the letter of the law with regard to completion of lecture courses, as he had been unaware of the changes to the regulations until he had arrived in Scotland,[110] while in March 1820 a candidate was allowed to take the diploma examination early because he had 'unexpectedly received an appointment in the Honourable East India Company'.[111]

Once the College diploma was accepted as qualification for surgeons' mates in the Navy, further demarcations were necessary, as the certificates awarded to these candidates had to be categorised as to the type of ship aboard which the individual was deemed competent to serve. In May 1797 a list of ship ratings and numbers of surgeons' mates who should serve on each type of ship was sent from the Navy Board (these ranged from five surgeons' mates on a first-rate ship, to one on a sixth-rate ship and none on a fire ship).[112] Thomas Lake was the first candidate to be tested under the new system and he was awarded a certificate of competence at the highest level, as first mate on a first-rate ship. Thereafter, each naval candidate's diploma was specific as to level of mate and rate of ship. By 1815 the separate military and naval diplomas were discontinued, and the full diploma taken by all candidates, and by 1816 it had been decided that all diploma holders would be known as Licentiates of the College.[113] Unlike the Fellowship examination, which saw very few failures or referrals, statistics for the first six months of 1820 (which was typical) indicated that thirteen candidates had failed their diploma examinations out of a total of ninety-nine (a failure rate of around 14 per cent).[114]

Parity with other bodies was quite another matter. The College had managed to win recognition for its qualifications for the East India Company (1799), Army surgeons' mates (1803) and assistant Army surgeons (1805). A petition was submitted to the Duke of York in November 1808 claiming parity for the Edinburgh diploma with that of the RCSEng in relation to full Army surgeons.[115] The petition was denied, re-submitted and again refused. It proved very difficult to convince the British authorities of the parity of the College's qualifications and this was a particular problem with the armed force. Success came eventually in 1813. Acceptance by the Navy took a little longer. In November 1828, David Hay wrote on behalf of the College to Lord Melville, including a copy of a document he intended to submit to the Commissioners for Victualling His Majesty's Navy, asking for Melville's views before transmitting the petition to the Board that the 'Diploma of the Royal College of Surgeons of Edinburgh may be recognised as a qualification for the rank of full surgeon in the Navy as it has been for the same rank in the Army since 1813' (the letter also included a query as to whether this was the right time for the College to submit a request to the Treasury for a 'grant of money' towards the building of the new Hall).[116] (One of the more amusing appeals to high political authority had come from James Russell, College President, in 1797, hoping that Henry Dundas would 'procure for those members of the Royal College of Surgeons of Edinburgh who keep carriages the same exemption from any increase upon the assessed taxes which has been granted to the Gentlemen of the medical profession in London'.)[117]

In time, and as the diploma became increasingly popular, it was less practicable for all candidates to attend the requisite lectures in Edinburgh. Gradually, over the years, a list of approved lecturers from beyond the city bounds was drawn up. Certified attendance at their classes would count towards the diploma requirements, and in 1811 it was decided that students could include study at Glasgow University as part of their approved curriculum.[118]

A development which would affect all qualifications, and one which reflects both long-term aims and more immediate external influences, was the awareness that if diplomas and fellowship qualifications offered by the College were to have credibility both at home and abroad, the College would not only have to examine rigorously but also be seen to impose minimum curriculum requirements. The Seal of Cause had encouraged the pursuit of strictly supervised apprenticeships, but was not specific as to exactly what experience the apprentice should have gained, or the knowledge he should have acquired before presenting himself for examination. By the end of the eighteenth century, though, steps had to be taken to present a publicly credible product. The College resolved that 'in order to prevent candidates who have not received a regular education from coming forward to be examined, no person shall be admitted as a candidate for the full diploma unless he produce certificates of his having studied at least two sessions in the University of Edinburgh or some other school of medicine'.[119] Candidates for Army and Navy diplomas would be obliged to attend for one session only. Relations between the College and the Boards of the armed services had been strained, the difficulties lying mainly in the areas of apparently poor candidates and of acceptability of the Edinburgh diploma as equal to a London equivalent. All of this once again can be seen to fit neatly into the theoretical standpoints of both Habermas and Jordanova, in terms of the pressures brought about by social change and increasing access to knowledge within the expanding public sphere of the Enlightenment period, together with, of course, continuing attempts to withstand encroachment by other Colleges.

During the first half of the nineteenth century the curriculum was steadily broadened, and the list of pre-examination requirements for the diploma became ever longer and much more recognisably akin to that of a medical school. In 1829 the optimium curriculum was:

Four winter sessions, including courses on:

- Institutes of Medicine or Physiology
- Practical Anatomy (5 months)
- Practical Chemistry (3 months)
- Clinical Surgery (5 months)
- Clinical Medicine (5 months)
- Surgery (two winter sessions, or one session and one on military surgery)
- 18 months' attendance at an approved hospital
- Midwifery (5 months)[120]

Candidates were also required to prove that they had received instruction in Latin, mathematics and mechanical philosophy. Latin standards had been criticised by the Army Medical Board in 1813, it being claimed that a number of Edinburgh-qualified surgical assistants had been unable to read prescriptions.[121] As a result of this criticism, an advertisement was inserted in the press to the effect that parents or guardians of potential students should ensure that they had received a good basic education, including Latin. Latin had been a requirement since 1505, but it took criticism from outside to spur the surgeons to publicise the need for the early acquisition of the language prior to undertaking surgical studies.

As mentioned, the diploma attracted candidates from all parts of the world, and this was the start of the American links with the College. The first American to hold the College diploma was William Lehre of Charleston, South Carolina, who gained the qualification on 20 September 1791.[122] From that point the transatlantic link was strengthened, not least with the foundation of the first medical school in America, in Philadelphia. Many American medical students at Edinburgh studied anatomy and the most famous of all, perhaps, Benjamin Rush, was in the anatomy class of Alexander Monro *secundus*.[123] Of those who would pursue a career in surgery, one of the most famous is Ephraim McDowell, the ovariotomist, who studied anatomy with John Bell.[124] The College's influence on the New World was multi-faceted. Many Americans chose to study in Edinburgh; many Scottish surgeons emigrated with their skills; and new institutions were built on the 'Edinburgh model'.[125] Similar links were, of course, made with Canada, Australia and other dominions and these have continued, though nowadays are very different, channelled mainly through scientific exchange, publications, Honorary Fellowships and overseas meetings.

Problems with diploma fraud did arise occasionally, and in 1809 the College had to deal with an allegation that a College diploma had been forged. The matter was reported in the minutes:

> They discovered that a student of the name of Waddel who was rejected a few months ago by the Examinators of this College had been guilty of forging a Diploma purporting to be one from the Royal College of Surgeons upon which they immediately applied to the Magistrates for his apprehension, and it appearing that Mr Sommerville the Engraver and Mr Paton the writing master were both implicated in the transaction, as well as a student of the name of Paxton who Waddell alleged had given his assistance in committing the forgery they were all brought before the Magistrates and severally underwent examination.[126]

The student concerned admitted the offence and the College 'out of clemency and compassion to this weak and unfortunate young man' decided not to take the matter further in his case, though expressing the view that Sommerville and Paton should be remitted to the magistrates for their part in the matter. Paton subsequently sent in a grovelling petition claiming that he had carried out the work in good faith, but now realised his mistake. It was decided to insert a warning notice in the newspapers about this event in the hope that any recurrence might be prevented.

### Fellowship

From 1709 to 1822 (when examination regulations changed and the records consequently provided less detailed information), the College Clerks noted the examination topics allocated to every candidate for full resident mastership/Fellowship, and these form the basis for the following discussion. During this period 182 candidates undertook surgical examinations for entry as masters (Fellows from 1778). Procedures which remained popular as examination topics throughout the whole period included trepanning, the removal of cataracts, treatment of lachrymal fistulas, and bandaging techniques. Some 24 per cent of candidates were tested on trepanning, while 14 per cent were allocated eye operations. Eleven candidates were tested on aneurysm, though it would be highly unlikely that any sufferer could hope to survive such a condition. Heroic surgery for aortic aneurysm could not have been contemplated (though various techniques and experiments were tried in the late eighteenth century, usually consisting of ligation of vessels proximal or distal to an aneurysm in the leg). Knowledge of the condition and the theory of surgical intervention were possibly the principal aims of the test. This topic appeared more frequently towards the end of the period.

Questions on the treatment of harelip appeared later in the eighteenth century (Thomas Hay, mentioned above, was tested on this procedure). The first candidate to be allocated this subject was John Willieson, who entered the College in 1769. His examination consisted of a discourse on gunshot wounds, questions on the bones of the face and lower jaw, *Material Medica* and the preparation of *diapalma* and Turner's cerate, together with the operation of harelip and the appropriate bandages.[127]

Though trepanning was a popular topic, and evidence for the procedure having been performed regularly survives from much earlier times,[128] there is little direct evidence of its being carried out by College Fellows, though its popularity as an examination topic would suggest otherwise. Indirect evidence that the procedure was still undertaken comes in the form of a gift sent to the College from Dr John Lorimer FRCPE, Medical Examiner to the East India Company, in February 1792.[129] The gift was a set of portable amputation and trepanning instruments, described as follows:

> The instruments differ little from those at present used by most practitioners but they are so placed as to be secured against injury from motion or the weather, and take up so little space that they may even be carried in the pocket; circumstances of great consequence to army surgeons in the field or on detachments; and the Dr imagined that they might be very convenient for country surgeons who cannot always get carriages. They are now used by all the Surgeons in the service of the East India Company. The breadth of the saw is exactly the diameter of the thigh bone of the Irish Giant,[130] and the length he has found to answer perfectly well. The handle he considers as an improvement, having less cross wood in it and giving an equally firm hold as the common one.

The instruments had been devised when Dr Lorimer was in America in the 1770s, and he considered that 'had they been in common use during the war...the Army would have derived considerable advantage from the surgeons having always with them the necessary instruments'. This would suggest that trepanning as well as amputation was still a common procedure, but its extent is impossible to determine.

Amputation, naturally, was a common topic, a technique which would be well practised by most surgeons, particularly in makeshift field hospitals behind battle lines. Given the Edinburgh surgeons' long tradition of expertise in military surgery and service to the crown and armed forces, it is not surprising that amputation and the treatment of gunshot wounds were considered to be important. It is not clear from the records, but to be assumed, that the particular techniques of amputation examined would be in line with current fashion as to guillotine- or flap-type amputations, and the use of ligatures or cautery to stem bleeding.[131]

Nine candidates were tested on the surgical management of empyema, though none after 1760. Surgical treatment of this condition seems to have developed more generally in the nineteenth century,[132] but one seventeenth-century Edinburgh surgeon, Archibald Pitcairne (who had joined the Incorporation after a dispute with the RCPEd), approved of some degree of surgical intervention. In a letter to Dr Gregory in Oxford about the case of Mr James Hay, who was suffering from acute empyema, he outlined his opinion on the correct treatment to be adopted:

> I think ane aperture should be made not far from the backbone to let out the matter of his empyeme and kept open as a cauter. Meantyme I highly approve of your designe of giving him the peruvian bark, and am very pleased with his getting the bath [presumably Bath] water. All I can say is that he should use the bath water sometyms and ane ass-milk diet, or a woman's by sucking, and in the spring to go to Aix-la-Chapelle or Montpellier.[133]

Though the claim is made here that examinations were as comprehensive and searching as possible, an amendment to the regulations in 1822 may be cited as a contradiction, at least in terms of the status and reputation of the FRCSEd. After discussion, it was agreed that there would henceforth be only three sessions, comprising one on general surgery, one on botany and *Materia Medica*, and the third on the subject of the candidate's probationary essay.[134] The final session on operations was discarded, and since the candidate would have detailed knowledge of his essay topic, this does seem to have been something of a reduction in rigour and difficulty (though it was perhaps felt that the trend would be for apprentices to have gained the College diploma prior to final examination, and thus to have already covered a broad curriculum). It would not be too long before possession of the diploma was the only prerequisite prior to election to the Fellowship.

Perusal of the topics chosen by some of the candidates for their probationary essays gives good illustration of the sorts of topics which were popular in the first third of the nineteenth century. They included:

| | |
|---|---|
| Retention of urine | Gangrene |
| Pathology of the mamma | Popliteal aneurysm |

Chronic abscesses

Neuralgia

Syphilitic inflammation of the iris

Tetanus

Caesarian section

Artificial pupil

Amputation in cases of
 external injury

Bronchocele

Infanticide

Paracentesis thoracis

Arch of the aorta
 (dedicated to Robert Knox)

New blood vessels

Spina bifida

Foreign bodies in the air passages

Feigned and factitious diseases

Viability of the fetus

Lateral operation for the stone
 (John Gairdner, dedicated to
 Charles Bell)

Powers which move the blood

Amaurosis

Dislocation of the processus dentatus

Venereal diseases

Bronchotomy

Use of mercury in syphilis

Lateral curvature of spine
 (Robert Knox, 1825)

Action of remedies (antiquarian)

Injuries of the head
 (dedicated to Robert Liston)

Carbuncle

Male urethra

Medical jurisprudence of
 blows and contusions

The length and scope of these dissertations varied considerably. Some were over 100 pages long; others less than 20. Some appeared to be summaries of current knowledge rather than a reasoned argument or potential contribution to knowledge. They covered a wide variety of the very general and the specialised. Some of the topics suggest a 'research-type' dissertation, rather than one based on surgical techniques. A few of the essays give a hint that orthopaedics was a popular area. In 1823 James Combe submitted an essay on diseases of the hip; in 1825 Robert Knox wrote on 'causes and treatment of lateral curvature of the human spine'; William Sharpey's essay, submitted in 1830, considered the 'pathology and treatment of false joints'; while Patrick Newbigging offered his thoughts on spina bifida in 1833. Thomas Tytler wrote on injuries of the spine for his examination in August 1841, but died less than a month later and was thus prevented from contributing further to what seems almost to be the first germs of a specialty, or at least consideration of the possibility that treatments could be developed for these conditions.

These were all useful topics, showing an interest in skeletal pathology and deformity. Old habits died hard, though, as witnessed by the dissertation presented by David Johnstone in 1823, entitled 'use and effects of mercury in the treatment of syphilis'. Mercury-based ointment was allocated regularly as one of the prescriptions to be made up by candidates, and though its dangers had long been recognised, and its iatrogenic effects were distressing for the patients, it was still considered to be an essential element in the treatment of a range of conditions, from gout to madness.

Care was taken to ensure that the writings of potential College Fellows did not cause public offence. The content of some probationary essays was questioned, and on occasion a candidate asked to alter or remove certain passages before final acceptance of the work. On such instance occurred in July 1823, during the examinations of John McIntosh. He submitted a probationary essay on childbirth, in which he had made reference to the recent death in childbirth of Princess Charlotte – the popular daughter of the Prince Regent, later King George IV – who had died following complications after giving birth to a stillborn child. There was much controversy about her medical care, which had been given principally by a man-midwife. The events, of course, made headline news and claims were made of medical misman-agement, including the decision not to use forceps when these were, apparently, required because of the position of the child. The following was noted in the College minute books:

> Dr Hay moved that previous to Dr McIntosh's being received on trial on the subject of his Essay, he should be desired to cancel certain passages therein viz. 1. The following passage occurring on page 6th. 'It is now well known that to this last cause the death of the Princess Charlotte is to be ascribed – an event which no human foresight could have anticipated; an event which is not more to be deplored from the national calamity it inflicted, than from the disgraceful feelings it produced in the minds of some accoucheurs which led them into an unjust persecution of the amiable and distinguished individual who had the principal charge on that interesting occasion – a persecution which has not even ceased with the life of him who fell a victim to its virulency – a persecution which I shall never cease to hold up as scandalous and infamous, because it was gratuitous as well as unjust and unworthy of a liberal profession' and the following passage from the bottom of page 8th. 'Some accoucheurs I am aware object to this simple manner of operating, because they will object to anything which strips this part of the profession of any of its mummery, or which will enable a general practitioner who happens to know little of the practise of midwifery to act as effectually as the most experienced accoucheur'.[135]

The College clearly objected to such inflammatory statements being made by an examination candidate, and after discussion the candidate was persuaded to remove the offending passages, the latter of which seemed to claim that any 'general practitioner' could carry out some of the duties undertaken by those qual-ified in midwifery.

A more difficult problem came to light some years later when John Sibbald's essay on 'Extraction of the placenta' aroused some disapproval. The problem was that he had already been deemed to have satisfied his examiners and had been admitted as a Fellow. The College could do little else but to advise that the contents of the essay should not be publicised too widely.[136]

In summary, between 1790 and 1830 the main changes to the examination reg-ulations were:

1798   All diploma candidates to attend a course of anatomy lectures and demonstrations, and should attend at a public hospital for one year. Knowledge of pharmacy to be demonstrated.

1806    Candidates who had not served an apprenticeship must attend three sessions of classes, together with classes on pharmacy and *Materia Medica*.

1808    Candidates who had not served an apprenticeship must have attended classes on anatomy, chemistry, botany, institutions and theory of medicine, practice of medicine, principles and practice of surgery, clinical surgery, midwifery and *Materia Medica*, together with hospital attendance. Apprentices had to attend similar courses, but for two years only.

1822    The FRCSEd examination was reduced to three days, comprising general anatomy and surgery, *Materia Medica*, pharmacy and prescriptions, and a final test on the subject of the candidate's pre-circulated probationary essay.

1822    All diploma candidates now had to provide proof of attendance at classes for three sessions.

1828    All candidates had to produce evidence that they had participated in dissection of the human body.[137]

As a result of these decisions, both apprentices and candidates for the diploma spent a fair proportion of their training attending formal classes at the University or extra-murally. The process was in part reaction to events or criticisms, but whatever the motivation, the results were probably to the benefit of the patients, as well as giving an 'academic' aspect to the College. Indeed, the curriculum by this date bore more than a passing resemblance to that for the medical degree at the University. A parallel can be seen here with the situation in France, although there were some differences. In 1772 an attempt was made to abolish the French apprenticeship system, with the order that thenceforth trainee surgeons should act as assistants to master surgeons for three years, but also spend one year (later increased to two years) in a town which offered an academic course in surgery. The French apprenticeship system was partially reinstated in 1784 after protests that 'riff raff' were pretending to be students and carrying out illegal surgery. What did remain, though, was a 'quasi national' system for training, and a system which involved academic study.[138]

## WHAT DID THE SURGEONS DO?

The procedures that the College Fellows were capable of undertaking were limited, but some direct evidence of what they were doing is necessary in order to sustain the history of the College in terms of the surgery carried out by its Fellows. One surviving record is 'Cases observed in the Edinburgh Infirmary in the year 1754–1755 by J. A. H. Reimaris'.[139] Some examples from this repay detailed reporting, if only to illustrate that nowadays many patients would have been cured without drastic surgery or amputation:

> John Byrne aged 55, fell down a stair about a fortnight ago, by which the wrist of his right arm was severely strained – an intense inflammation and swelling all up the forearm appeared immediately and was soon succeeded by a mortification which in a short time overspred the hole hand up as far as the wrist, but was there stopt by proper applications and the use of the cortex Peruv [Peruvian bark, a commonly used substance]. A consultation being held this day it was agreed the arm should be taken off without much delay. The arm was amputated by Mr Hay.

The last note was some eight days post-operatively, when it was noted that the stump was 'looking very well'.

Another patient, Andrew Elder, presented with symptoms of bladder stone and 'was sounded before some gentlemen and it being plain that there was a stone, it was agreed he should be cut . . . was cut this day by Mr Hay. The stone was not very large but hard'. 'Fomentation bags' were applied immediately, and the patient was discharged 'quite well' one month later.

A third patient, who would probably not require amputation in the modern era, was admitted with a knee injury. Above-knee amputation was carried out by Mr Bruce – 'the joint of the knee being opened there issued a collection of pus and the cartilages of the patella and condylii externa ossis femoris were arroded'. Recovery took two months, but the patient was discharged well.

Some insight into gynaecological procedures comes from surviving evidence from patients who had undergone Caesarian section while alive. This procedure was relatively rare at this time, though removal of infants from recently deceased mothers had long been performed. Examination of the skeletal remains and other evidence has allowed some insight into the live Caesarian operation performed by College Fellows during the eighteenth century. The first recorded, in 1737, was performed by Robert Smith, and others were carried out by Alexander Wood (date not known), Thomas Young (probably 1760s), William Chalmer (1774) and John and Charles Bell (1800). Of the eight cases for which details are known, all of the mothers died, but three of the infants survived.[140] This is clear indication that the Incorporation, through its masters and their contacts with the RIE as well as their academic publications, was involved in surgical risk-taking as well as finding better explanations for successes and failures. While Alexander Hamilton, Professor of Midwifery, was widely published, no less important are the surviving manuscript lecture notes of Thomas Young, who carried out two of the operations in question, and was Deacon of the Incorporation from 1756 to 1757, before graduating MD in the early 1760s.[141]

A record of operations performed in the RIE between 26 November 1836 and 30 April 1837 included around fifty cases dealt with by the attending surgeons.[142] An operation for hydrocele was carried out by Robert Lizars on 8 November 1836, by means of 'the Common Method persued by Mr Lizars of puncturing and afterwards injecting the port wine mixture'. Some months later, on 19 February 1837, Alexander Watson treated a similar condition, by the 'new method of introducing a needle so as to allow drops of the fluid to escape', following which 'a blister was applied to the scrotum', demonstrationg a willingness to try out new methods.

A departure from usual practice was noted in a burns case treated by James Syme, the patient being 'a man with leg dreadfully burnt', which was 'amputated below the tubercle of tibia leaving also remains of fibula, the posterior flap being made very large so as to allow for contraction. Mr Liston has been in the habit of removing the whole of the fibula but inflammation of the joint is generally the consequence' – an example here of surgeons disagreeing on the details of certain procedures. Consideration of method is also demonstrated in a case of 'amputation of forearm below insertion of pronator radii teres. Mr Syme recommends amputating pretty high so as to have sufficient for a good flap. Some however in diseases of the hand amputate at the wrist joint'.

These records also indicate graphically the suffering of the patients, before the days of general anaesthesia. On 19 February 1837, Mr Watson operated on a 'man who had his right leg removed on the 13th by Mr Syme [and] had part of his foot removed today. The plantar surface of the foot was so mortified that a dorsal flap was made which will barely cover the astragolus and calcaneum, the neck of the tarsus having been removed'. A few days later the records note a 'woman rather advanced in years with carcinomatous tumour of mamma. The two semilunar incisions having been made it was dissected out quite easily. It presented the true carcinomatous characteristics. Two arteries were only tied. A wet piece of lint was then applied to the wound'.

Further evidence of the very general and wide-ranging surgical competence of the early-nineteenth-century surgeon comes from a publication outlining surgical cases treated by Robert Liston between 1818 and 1821. Some of Liston's more memorable operations have been described elsewhere,[143] but in this publication Liston describes cases of stricture of the urethra; aneurysm, with a full description of the treatment of several individuals; fracture of the femur ('it is necessary to keep the parts steady and in apposition during the time required for their consolidation'); tumours of various sorts and in various locations; operations on diseased bones; and polyps of nasal antra.[144] These were genuine general surgeons, and could turn their hand, with greater or lesser success, to most surgical requirements. Many of the surgeons involved held high office in the College, thus clearly strengthening the links between the organisation and the practical work of its Fellows.

### Relations with the physicians

Although there were serious disputes about arrangements at the RIE, by the turn of the nineteenth century there was rather more co-operation, or at least less overt antagonism between the surgeons and physicians, but various attempts would be made subsequently to try to bring about closer relations, if not union. An anonymous document dated 1821 and entitled *Remarks on the Expediency and Practicality of a Union of the Royal Colleges of Physicians and Surgeons* demonstrates clearly

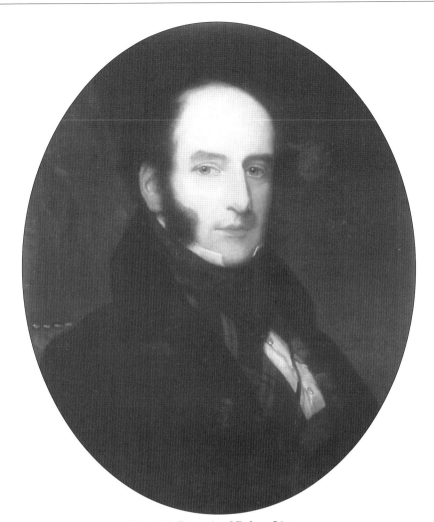

*FIG. 4.7* *Portrait of Robert Liston.*

what problems were to be overcome. The distinctions between physicians and surgeons are described as follows:

> The Physician is a graduate; takes precedence over the surgeons and obtains a guinea as the fee of his visit; while the surgeon is a tradesman, and is paid like other mechanics at the end of the year; the physician uses his head in the investigation and cure of diseases, while the surgeon requires chiefly manual skill in the use of his instruments; the physician cures internal diseases while the surgeon takes charge of outside ones.

The author admits that some of the conditions treated by physicians were trifling, 'tho' gravely entertained by our patients'.[145] Despite these differences, though, by that date it was claimed that half of the Fellows of the College of Surgeons had an MD degree, and also that 'physicians treat Porrigo as frequently and as well as

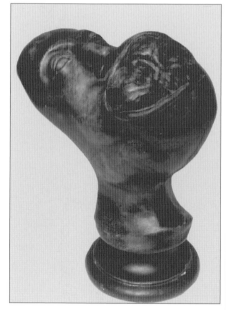
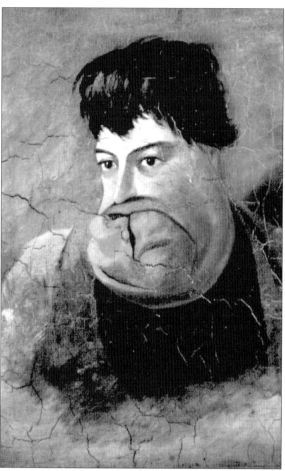

*FIG. 4.8  Illustrations of osseous tumour excised by Robert Liston.*

surgeons do pneumonia; physicians act frequently as accoucheurs and then require the possession of delicate manual skill as much as of intellectual knowledge'. Union would ensure that the 'idle debates about precedency, so dishonourable to the profession and so injurious to their patients would be for ever at an end'.[146] The evidence from the required curriculum and examinations does confirm that surgical apprentices learned very much the same things as medical students, and each group took courses at the University, while many medical students took the Licentiate Diploma of the College. This was not enough to bring the two bodies closer, and the matter was not taken further.

## MUSEUM AND LIBRARY

By the end of the seventeenth century the Incorporation was on surer foundations, and a library and museum collection had been instituted. By the middle of the eighteenth century, though, the College was in serious difficulties and facing impending demise. As a result, most of the library collection and the curiosities were transferred to the University of Edinburgh in 1763. Only two museum items seem to have been retained within the Incorporation, both of which were contributed by famous names. One is a dissection by Archibald Pitcairne, dated 1702, and the other is by Alexander Monro *primus*, in 1718, before he qualified as a master surgeon, and before he was appointed Professor of Anatomy by the Town Council (see Figure 3.8).

Given the College's academic aims, it was natural that consideration would be given to re-establishing and boosting the museum collection. It was stated that 'it would greatly facilitate the teaching of surgery and prove useful as well as creditable to the College to form a Museum of morbid preparations, casts and drawings of diseases and that all the members of the College should be requested to give their assistance in promoting this very necessary part of the plan by supporting it with all such articles of this kind as may be in their power'. At this point also, it was decided to appoint curators and form a Museum Committee, a body which lasted until it was subsumed within a broader remit at the end of the twentieth century, when the management and committee structure of the College was reorganised.

As noted in a publication by the College Museum,[147] the provenance of the early collection is difficult to establish, but it is most likely that specimens were provided from the private collections of anatomists, as it was usual for these individuals to have collections of suitable preparations for the purposes of teaching the students. In his capacity as the College's own Professor of Surgery, John Thomson, along with the curators, had the responsibility of cataloguing and maintaining the collection, as there was, at that point, no provision for laboratory assistance to look after the specimens. It is clear from the surviving catalogues that successive curators were variably conscientious in the discharge of their duties, so that on some occasions only minimal information is given about the specimen or its origins.

The arrangements were further strengthened in 1814, when the College introduced the formal appointment of Keeper of the Museum, with responsibilities detailed in the minutes, including giving 'an accurate history of all the diseases to which morbid specimens may refer, as far as he is able to procure it'. The first incumbent of this post was J. W. Turner, appointed in 1816. As the collection grew, more formal arrangements for its conservation and expansion had to be made, and a Museum Committee was formed, which was answerable to the College Council. Clearly this was a much better start and seemed to be predicated on better forward planning than in the 1690s, when the Incorporation merely wanted to gather in some curiosities. This word curiosity bears consideration too. At the time, that is really just what these items were – curious. A century later they were being described in very different terms. They were still curious – though they at least aroused the curiosity of the surgeons because of their demonstration of abnormal pathology rather than their mere interest as anatomical or pathological oddities or aberrations, though curiosities did continue to come in. So it may be said that these more formalised curiosities stimulated the academic and intellectual curiosity of the surgeons, a curiosity which, when established on a formal basis, would serve to further the cause of advancing knowledge in pathology, morbid anatomy and surgery. This is another good example of changing discourse over time, though just because these items were referred to as curiosities rather than items for serious

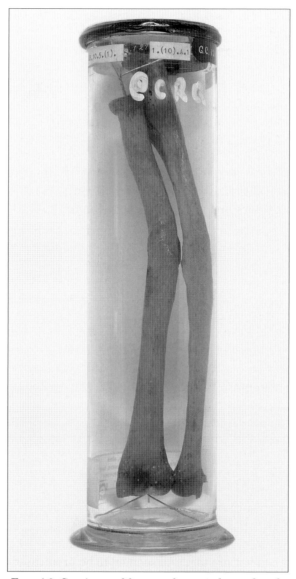

***FIG. 4.9*** *Specimen of forearm fracture donated to the*
*College Museum by John Thomson (1804).*

analysis, this does not detract from the fact that the collection was thought to be
necessary for the academic and intellectual progress of the Incorporation.

The cataloguing of specimens and general organisation of the Museum and its
collection became more regularised, though the problem of housing and storing the
ever-increasing collection would not be even partly solved until the advent of the
Playfair Building, which opened its doors in 1832. The 1820s and 1830s have been
described as 'the years of expansion'. This fits in well with the general background
of expansion in the teaching of anatomy, particularly in the extra-mural school,
and particularly by those anatomists with a focus on the teaching of anatomy as

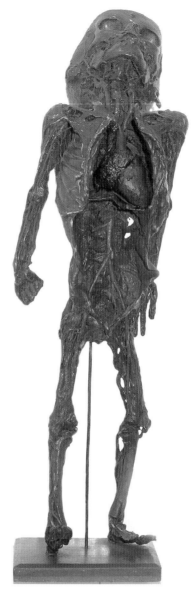

**FIG. 4.10** *Dissected specimen donated to the
College Museum by John Barclay.*

an aid to surgery rather than as an end in itself. By this time the reputation of the
Monros as teachers was on the wane, and it fell to teachers such as John Barclay
and the Bell brothers to advance the cause of surgical anatomy. As described by
Lawrence, this was the 'end of the old thing'[148] as far as anatomy was concerned,
and for the immediate future the vanguard of anatomy would be outwith the university walls, and much more within the ambit of the College, though the formal
School of Medicine of the Royal Colleges would not be set up until 1895. So it was
not just a question that the College wished to expand its collection of anatomical

specimens. As always the context of the time was crucial. The foremost anatomists of the day were taking anatomy forward in new directions, directions aimed at assisting surgery as well as elucidating body structures and functions. In these circumstances, therefore, it is not at all surprising that this period saw considerable and ongoing expansion in the museum collections. Much of the material was gifted to the College by some of these teachers, and in particular the collection of John Barclay was crucial to the expansion of the collection with specimens of wide pathological interest. Many of these items survive in the current museum collection held by the College. (Barclay was awarded an Honorary Fellowship by the College in 1821, in recognition of the gift of this substantial collection.)

Barclay was one of the most significant anatomical teachers of this period, not only in the area of human anatomy, but also in the field of comparative anatomy. His collection was donated to the College with the considerable stipulation that a new hall should be built to house it, and that the collection should retain his name. He informed the College that he wished to have his collection 'deposited with some learned and respectable Society or body of men who could estimate its value and render it useful to themselves and others'.[149] The College was quick to accept this bequest, though it could not be transferred immediately because of the lack of suitable accommodation. After temporary residence in a local house acquired by the College for the purpose, the items were transferred to the College in 1832 (see the account of the Playfair Building in Chapter 7). There is some ambiguity about Barclay's alleged partnership with Robert Knox at this point, but whatever the case, the College did gain both a new hall and an important anatomical collection.

This would not be the last such collection acquired by the College, and indeed the College a few years previously had tried to buy an entire collection from abroad, that of Dr Meckel of Halle. Despite protracted negotiations and the willingness to expend a considerable sum from College funds, the transaction fell through when the collection was withdrawn from sale by the relatives of Dr Meckel. The significance of this failure, though, was that it demonstrated that the College saw it as of considerable importance to be able to acquire such items. Shortly thereafter, William Cullen, great-nephew of the famous physician of the same name, offered to purchase pathological material in Paris, and a considerable sum was pledged by the College for that purpose. Unfortunately this mission proved fruitless as Cullen suffered a stroke and returned with only a few specimens.

Over the years a number of collections did come the way of the College, as well as large numbers of individual specimens donated by College Fellows. Among these was the important collection of Charles Bell, another of the noted extra-mural anatomists who, together with his brother John, was forced out by the Edinburgh establishment and had set up teaching establishments in London. The College bought the Bell collection in 1825 at a cost of £3,000, a considerable sum at the time. These collections formed the core of the College collection, and are still the core of the historical pathology housed in the Museum. That is not to say, however, that the collection of curiosities did not proceed apace. It is sometimes assumed that when an organisation becomes focused on more 'modern' or scientific aspects of a subject, it immediately loses interest in or concern with the unusual or unexplainable, or just plain odd. The nineteenth century was a period in which it was still possible to bring in shrunken heads without creating a stir in the consciences of observers.

There is no room here to detail the minutiae of cataloguing, storing and conserving the collection, but suffice to say that as it grew, it demanded care, control and supervision. It was necessary not only to have a proper and full catalogue list of the specimens and their nature and provenance, but also to put in place arrangements for responsibility. These arrangements saw the formalisation of the appointment of Curator and the setting up of a museum committee which had overall responsibility for the care and continuity of the collection, and for making it available for consultation by Fellows, medical students and other interested individuals. Interestingly for the historian, the first individual appointed as Conservator was none other than the notorious Robert Knox, of Burke and Hare notoriety. He was appointed Curator of the Barclay collection in 1825, not without some opposition, notably from James Syme, a rival to Knox for the attentions of extra-mural anatomical students. Once the Barclay collection came to the College in 1828, and Knox had been appointed Conservator of the full collection, the current Keepers of the Collection resigned their posts and were then appointed Curators. The precise implications of the two terms are unclear.

The College Library, which had been lost in 1763, was resurrected in the early part of the nineteenth century, and boosted considerably by the donation by his daughters in the late 1840s of over 1,000 volumes belonging to the late Dr Abercrombie, as well as by the growing numbers of medical periodical publications (see Chapter 5).

## PUBLIC HEALTH AND PUBLIC SPIRIT

Since before the foundation of the Incorporation the surgeons had been consulted by the Town Council on medical matters, and this continued throughout the Enlightenment period – indeed it would increase as the squalor of the nineteenth century brought about serious urban disease and deprivation. In December 1781, for example, the College was asked to give its view on the health risks of slaughterhouses. The response was that the College had 'no difficulty in declaring that all nuisances must be in some measure pernicious to health, and that the slaughtering houses in particular from their tendency to corrupt the different kinds of meat hanging in them are noxious not only to those in the neighbourhood but to all the other inhabitants'.[150]

Shortly thereafter the debate on inoculation occupied the surgeons' minds, and would do for the next half-century. They were in favour of 'gratuitous inoculation of the poor', but wanted to do it 'in the cheapest and easiest manner'[151] (see Chapter 5). There was something of a dichotomy here between making something available and making it compulsory, no matter how much good it may have done. Enforcing or enabling general public health, in which the College could participate without compunction, was one thing. Enforcing a procedure that was widely believed to be against the will of God was quite another. What is clear from the College records, though, is that it supported strongly general 'cleansing' and charitable measures, and would do so throughout the nineteenth century, and particularly during periods of epidemic disease such as cholera.

Even the most eminent and famous Fellows of the College were not without social conscience, and this was seen, for example, in the area of the provision of medical services to the poor. Until the passing of the new Poor Law in 1845, poor relief was in the hands of the kirk and sundry voluntary organisations. The various *Reports of the Royal Public Dispensary for the City and County of Edinburgh* afford some illustration of this. The report for the year 1822 indicates that nearly 17,000 individuals had been vaccinated, 42,000 prescriptions had been dispensed by the apothecaries, and that 'though at considerable expense', the provision of 'steel bandages was made to the ruptured poor, who are thereby enabled to gain a livelihood for themselves, in place of being a burthen upon the public'.[152] It had also been decided to appoint a surgeon and physician for each parish of the city, and on the list was George Ballingall, who would achieve great fame in the field of military surgery. Twelve surgeons were also listed among the financial contributors to the institution. By 1831 the managers of the Dispensary included Liston and Lizars, and in 1837 James Syme also served in that capacity. By 1845 the 'trusses are given at half price, on a certificate of the presence of Hernia, from one of the Medical Officers in attendance'.[153] The College supported the widows and dependants of Fellows, mainly through the Widows' Fund, but it was also involved in nominating inmates to the Trades Maiden Hospital and in giving donations to distressed individuals or groups in times of hardship.

The period covered in this chapter is one in which the political strength of the medical profession was perhaps at its greatest, as it was often the first to be consulted by government on matters affecting the general public, and by the 1850s was 'a significant feature of the machinery of the British state'.[154] The College was part of this. Its political face changed according to circumstance, but was, none the less, still significant.

## CONCLUSION

The period reviewed here was a little paradoxical. During a long period of severe financial difficulty, the Incorporation and College nevertheless managed to make considerable progress in a number of areas. The achievement of the status of Royal College helped in no small way to confirm that the surgeons were a group set apart from the other trades; the significant developments in examinations and curriculum enhanced the academic nature of the teaching; surgeons attended the RIE, gaining valuable experience in hospital medicine; teaching was offered to apprentices and students; and one positive outcome of the protracted difficulties with the University and the RIE was that the surgeons became highly experienced in the use of legal opinion to assist their ends, the influence of Henry Dundas being of particular importance. The diploma examination proved to be of great financial benefit to the College once numbers of candidates began to increase rapidly after 1815. Between 1821 and 1830, examination fees comprised 22 per cent of the entire income of the College; from 1831 to 1840 the figure was 48 per cent, and between 1841 and 1850 no less than 62 per cent of the entire disposable funds came from this source.

At the same time, though, the library was lost to the University, parts of the buildings had to be disposed of and membership was relatively slow to increase. Despite the problems, though, it does seem clear that this period was more outward-looking. Some things may have happened because of outside influences or pressures, but by the turn of the nineteenth century the College was beginning to regain its firm foundations and was able to move forward with some confidence. At the end of the period covered here the College was about to move into its impressive new building (see Chapter 7) with all the symbolism which that would offer. The nation itself was beginning to recover from the economic depression which had followed the end of the Napoleonic Wars, and as the nineteenth century progressed into the reign of Victoria and the flourishing of Scottish industrial power and global outreach, so the College would face further challenges to its survival, particularly those of large-scale government, medical reform and the revolution in surgery which would come with anaesthetics and antiseptics. If influences can be seen in terms of concentric circles, outer circles continued to be added to the spheres affecting or affected by the College. In terms of the Habermasian approach, this was the peak of the influence – or alleged influence – of the 'bourgeois public sphere'. It is clear that the College, both corporately and individually, was affected by – and in its own way affected – the general public sphere as well as its primary concern, the medical sphere.

## NOTES

1. Petition for Royal Charter, 1778.
2. Hook, A. and Sher, R. B., *The Glasgow Enlightenment* (East Linton, 1995); Geyer-Kordesch and Macdonald, *Physicians and Surgeons in Glasgow*, pp. 154–91.
3. The historiography of the Enlightenment is vast. There are good accounts in: Allan, D., *Virtue, Learning and the Scottish Enlightenment* (Edinburgh, 1993); Campbell, R. A. and Skinner, A. S. (eds), *Origins and Nature of the Scottish Enlightenment* (Edinburgh, 1982); Chitnis, A. C., *The Scottish Enlightenment. A Social History* (Edinburgh, 1976); Emerson, R. L., 'Science and moral philosophy in the Scottish Enlightenment', in M. A. Stewart (ed.), *Studies in the Philosophy of the Scottish Enlightenment* (Oxford, 1990), pp. 11–36; Porter, R. and Teich, M. (eds), *The Scottish Enlightenment in its National Context* (London, 1981); Wood, P. (ed.), *The Scottish Enlightenment. Essays in Reinterpretation* (Rochester, 2000). For recent coverage of the medical and scientific aspects, see Withers, C. J. and Wood, P. (eds), *Science and Medicine in the Scottish Enlightenment* (East Linton, 2002).
4. Geyer-Kordesch and Macdonald, *Physicians and Surgeons in Glasgow*, pp. 153–66.
5. College Fellows such as James Russell were members of the Philosophical Society. See Emerson, R. L., 'The Philosophical Society of Edinburgh 1768–1783', *British Journal for the History of Science*, 18 (1985), pp. 255–303.

6. There is a full account of the development of the New Town in Youngson, A., *The Making of Classical Edinburgh* (Edinburgh, 1967).

7. Devine, T. M., *The Scottish Nation 1700–2000* (Edinburgh, 1999), pp. 140–1.

8. See Colley, L., *Britons. Forging the Nation, 1707–1837* (Yale, 1992), for controversial discussion of the nature of Britain and its identity.

9. Brockliss and Jones, *Medical World of Early Modern France*, p. 521.

10. Stott, R. M., 'The Incorporation of Surgeons of Edinburgh and medical education and practice in Edinburgh 1696–1755' (unpublished Ph.D. thesis, University of Edinburgh, 1984), p. 86.

11. Many claims by the College referred to justice in terms of 'custom, utility, economy and popular demand'. Ibid., p. 349.

12. ECA, Macleod D104, 19 March 1742. Eccles was fined £10 for having the body in his possession.

13. College Minutes, 31 March 1773. Though techniques for treating harelip were well known, it did not appear as an examination topic until 1769, when John Willieson was examined on the operation (College Minutes, 28 April 1769).

14. Colston, J., *Incorporated Trades of Edinburgh*.

15. Rivalries were, and apparently still are, such that heated debates would take place as to whether surgeons or physicians should take precedence on civic or national occasions.

16. College Minutes, 19 January 1778.

17. College Business Papers, 23 March 1778.

18. Ibid., 9 May 1778.

19. College Minutes, 22 May and 10 August 1778. It was also noted on the latter occasion that because of the well-planned course of education undergone by surgical apprentices, they were entitled to 'be considered as a literary society and not in the line of mere mechanicks'.

20. Ibid., 17 March 1769.

21. Creswell, *Royal College of Surgeons*, pp. 162–3. Hay was presented with an inscribed plate in appreciation of his efforts relating to this legislation.

22. College Minutes, 5 December 1813.

23. Geyer-Kordesch and Macdonald, *Physicians and Surgeons in Glasgow*, pp. 353–4.

24. College Minutes, 8 April, 31 May and 24 June 1763.

25. NAS, GD214/60/9, 'Papers relating to the dispute between the University and the Royal College of Surgeons regarding the use of the University Library' (1825–8).

26. EUL, Da31.5, Senatus Minutes, 29 March 1764. The Committee appointed to discuss the matter comprised the Principal, Alexander Monro *secundus* and physician William Cullen.

27. NAS, GD214/60/1–5.

28. The beginnings of the present College library date from 1845, when the Misses Abercrombie presented the College with around 1,000 books which had belonged to their father.

29. College Minutes, 12 September 1793. Further amendments formalised in 1804, 1816, 1826, 1833, 1840, 1852.

30. *Laws and Regulations of the Royal College of Surgeons* with *Chronological Lists of Members, Presidents, Deacons and Honorary Members* (Edinburgh, 1793).

31. For a discussion of apprenticeship, see Dingwall, *Late Seventeenth Century Edinburgh*, pp. 186–96.

32. Strachan, J. M., 'The non-resident Fellowships of the Royal College of Surgeons of Edinburgh', *EMJ*, II (1856–7), p. 475.

33. Ibid., pp. 571–2.

34. Loudon, I., *Medical Care and the General Practitioner 1750–1850* (Oxford, 1986), pp. 189–207.

35. Cook, H. J., 'Boerhaave and the flight from reason in medicine', *Bull. Hist. Med.*, 74 (2) (2000), pp. 221–40.

36. For a full account of the foundations of the Infirmary, see Turner, A. L., *Story of a Great*

*Hospital. The Royal Infirmary of Edinburgh, 1729–1929* (Edinburgh, 1937), pp. 39–67.

37. There is a narrative account of its foundation in Thin, R., 'The old infirmary and earlier hospitals', *BOEC*, 15 (1927), pp. 135–64.
38. Such as Cullen, W., *Synopsis Nosologiae Methodicae* (Edinburgh, 1772).
39. For a comparison of clinical teaching in Edinburgh with other European cities, see Risse, G., 'Clinical instructions in hospitals: the Boerhaavian tradition in Leyden, Edinburgh, Vienna and Pavia', *Clio Medica*, 21 (1987–8), pp. 1–19.
40. The nature of the consultation has changed over time, and is seen by Lawrence as one of the key factors in assessing the role of practitioners. Lawrence, C., *Medicine in the Making of Modern Britain* (London, 2000), p. 3.
41. NLS, MS 3774, Medical Casebook, 1733–5, 84.
42. *Caledonian Mercury*, 27 February 1725.
43. College Minutes, 11 August 1741.
44. Ibid., 2 May 1729.
45. Ibid., 3 August 1732. The document to be laid on the physicians' table was entitled 'Observations upon Pharmacopoeia Edinensis by the Incorporation of Surgeon Apothecaries of Edinr in compliance with a letter from the Royal Colledge of Physitians dated 20 July 1732'.
46. Ibid., 20 April 1736.
47. Thin, 'The old infirmary', p. 148; Kaufman, M., *Medical Teaching in Edinburgh during the 18th and 19th Centuries* (Edinburgh, 2003), p. 42.
48. See account in Creswell, *Royal College of Surgeons*, pp. 208–18.
49. College Minutes, 2 August 1738.
50. LHSA, LHB1/1/2, Minutes of the Managers of the Royal Infirmary of Edinburgh, 1 November 1742.
51. Ibid., 26 December 1751.
52. Ibid., 11 February 1749.
53. Ibid., 1 October 1792.
54. Ibid., 2 January 1758. The surgeons were ordered not to operate until they had given reasons to the managers. Permission was granted to operate in private the next day.
55. Ibid., 1 September 1758.
56. Steedman, J., *History and Statutes of the Royal Infirmary of Edinburgh* (Edinburgh, 1768), p. 64.
57. This complaint was made by John Kennedy, a past Deacon, who refused to take part in the arrangements with the Infirmary. Creswell, *Royal College of Surgeons*, pp. 218–19.
58. College Minutes, 9 July 1776.
59. LHSA, LHB1/1/2, Minutes of the Managers of the Royal Infirmary of Edinburgh, 19 January 1742.
60. Ibid, 3 April 1769.
61. Ibid., 7 April 1794.
62. Ibid., 14 August 1786.
63. It was proposed that: there would be two ordinary surgeons; the next two on the rota would attend as often as they could in order to offer advice and further opinions; three consultants would give advice and help to treat emergencies; any surgeon could offer an opinion on any particular case; operations would be performed by the ordinary surgeons; ordinary surgeons would report on cases to surgical students and apprentices; ordinary surgeons would be allowed to give clinical lectures; consultants would ensure proper maintenance of instruments. See Thomson, J., *Outlines of a Plan for the Regulation of the Surgical Department of the Royal Infirmary Submitted to the Consideration of the Managers of that Institution* (Edinburgh, 1800).
64. For a full account, see Creswell, *Royal College of Surgeons*, pp. 221–7; Turner, *Story of a Great Hospital*, pp. 125–30.
65. Creswell, *Royal College of Surgeons*, p. 228.

66. College Minutes, 23 January 1819.

67. Ibid., 19 March 1822.

68. Ibid., 1 May 1777.

69. ECA, Council Records, 6 August 1777. The claim was made that the actions of the Monro camp were 'evident marks of a design to monopolise every branch of medical instruction, which attempt if successful may have a destructive tendency to the University of which you are the patrons'.

70. *Edinburgh Advertiser*, 12–16 January 1784.

71. EUL, Senatus Minutes, 28 May 1802.

72. Thomson joined the College in August 1793, having successfully negotiated examinations comprising a discourse on fracture of the patella, tests on the anatomy and diseases of the head, preparation of mercury ointment and spirit of hartshorn, and examination on the techniques of amputation.

73. EUL, Da.31.5, Senatus Minutes, 30 November 1801.

74. *Edinburgh Advertiser*, 19 November 1805.

75. College Minutes, 2 December 1816.

76. EUL, Senatus Minutes, 11 October 1804.

77. See Barfoot, M., 'To ask the suffrages of the patrons: Thomas Laycock and the Edinburgh Chair of Medicine 1855', *Med. Hist.*, supplement no. 15 (1995).

78. College Minutes, 28 October 1819. There is a full account and analysis of Thomson in Jacyna, S., *Philosophic Whigs: Medicine, Science and Citizenship in Enlightenment Edinburgh* (Edinburgh, 1997).

79. Creswell, *Royal College of Surgeons*, p. 247.

80. Wood was a larger-than-life character, who served as Deacon in 1762–4, was apparently the first user of an umbrella in Edinburgh and was said to have been accompanied on his rounds by a pet sheep. Rix, K. J. B., 'Alexander Wood (1725–1807): Deacon of the Incorporation of Surgeons, Surgeon-in-ordinary, Edinburgh Royal Infirmary, and "Doctor of Mirth"', *Scottish Medical Journal*, 33 (1988), pp. 346–8.

81. Kaufman, M. H., *The Regius Chair of Military Surgery in the University of Edinburgh, 1806–55, Clio Medica* 69 (Amsterdam, 2003), pp. 47–8.

82. Ibid., p. 51. Bell's views appeared in *Memorial Concerning the Present State of Military and Naval Surgery. Addressed Several Years ago to the Right Honourable Earl Spencer; First Lord of the Admiralty; and now Submitted to the Public* (Edinburgh, 1800).

83. Records show that of the 1329 entrants to the naval medical service between 1807 and 1824, 201 were Licentiates of the Edinburgh College, and may well have been taught by Thomson. Ibid., pp. 80–1.

84. Ballingall was also noted for his collection of specimens. See Kaufman, M. H., Purdue, B. N. and Carswell, A. L., 'Old wounds and distant battles: the Allcock-Ballingall collection of military surgery at the University of Edinburgh', *J. Roy. Coll. Surg. Edinb.*, 41 (5) (1996), pp. 339–50.

85. Thomson, J., *Report of Observations Made in the British Military Hospitals in Belgium after the Battle of Waterloo; with Some Remarks upon Amputation* (Edinburgh, 1816).

86. Ballingall, G., *Outlines of Military Surgery* (Edinburgh, 1838) and many subsequent editions.

87. For a very detailed account of cases treated in this period, see Kaufman, M. H., *Musket-Ball and Sabre Injuries from the First Half of the Nineteenth Century* (Edinburgh, 2003); see also Kaufman, M. H., McTavish, J. and Mitchell, R., 'The gunner with the silver mask: observations on the management of severe maxilla-facial lesions over the last 160 years', *J. Roy. Coll. Surg. Edinb.*, 42 (1997), pp. 367–75; Kaufman, M. H., 'Clinical case histories and sketches of gun-shot injuries from the Carlist War during the period between May 1836 and December 1837, *J. Roy. Coll. Surg. Edinb.*, 46 (2001), pp. 279–89; Kaufman, M. H., *Surgeons at War: Medical Arrangements for the Treatment of the Sick and Wounded in the British Army During the Late 18th and 19th Centuries* (Westport, 2001).

88. *Edinburgh Advertiser*, 24 September 1771. Rae had a particular interest in dentistry.
89. Lawrence, C., 'The Edinburgh Medical School and the end of the "Old Thing" 1790–1830', *History of Universities*, 7 (1988), p. 262. See also Lawrence, C., 'Alexander Monro *primus* and the Edinburgh manner of anatomy', *Bull. Hist. Med.*, 62 (1988), pp. 193–214.
90. *Edinburgh Advertiser*, 3 October 1800.
91. RCSEd, Benjamin Bell Papers, 'Reminiscences', unpublished typescript, p. 55.
92. NLS, Ry.1.3.1(1), *Letter to the Lord Advocate Disclosing the Accomplices, Secrets and Other Facts Relative to the Late Murders; with a Correct Account of the Manner in Which the Anatomical Schools are Supplied with Subjects* (Edinburgh, 1829). The document purported to give evidence from David Paterson, who worked as museum keeper in the service of Knox, and had 'management of that traffic [bodies]'.
93. NLS, Ry.1.3.1(2), Aristides, *Letter to Sir William Rae of St. Catharines, Baronet, Lord Advocate of Scotland* (Edinburgh, 1829).
94. Full account in Creswell, *Royal College of Surgeons*, pp. 187–9.
95. Quoted in ibid., p. 189.
96. Ibid., p. 190.
97. See Dingwall, H. M., '"To be insert in the mercury". Medical practitioners and the press in eighteenth-century Edinburgh', *Social History of Medicine*, 13 (1) (2000), pp. 25–42.
98. College Minutes, 20 March 1737.
99. Ibid. Entry undated but appears at the start of the volume covering the year 1738 onwards. Following the establishment of the Medical School at the University in 1726, apprentices began to take courses there.
100. Geyer-Kordesch and Macdonald, *Physicians and Surgeons in Glasgow*, pp. 251–4.
101. College Minutes, 20 November 1751. A committee was set up to examine the candidate. In France by the 1780s midwives had been 'brought completely under the umbrella of the corporative community'. Brockliss and Jones, *Medical World of Early Modern France*, p. 491.
102. College Minutes, 2 March 1757.
103. Ibid., 20 November 1769.
104. Ibid., 1 May 1777. A further sum of 100 merks was payable by any individual who chose to settle and practise in the local area.
105. See Rosner, L., *Medical Education in the Age of Improvement. Edinburgh Students and Apprentices 1760–1826* (Edinburgh, 1991) for a detailed account of medical students and apprentices at that time.
106. Numbers of these particular diploma holders were small, around 20 surgeons out of some 1,300 diplomas awarded between 1770 and 1815.
107. College Minutes 8 October 1788. A further minute, dated 24 March 1789, appointed the Deacon's Council to act as a committee to monitor the forthcoming consideration of the matter in the House of Commons. A letter from Henry Dundas, dated 24 July 1789, indicated that he had represented the interests of the surgeons during the passage of the Bill through the House of Commons.
108. College Minutes, 8 March 1790.
109. Ibid., 13 February 1792.
110. Ibid., 28 March 1809.
111. Ibid., 7 March 1820.
112. Ibid., 15 May 1797.
113. Ibid., 15 May 1816. The matter had been considered in 1805, but the title of Licentiate rejected on that occasion.
114. Ibid., 1 August 1820.
115. Ibid., 11 November 1808.
116. NAS, GD51/2/697/1, Letter from David Hay to Lord Melville, 23 November 1828.
117. NAS, GD51/5/649, Letter from James Russell to Henry Dundas, 7 December 1797.
118. College Minutes, 2 April 1811.

119. Ibid., 11 September 1794.

120. College Minutes, 15 May 1829.

121. Ibid., 7 May 1813. The Army Board complained that a number of candidates had appeared who 'are very young and very indifferently qualified being so destitute of a due degree of preliminary education as to be unable to translate the Pharmacopoeia or to read the Latin directions to prescriptions'. It was also resolved to legislate to the effect that candidates could not be admitted to the diploma under the age of 21 years. Matters did not improve immediately, though, as the surgeons noted in 1820 that a number of candidates were still deficient in Latin. A College sub-committee was asked to look into the matter of trying to raise standards. Ibid., 2 February 1820.

122. Lehre returned to America and practised as a physician in South Carolina, but died in 1799. Information provided by the South Carolina Historical Society.

123. Account of links in Rosner, L., 'Thistle on the Delaware: Edinburgh medical education and Philadelphia practice, 1800–1825', *Social History of Medicine*, 5 (1) (1992), pp. 19–42.

124. A saucer belonging to McDowall was donated to the College in 1994.

125. See Girdwood, R. H., 'The influence of Scotland on North American medicine', in D. Dow (ed.), *The Influence of Scottish Medicine* (London, 1986), pp. 31–42.

126. College Minutes, 28 March 1809.

127. Ibid., 28 April 1769.

128. Comrie, *History*, i, pp. 26, 27, 31, 233.

129. The gift was transmitted to the College by Mr William Robertson, surgeon to the 42nd Regiment of Foot.

130. Patrick Cotter, alleged to have been around eight feet tall. Born in Kinsale in 1760, he died of liver disease in 1805. He had spent his life travelling the country, claiming that he was descended from the ancient, gigantic Irish kings.

131. For a general historical outline of surgical procedures, see, for example, Wangensteen, O. H. and Wangensteen, S. D., *The Rise of Surgery: From Empiric Craft to Scientific Discipline* (Minnesota, 1979).

132. Ibid., pp. 188–94.

133. Johnston, W. T., *'The Best of Oure Owne'. Letters of Archibald Pitcairne, 1652–1713* (Edinburgh, 1979), p. 156. Perhaps the most shocking aspect of this proposed treatment, to twentieth-century sensibilities at least, is the inference that the work of the wet-nurse may not have ended with the weaning of the baby. Asses' milk was prescribed for many conditions at the time, particularly scurvy, and peruvian bark (cinchona) was used to treat many ailments.

134. College Minutes, 11 November 1822.

135. Ibid., 4 July 1823. See also Holland, E., 'The Princess Charlotte of Wales. A triple obstetric tragedy', *British Journal of Obstetrics and Gynaecology*, 58 (6) (1951), pp. 905–19.

136. College Minutes, 20 October 1829.

137. Ibid., 1 August 1798; 3 February 1806; 15 March 1808; 15 October and 11 November 1822; 1 April 1828. Nowadays medical students in Edinburgh do not dissect at all, a development which would have horrified the early masters of the Incorporation.

138. Brockliss and Jones, *Medical World of Early Modern France*, p. 490.

139. EUL, Dc3.93, Cases observed in the Edinburgh Infirmary in the year 1754–1755 by J. A. H. Reimaris'.

140. Kaufman, M. H., 'An early Caesarian operation (1800) performed by John and Charles Bell', *J. Roy. Coll. Surg. Edinb.*, 39 (1994), pp. 69–75; Kaufman, M. H., 'Caesarian operations performed in Edinburgh during the eighteenth century', *British Journal of Obstetrics and Gynaecology*, 102 (1995), pp. 186–91.

141. Hamilton's publications included *Elements of the Practice of Midwifery* (London, 1775) and *Outlines of the Theory and Practice of Midwifery* (Edinburgh, 1784), while Young's lecture notes cover his courses during the 1770s, and are preserved in various locations (see Kaufman, 'Caesarian operations', p. 191).

142. EUL, Dc2.76/24, Operations performed in the theatre of the Royal Infirmary.
143. Kaufman, M. H. and Royds, M. T., 'Excision of a remarkable tumour of the upper jaw in 1834 by Robert Liston', *Scottish Medical Journal*, 45 (2000), pp. l58–60.
144. EUL, P46/4/1–7, Cases described by Robert Liston.
145. EUL, SB.6104/5/5, *Remarks on the Expediency and Practicality of a Union of the Royal Colleges of Physicians and Surgeons in Edinburgh* (Edinburgh, 1821), p. 5.
146. Ibid., p. 13.
147. Tansey, V. and Mekie, D. E. C., *The Museum of the Royal College of Surgeons of Edinburgh* (Edinburgh, 1982).
148. Lawrence, 'Edinburgh Medical School'.
149. Tansey and Meikie, *Museum*, p. 5.
150. College Minutes, 19 December 1781.
151. College Business Papers, Report of the Committee on the Subject of the gratuitous inoculation of the poor, May 1782.
152. *Report of the Royal Public Dispensary for the City and County of Edinburgh* (Edinburgh, 1822), p. 1.
153. *Report of the Royal Public Dispensary for the City and County of Edinburgh* (Edinburgh, 1845), p. 6.
154. Lawrence, *Medicine in the Making of Modern Britain*, p. 55.

# 5

# The College in transition: medical reform to NHS, c. 1830–1948

Let the Medical Corporations be compelled to submit to all such regulations as the welfare of the public requires, let their privileges in particular altogether cease to be exclusive and local in their character, but let not an apparatus, so capable of being beneficially employed, be gratuitously and inconsiderately annihilated.[1]

## INTRODUCTION

The nineteenth century was a period of considerable change in Scotland. The rise of the large cities, particularly Glasgow, and the ongoing changes in the demographic map meant that medicine and its organisation had to change also. Large populations required large hospitals; large hospitals required better organisation and staffing. College Fellows were involved as practising surgeons and as members of hospital boards, government bodies and other supervisory and policy-making organisations. This was the heyday of Empire, and Edinburgh-trained surgeons took their skills to all parts of the world. Scotland was the industrial capital of the world and wielded industrial machinery and economic power out of all proportion to its very small size. It was against this background – a complex amalgam of power, poverty and political change – that the College acquired its current home, participated actively in the push for medical reform, and gradually began to embrace the surgical possibilities afforded by the advent of anaesthesia and antisepsis. This was the period when it has been claimed that science became the 'third estate' of medicine. The surgical careers of College Fellows were affected by the rise of the laboratory sciences, and Fellows themselves contributed to scientific research. This was the great age of Pasteur and Koch, Lister, Billroth, Charcot and Simpson, so that 'science did matter to doctors collectively even if it could be neglected by them individually.'[2]

The middle and later parts of the nineteenth century saw a number of new directions for the College. The diploma examination was a welcome source of income as well as enhancing the reputation of the College worldwide, and from 1815 became its major examining activity, especially during the period 1850–85 when the Fellowship examination was discontinued. The issue of medical reform occupied the energies of the College for much of the first half of the century, and there was unusually close co-operation among the British medical colleges to try to influence the shape of any legislation.

The First World War stimulated advances in peacetime surgery (and also, importantly, record-keeping), and following the end of hostilities in 1918, continued attempts were made to improve the social conditions of the population. Schemes were introduced for national insurance, and the attention of many in the wider field of medicine was drawn to the topic of improving general health, in particular that of women and children. A recent book on health policy in Scotland between the wars gives very detailed coverage of these aspects, and highlights the roles of central and local government in these areas.[3] It has been claimed that the introduction of National Health Insurance in 1913 'effected a major extension of state authority into private life'.[4] Though the College may not have been directly involved in this extension, there were implications for the health services in general and, therefore, for the College and its Fellows. Following the cessation of hostilities in 1945, the Labour government swept to victory and one of its first measures was to ensure the passage of legislation enabling the NHS, consequent on the Beveridge Report.[5] The 'free at the point of need' pledge epitomised the aims of the Labour administration to provide comprehensive health care for the whole population. The College was involved, both collectively and individually in the organisation and operation of the NHS, primarily in the hospital setting.

During periods of war many individual Fellows and Licentiates of the College gave distinguished war service; many surgical techniques evolved out of the improvisation demanded by the need to deal with large numbers of casualties in difficult operating circumstances. The technical possibilities of surgery were influenced by the effects of war; they always had been, but in the modern era these techniques were increasingly developed and applied in a peacetime context, thus perhaps removing any lasting boundary or distinctiveness between military and general surgery.

The social construction of the College between and including two world wars was characterised and shaped by influences different from those either before or since. The geographical distribution of the Licentiates, for example, changed to include many more individuals from mainland Europe who had been forced to emigrate as a result of ethnic persecution; the numbers of female TQ candidates rose towards the end of the Second World War, and these and other factors were important in focusing the attention of the College on educational provision and preparation for the considerable impact which the NHS would have on Fellows and their rights and abilities to practise within the new setting.

In terms of surgical possibilities, of major importance also were the slow acceptance of anaesthesia in surgery, together with the equally important and equally controversial evolution of antisepis and the means to control infection. Though

Fellows had long had the knowledge to carry out complex surgical procedures, the lack of anaesthetics and the prevalence of post-operative infection and shock had hindered greatly their ability to put this knowledge into useful practice. The ability to perform new techniques successfully meant that the College would have to teach and examine them as part of the diploma and Fellowship examinations. The combination of new circumstances, including larger hospitals, the emergence of specialist hospital surgeons and better chances of patient survival had implications for the academic side of surgery. The theoretical aspects of surgical advances were published in medical journals and debated widely in the flourishing medical societies. The role of the *Edinburgh Medical Journal* and similar publications was of particular importance in this time of rapid scientific advance.

What the more modern volumes of the College minutes tend to reveal is an increasing need to clarify and develop more and more detailed examination regulations, and to ensure that standards of training were maintained. The College was represented on many medical, surgical and peripheral boards and committees, reflecting the increasingly organisation-driven, or committee-driven, nature of progress in all areas of medicine, surgery and other areas with which the College would be concerned.

This chapter will look at the continuing and new influences on the College in this period of significant change in the organisation and supervision of medical training and practice, and in the provision of health care. The key areas of medical reform, the increasing importance of higher surgical training, and developments in surgery form the core of the chapter.

## GENERAL COLLEGE AFFAIRS

Relations with the Town Council were still useful, but seen as a disadvantage by the College, which wished to divest itself of all of the trappings of the early craft. It had been brought into existence by the Town Council, but times had changed. From the time of the Royal Charter in 1778 the title of President replaced the historic designation of Deacon, but it was not until the Burgh Reform Act of 1833 that the College was able to choose its own President without Town Council confirmation. By 1843 discussions were underway on the subject of a new charter which would enable it to separate itself finally from the Town Council. This was achieved in 1851 and, with it, the final severance of the historic links with the Town Council.

In 1861 consideration was given to the duties and expenses of the College secretary, and it was proposed to rearrange administration to the extent that a law agent would be engaged to carry out legal business and a Clerk to organise minutes and examinations, while a Fellow would be appointed as Honorary Secretary to cater for the 'surgical' aspects of affairs, particularly concerning the many changes which were being made to examination regulations.[6]

In the tradition of the times, the College was quick to send off loyal addresses on every possible occasion, whether in the form of congratulation or condolence. It may appear to the modern eye that the language was a little over-grovelling, but this was entirely consonant with the elaborate nature of Victorian life, society, artefacts, literature and formal public discourse. Just one example of this will suffice – a quote from the address marking the death of Prince Albert.

The Royal College of Surgeons of Edinburgh desires to express its sincere and heartfelt condolence with your Majesty on the great and irreparable loss which your Majesty and the nation have sustained in the death of the Prince Consort – a Prince who in every relation of life has earned universal esteem, whether regard be had to the wisdom, prudence and ability which he has displayed in the exalted but difficult position close to the throne which he has for so many years occupied, to the devotion with which he has given support and comfort to your Majesty in the exercise of your high functions, to his affectionate and judicious training of the Royal offspring, or to the constant discriminating and effective patronage which he has extended to the cause of science and the arts – services which will cause his memory for ages to remain embalmed in the hearts of a grateful nation.[7]

Closer to home, and very much in tune with emerging civic pride, when asked its opinion on plans for a Roads and Streets Bill to improve the thoroughfares of Edinburgh, the response was that 'the improvements contemplated in the Bill would be to the advantage of the public'.[8] The College also gave its opinion on matters such as road improvements and street lighting, nuisance removal and vaccination. Concerning more medical matters, strong opposition was expressed to proposed amendments to the Lunacy Bill, which would have removed medical representation, making the points that lunacy was a medical disease, that patients were treated in hospitals supervised by doctors, and that the functions of the Board would be impeded without medical input.[9]

A significant event was, of course, the 400th anniversary of the College in 1905. This was a most prestigious occasion, on which no less than thirty-six of the world's greatest surgeons were awarded Honorary Fellowships. Among those was Lord Lister, who holds the unique distinction of being both Fellow and Honorary Fellow, as well as being the first surgeon to be elevated to the Peerage. The occasion was marked with solemn worship in St Giles' Kirk, together with dinners and speeches, fraternal greetings being received from other Colleges and medical institutions worldwide. In a publication to mark this occasion, John Smith (who had been College President in 1883) remarked: 'May it not without exaggeration be affirmed that the genesis and development of the Royal College of Surgeons of Edinburgh are of sufficient note to constitute one of the many landmarks in the history of Scotland?'[10] Considerable expense was also required for the major modifications carried out to the College buildings at this time (see Chapter 7) and for dealing with problems relating to employees.[11]

Relations with the RCPEd, though much more cordial than in earlier times, were still strained on occasion, and in the early years of the twentieth century the question of precedence was hotly and expensively debated and taken to law. The

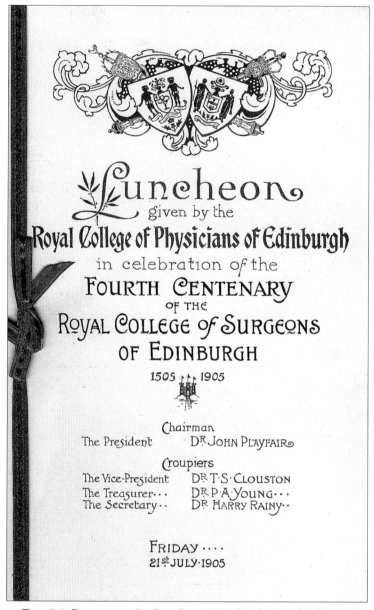

**FIG. 5.1** *Programme for Luncheon given by the Royal College of Physicians of Edinburgh to mark the 400th anniversary of the College in 1905.*

Lyon King of Arms had ruled in 1901 that when the corporations presented loyal addresses, the RCPEd should have precedence. By 1911 the College was trying actively again to reverse the situation. Further appeal was made to the Lyon Court, and when this was rejected the College approached the Court of Session, which ruled that the Lyon Court did have powers to decide the matter. Meanwhile the RCPEd petitioned the King, and the College followed suit, but after much debate and further royal petitions, the matter was lost, the minutes noting sombrely that the College had done all it could in the matter.[12]

As always, impending national legislation which threatened the independence of the medical profession was viewed with considerable nervousness, and this was the case with the National Insurance Act, which came into force in 1911. The College President intimated in a communication to the Prime Minister and Chancellor of the Exchequer that while the College sympathised with the objectives of the Bill, it wished to express the 'very strong feeling that this Bill ought not to be pressed forward in the present session in order that the public and very specially the medical profession, may have time to thoroughly consider the provisions contained in it'.[13] In other words, potential detriment to the College must be identified and opposed at all costs. Opposition centred on the perception that general practitioners would have increased powers under the scheme, with a concomitant reduction in the influence of consultants, who at the time had lucrative relations with the Friendly Societies.[14] Once the Act passed into law, the Scottish corporations set up a Scottish Medical Insurance Committee, and the College voted £500 to cover any future action that would be necessary.[15]

At the same time, and concerning one of the College's own eminent Fellows, the death of Lord Lister in 1912 produced international reaction as well as stimulating plans for permanent memorials in Edinburgh, Glasgow and London. A communication was received from the German Ambassador, expressing the 'condolences of the Imperial Chancellor and of the Prussian Government . . . to the institutions of which the deceased man of science was President'.[16] The College immediately set about discussing how best to commemorate Lister, and plans were set in train for the commissioning of a marble bust, to be displayed in the College, and also, on a much grander scale, for the establishment of a Research Institute in combination with the University of Edinburgh and the RCPEd. Once it was accepted that Glasgow and London wished to act independently in this matter, the College set up a Lister Committee to carry the plans forward, though this would not be without considerable difficulty.[17]

To summarise, these 'miscellaneous' affairs illustrate both continuity and change in the general interests of the College. There was continuing deference to royalty, interest in public health and medical politics, and the commemoration of a famous Fellow. There was also, though, concern with national legislation and its impact.

## Financial matters

During the first half of the nineteenth century, the College was involved in considerable expenditure in two main areas – its political activities in the period leading up to the Medical Act of 1858 and the Playfair Building. The building cost rather more than anticipated (see Chapter 7), while the political storms surrounding successive medical Bills meant that the College incurred considerable expenses in obtaining legal opinion and sending representatives to lobby London politicians or take part in conferences with the other medical corporations. The heavy financial cost to the College is illustrated in a minute of 4 February 1861, noting that expenditure on this problem from 1855 to 1858 alone was almost £1,000.

Once the Medical Act was in place, and recovery made from the expenses of the Playfair Building, the College's financial situation was relatively stable, with a projected surplus of £1,018 in May 1863. Advice from the finance committee, with a sideswipe at the government, was:

> Now as this statement is of a very satisfactory description, and as the knowledge of the existence of a surplus, of whatever amount, has a tendency, well known to the Chancellor of the Exchequer, to generate a multitude of schemes for getting rid of it, I think it may not be amiss to advise the College, that if they really wish to escape from the evil of debt in future, a considerable surplus is a thing necessary to this end, and to their future pecuniary independence and, moreover, that it appears to be a thing at present attainable, if the Fellows of the College can only be brought to see its importance, and to regulate their votes on money questions, with a view to its attainment.

Achieving a 'considerable surplus' was, though, not easy and not often forthcoming, and indeed concern was expressed in the 1870s about a relative fall in diploma income. On reporting a projected surplus of only £157 in early 1870, the minutes state that 'troublous times may be approaching this as other Colleges. As the College has never hesitated to keep itself at whatever cost abreast of the progress of the profession, and will never act otherwise, it can therefore with a good conscience (if corporations can have consciences) maintain its rights and privileges against all comers from whatever quarter these may be assailed'.[18]

The College has always depended on fees of various sorts for its financial survival, and this was no less the case in the nineteenth century. Ever mindful of this, it was stressed that 'a prosperous state of revenue even with receipts beyond what can be reasonably expected, can only be maintained by a wise and rigid, though not a niggardly economy' – and the recommendation was made that a semi-permanent finance committee be set up to maintain the College in as good a financial position as possible. It was also decided that a 'peremptory circular' be sent to Fellows in arrears of fines or other dues.[19] From that point it was a regular feature of the minutes that detailed financial statements and forward projections were made, together with summaries of diplomates and numbers of Fellows. By the late 1860s there was an average of 14.4 Fellows entering each year. The Licentiate diploma was a considerable source of income, as demonstrated in Table 5.1.

The Widows' Fund, which had been set up in the 1770s, generated considerable income and supported large numbers of widows, some of whom outlived their husbands for many years. The Fund, though, became a burden to the Fellows, and eventually the requirement that new Fellows must subscribe to it was discontinued. By the 1830s, when the College was still in financial difficulties, it was felt that the existence of the Fund was 'injuriously limiting the number of candidates for the Fellowship'. It seemed that the only way to solve the problem and to boost the Fellowship of the College was to close down the Fund, a move which would require a further enabling Royal Charter. The appearance of private insurance companies would cater for any need in this area, and at the same time any legislation could deal with separation from the Town Council. A third purpose, that of creating a Royal College of Surgeons of Scotland, would not come to fruition, and has not yet done so. This proposal sparked furious reaction from the FPSG, which immediately made a counter-bid for its own Collegiate status. Without this controversial clause, the new Charter was granted in May 1851 (13 Victoria Cap. xxiii). This was not the end of the Fund, though. Further legislation in 1860 (23 & 24 Victoria Cap. clxxvi) restricted the diminishing number of Fellows entitled to join the Fund, the aim being to bring about its natural demise, and the final list of contributors for 1890 comprised only twelve.

**Table 5.1 Percentage of College cash income from diploma fees, 1820–70.**
(Source: *States of the Affairs of the Royal College of Surgeons of Edinburgh and of the Widows Fund with Lists of Members, Office Bearers, Acts of Parliament etc.*)

| Year | Total income (£) | No. of diplomas | Income from diplomas (£) | % of total College income |
|------|------------------|-----------------|--------------------------|---------------------------|
| 1820 | 3170 | 123 [10] | 683 | 33.66 |
| 1830 | 3073 | 190 [33] | 923 | 41.67 |
| 1840 | 1527 | 161 [25] | 927 | 66.56 |
| 1850 | 1003 | 102 [15] | 712 | 70.15 |
| 1860 | 1652 | 98 [8] | 858 | 54.49 |
| 1870 | 1465 | 118 [0] | 784 | 66.99 |

[number of candidates referred]

Reports on the affairs of the Fund give some insight into the mortality pattern of the Fellows. In the period 1844–68, for example, mortality up to the age of 60 was higher than predicted (26 as compared to predicted 15.662), but above that age the death rate fell to within the expected range. The reason given for this was that 'at this period a Medical man is exposed to all the labour and risk of active practice, and many constitutions will, no doubt, yield to the unfavourable influences brought to bear upon them'.[20] The list of Fellows for 1844 contained ninety-three names, the most senior of whom, Henry Johnston, had entered in 1791. By 1869 this had risen to 240, with John Gairdner at that time the 'father of the house', having entered in 1813, confirming that this high early mortality had not prevented a steady increase in the number of Fellows (and consequent increase in income).[21] The sharpest increase seems to have been from 120 in 1858 to 155 in 1859 – though the latter list contained Army and foreign surgeons. Henceforth membership of the Fund was not a prerequisite for entry, and this measure seems to have had the desired effect. What is also informative from the Fellows' list for

1830 is that of the ninety-nine Fellows, no less than sixty-one also possessed an MD degree.

## Wartime and the College

The College records say very little about war – any war, and there are few references to the general impact of war, the effects on the College or the experiences of its Fellows and Licentiates. Most of the references are to delays in organisational change occasioned by war, or donations to charitable causes. Many Fellows and Licentiates gave distinguished service, and three Licentiates were awarded the Victoria Cross – William Sylvester (Crimea, 1855), Valentine McMaster (Indian Mutiny, 1857) and Campbell Mellis (Andaman Islands Expedition, 1867).[22] However

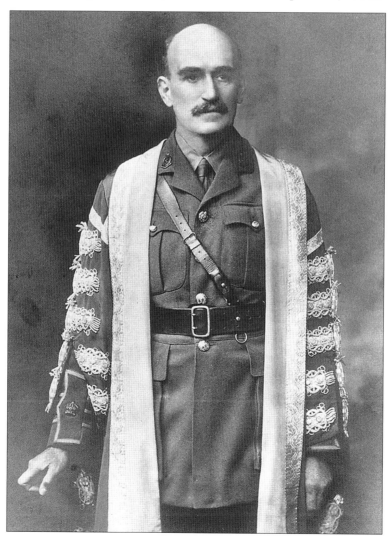

*FIG. 5.2* Photograph of Sir James Hodsdon, College President 1914–17, *in military uniform.*

meritorious was the war service of individuals, though, the impact on the College as an institution was mainly to delay corporate decisions or actions. The first mention of the 1914–18 war in the College records concerned its agreement in 1914 to 'give Venereal Lectures to the troops stationed around Edinburgh', and to the vote of £500 for 'patriotic and charitable purposes, giving preference to treatment of the sick and wounded.'[23] One step which was taken, though, was to issue a circular to Fellows and Licentiates in May 1915, communicating the urgent need for medical officers for the Army. Over 4,800 copies were sent out, and the replies indicated that large numbers 'were already engaged in Naval or Army medical service; as combatants; in Red Cross work; relieving practitioners eligible for war service; offering part-time service'.[24] On 15 December 1915 the accounts for extra-ordinary expenditure included £49 for 'insurance against air craft bombardment', and on 18 December 1918 the death of C. H. Creswell was noted, and appreciation expressed of the 'conscientious performance of his duties . . . to the valuable services which he had rendered in the Library and to the great interest which he had taken in the old documents of the College'. At the same meeting the President noted that during the hostilities 'the work of the Surgical Profession had contributed largely to the success of our Arms, and the part played by Fellows and Licentiates would redound to the credit of the College for all time.' At the end of the conflict the College awarded Honorary Fellowships to the heads of the Armed Services.

The College was no less patriotic during the Second World War. In July 1940 it was agreed to invest £1,000 of College funds in Defence Bonds and £10,000 in National War Bonds,[25] while regular contributions were made to the British Red Cross Society. Some disruption to teaching in the School of Medicine was noted, it being impossible to run classes for the Diploma in Public Health, as the MOH was 'too much occupied with other work to spare sufficient time for adequate instruc-tion'. It was also mentioned, though, that considerable numbers of students from the south of England had come to Edinburgh to complete their studies, and that they had 'expressed themselves as more than satisfied' with the teaching that they had received.[26]

The wartime role of medical institutions is complex. Scope for corporate action was confined mostly to financial support and modifications to teaching and exam-inations, while the surgical consequences were catered for by individual Fellows in the field and in military hospitals at home and abroad. The extension to peacetime of surgical techniques developed during conflicts, though, linked to the emergence of surgical specialties, stimulated the College towards new training initiatives, research and examinations.

## THE COLLEGE AND POLITICS

### Medical reform – a watershed for College and nation

The College has always been involved in politics, but by the mid-nineteenth century the main focus was on relations with government, though contact with influential individuals was still crucial. The question of standardisation of medical training and the introduction of compulsory national registration occupied the mind of the College for most of the first half of the nineteenth century. It arose for a number of reasons, some of which were not at first sight directly related to education. After 1815, practitioners without a qualification from the London Apothecaries were debarred from taking up appointments in English institutions – appointments which carried remuneration. Many complaints came from College Fellows and Licentiates who had been informed that Scottish qualifications were not sufficient. While the ultimate aim and eventual achievement was national registration and control of medical education, the initial stimulus, as with many other aspects of medical life, was problems with one piece of legislation. By the early 1830s, the clamour for medical reform was becoming louder on the part of politicians as much as the medical profession itself, and the British medical corporations began to discuss means whereby it would be possible 'to restore regularly bred surgeons to their lost privileges'.[27] From that point on there was unprecedented contact and co-operation among the Colleges, though not always with a united or common purpose.

### The College and London

Correspondence between the Edinburgh and London surgical corporations took place regularly, the aim being to maintain historic privileges as well as secure the best political outcome. Petitions were submitted to parliament and MPs lobbied, particularly at key points when one or other of the many failed medical Bills was under discussion in parliament. A conference took place in London in April 1838, ostensibly to debate the Irish Medical Charities Bill, but also 'general matters of medical education'. Preliminary agreement was reached among the British Colleges on the outline structure of the ideal training programme and curriculum – the only disagreement being in relation to the status and examination of pharmacy. Subsequent correspondence between London and Edinburgh showed that all was not sweetness and light, though. The RCSEng was very wary of regulations being enshrined in law, as 'it would make each college appear unable to be self-regulating or self-policing' (key features of the self-image of professional bodies).[28]

Further debate took place over the draft Bill submitted by Mr Warburton in 1840, which proposed to establish a College of Medicine, which would allow its Fellows to 'hold any medical appointment whatsoever in any part whatsoever of the United Kingdom'.[29] The Scottish and Irish Colleges appear to have been correct in their suspicion of the real motives of the RCSEng, though, as the records of the latter institution show that it was in regular communication with the Apothecaries and the London physicians, with the hope that these three bodies could 'cordially unite' in setting up a standard curriculum.[30] This was despite the expression of warm appreciation of the Edinburgh College, which had been 'characterised with uprightness, honor and good faith'.[31]

Shortly after this, in January 1842, Sir James Graham's Bill was tabled for discussion, and he had communicated with the RCSEng in advance of consulting the other Colleges, stating that he was 'unwilling to communicate with the Medical Authorities in Scotland and Ireland, until I have obtained knowledge of the sentiments and wishes of the College of Physicians and of the College of Surgeons in London'.[32] An olive branch was proffered eventually, as it was decided by the RCSEng in 1852 that Edinburgh Licentiates could be admitted to the RCSEng *ad eundem*, despite the view that the 'Anatomical and Physiological instruction is somewhat indifferently conducted' (in Edinburgh).[33]

Graham's Bill came to nothing, but the three London bodies continued to maintain contact, and two additional factors came into the reform equation – the Council of General Practitioners, and the Provincial Medical and Surgical Association (a forerunner of the BMA). It has been claimed that the elite of the profession could no longer ignore the lower echelons who were forming societies to protect their interests and act on their behalf, and from that point the medical societies of various sorts had a significant political role to play in the politics of medicine.[34] Over the next few years successive Bills were tabled by, among others, Mr Hastings, Lord Palmerston, Mr Brady and Mr Headlam, though contacts with London were less frequent than they had been earlier in the process. A further conference did take place in March 1856, attended by Andrew Wood on behalf of the College, and a new petition against the proposals was agreed, the main objection being that the proposed Medical Council would be composed of 'discordant elements'. Later that year draft articles of agreement were drawn up, covering the proposed Council, lists of Fellows, and examinations. By the time of Lord Elcho's Bill in 1857, the RCSEng noted that 'the several corporations were still acting with the utmost unanimity and good faith'.[35]

### The College and Dublin

Scrutiny of the records of the RCSI for this period reveals concerns very similar to those enunciated in page after page of the College minutes, in terms particularly of fears of encroachment by the RCSEng. The details of the negotiations and political activities of the Scottish and Irish Colleges have already been outlined in detail in the recent history of the RCPSG,[36] but it is useful to consider what was being said in Dublin.

In February 1838 the RCSI formed a committee prior to negotiations with the RCSEng 'for the enactment of a standard of professional education'.[37] Negotiations with Edinburgh were set up the following month and draft proposals outlined for a common programme of medical education. In view of the protracted difficulties in reaching reciprocity agreements in the twenty-first century, some of these proposals seem far-sighted indeed, as they included plans for an agreed curriculum among the three Colleges, together with standardisation of fees and examinations. The Edinburgh contact at that point was Douglas MacLagan. (An aside in the RCSI minutes at that point gives a reminder of the less political functions of the surgical colleges. In the midst of the heavyweight discussion on medical reform appears the note of purchase of a skeleton, 'in which almost every joint of whose body was rendered immoveable by anchylosis', and 'great expense and risk were incurred in disinterring it and procuring it from the Isle of Man').[38]

Amidst fears of the alleged imperial aspirations of the RCSEng, Dublin voted 'the strongest expression of the confidence felt by this College in the good faith of the Royal College of Surgeons of Edinburgh'. Indeed, George Ballingall was awarded Honorary Membership of the RCSI shortly thereafter. One doubt held in Dublin, though, related to the lack of a formal institution for pharmacy in Scotland, which had resulted in every surgeon being a qualified pharmacist. It took the view that there should be a Pharmacy institution in 'every metropolis in the Empire'.[39]

During the subsequent years of protracted negotiations and failed parliamentary Bills, the same concerns made a constant thread through the records of both Colleges – the problems of licensing, especially for posts in charity institutions; the recognition of hospitals, the outline of any proposed curriculum, and, not least, the powers – real or perceived – of the RCSEng. Dublin petitioned parliament in 1854 on the topic of conditions for Navy surgeons at the same time as did the Edinburgh College and despite appearing to offer at times more cordial sentiments towards the RCSEng, Dublin strongly opposed any central governing council being based in London, stating that this would be 'in the highest degree objectionable'.[40]

As the final Bill took shape and passed into law, the intercollegiate contacts declined, and attention in Dublin passed, as it did elsewhere, to matters of participation in the GMC and implementing the new legislation and regulations for registration and supervision that the Bill contained. It is clear, though, that for most of the period leading up to 1858, the RCSI aligned itself much more strongly with Edinburgh and Glasgow than it did with London.

## The College and Glasgow

While the main thrust of the relationships and conflicts involving Edinburgh, London and Dublin centred on the question of corporate power and the rights of individual practitioners, the problem facing the Glasgow Faculty was much more one of survival and inclusion. The FPSG was frequently omitted in draft Bills, and it had to withstand proposals to amalgamate with the Edinburgh College. From the Glasgow perspective the Edinburgh College seemed at times to be no more of a 'friend' than London or Dublin, and while initial moves may have been made with the general 'British' aim of giving status, regularity and supervision to general practitioners, particularly in England, where there was a 'vacuum of supervision', the FPSG quickly had to fight for basic inclusion as a validating body and for a specific mention in successive draft Bills.[41]

During the initial flurry of activity and meetings in the early 1830s, as with the RCSI, there was a brief outbreak of co-operation when the Scottish corporations made a concerted effort against the provisions of the Apothecaries Act, with petitions to parliament and lobbying of MPs, and again with the Irish Medical Charities Bill. It is clear throughout, though, that the prime concern of the FPSG was to be seen as an equal partner, the view being expressed that 'we should force the door wide enough to let us all in'.[42] In order to counter the perception that Glasgow standards were inferior, the FPSG was encouraged in a letter from the College, under the hand of George Ballingall, to extend its curriculum and raise fees in order to be included in the terms of the Irish Medical Charities Bill, but this was refused, the FPSG claiming that opposition was to its 'cheap rate', not the quality of its curriculum.[43] Some months later, though, cordial relations seem to have been restored, as it was noted that the Faculty 'rejoice in the mutual good feeling which subsists between the University and the Royal College of Physicians of Edinburgh and the Royal College of Surgeons of Edinburgh, and beg to congratulate them on the liberal and enlightened manner in which they have discussed the important subjects of medical education and medical practice'.[44] By 1844, however, when proposals were made for a single Scottish college, this was opposed by the Faculty, which claimed bitterly that its members would become 'degraded into irregular practitioners'.[45]

The extent of the periodic animosity between east and west is seen in some of the remarks made in correspondence by the FPSG. In March 1853, for example, it expressed regret that the Edinburgh Colleges were making firm proposals without consulting it, making the point that 'we must all expect to yield a little to each other and the force of circumstances'.[46] The Faculty expressed its view that it could not 'but conclude that the good understanding and harmonious co-operation . . . must now be considered at an end'. On matters of mutual interest there was, generally, co-operation with the other Colleges, but there were occasional 'misunderstandings', which yielded copious correspondence and explanations, which became more intense as 1858 approached, and though the Faculty entertained the desire to 'cultivate a friendly and useful intercourse with their brethren of Edinburgh', it was of key importance that it 'must not forget the respect which they owe to themselves.'[47]

The sense of the relationships between Edinburgh and Glasgow at this time is that there was genuine co-operation, but tempered by a fear of exclusion or perceived inequality in Glasgow, and perhaps an over-confident tone taken by Edinburgh at times. The common enemy, though, was London, whether or not the perceived threat was over-stated.

### The College and the Edinburgh physicians

The RCPEd shared many of the views of the College on the subject of medical reform. There was a common suspicion of the motives of the RCSEng and, of course, the apothecaries, whose actions were seen as a 'useful instrument in repelling invaders from the north'.[48] The RCPEd participated in the conferences organised by the British corporations; it co-operated with the surgeons;[49] it petitioned parliament and lobbied MPs. There was some disagreement, though. When proposals were mooted in 1816 for a Bill to regulate the practice of surgery, the RCPEd had been opposed as it felt that the Bill would be 'injurious to them'.[50] It was considered that in Scotland there were few instances of patients suffering at the hands of unlicensed surgeons, and claimed that nineteen out of every twenty cases were medical, not surgical. A broader Bill to cover all branches of medicine was suggested, together with a joint examining board with the RCSEd.[51] Though the RCPEd perhaps supported the University of Edinburgh and its Medical Faculty more strongly than did the surgeons,[52] it was in complete agreement with the other British corporations on the general aims of standardising medical education and registering medical and surgical competence to practise.[53] Relations between the Edinburgh Colleges were not always harmonious either, though. It was noted in February 1854, during the debate surrounding Lord Palmerston's Bill, that copy correspondence from the RCSEd had been received 'not without surprise, with an intermixture of other feelings'.[54] On the whole, though, the RCPEd shared the aims of the College and generally offered support to intercollegiate proposals and strategies. By 1857 negotiations were eased a little by the fact that it was now possible to send 'telegraphic messages' to and from London[55] and agreement had been reached on how any supervisory medical council should be structured and organised.

## The final Bill

The whole episode surrounding the Medical Act and its provisions was one of enforced intercollegiate co-operation and each of the participating institutions had its own agenda of grievances and priorities. The eventual structure of the Act was shaped by some four decades of manoeuvring, petitioning, argument and counter-argument. Each institution wanted the same as the others, in general, but for different reasons.

One additional factor which is sometimes not taken into account is the general background of increasing state power, together with the effects on the franchise of the 1832 Reform Act. Sometimes referred to as the 'Great Reform Act', it afforded a very limited increase in the franchise, with some 217,000 new voters. Significantly though, this brought many medical and surgical practitioners into the electorate, and they were 'among the best-educated and most influential' of these extra electors, so that from that point until the next major electoral reforms of 1867, 'medical politics counted for more in the government of the country than ever before'.[56] The state was strong enough to be able to legislate for an entire profession – one which had been built on patronage and exclusivity, but which could no longer maintain aloof detachment from the ever-growing machinery of the state and desire of the public to see a reformation in medical and surgical provision. Like it or not, the College was part of this general change.

The Bill passed into law on 2 August 1858. One of the major derivatives was the setting up of the GMC,[57] which would become the national arbiter of standards in medical and surgical training, qualification and accreditation. In the wake of the Act it was stipulated by some organisations, including the Army, that medical personnel should gain separate qualifications in medicine and surgery. This resulted, after brief negotiation, in the setting up of the Double Qualification (DQ) (see below), awarded jointly by the College and the RCPEd. Now that the Act was in force the College turned its attention to the question of compliance with its regulations and meeting GMC training and examination requirements.

The provisions of the Medical Act did not, however, result in immediate acceptance of Scottish qualifications for posts in English Poor Law institutions. In December 1859 a letter was received from the secretary of the English Poor Law Board, stating that the matter relative to the value of the Diploma of the College as a qualification for English Poor Law appointments was still under consideration, and the 'answer having been considered unsatisfactory, it was remitted to the Presidents Council to keep the matter in view, and failing any more satisfactory communication from the Board before the beginning of the year, to renew the application for a decided answer on the subject'.[58] A few months later, confirmation was received that the Edinburgh surgical diploma would be acceptable as qualification for English Poor Law Board appointments, as would medical degrees from Scottish universities.[59]

In the short-term, it was found that the Medical Act was unwieldy and difficult to implement, in terms of ensuring comparability of qualification and regulations for licensing. These problems have been articulated in detail elsewhere,[60] but the major problem was confusion about what constituted a double qualification and, therefore, a licence to practise as both physician and surgeon. There were considerable problems with the GMC's desires for conjoint examining between corporations and universities, which was resisted by all of the corporations and, indeed, the universities in Scotland. Eventually, after much debate and a plethora of proposals – as had been the case with the original Medical Act – the Medical Act Amendment Act was finally passed on 25 June 1886. This Act effectively ended the struggle – temporarily – for single-portal entry and training; this would have to await the changed days of post-1945 Britain.[61]

The College had fought doggedly for centuries to maintain its privileges in relation to its licensing rights. The second half of the nineteenth century and the first half of the twentieth saw not defeat, but a changing set of medical and political spheres in which it had to operate. The College had always been politically active, but the means by which it could wield political influence were changing. A recent survey of medical links with parliament in the Edwardian and inter-war period demonstrates that some 27 of 159 medical candidates were elected to parliament; this did not result in a cohesive medical group or policy within parliament, and is described as a 'less than successful experiment in pressure group politics'. Politics in the modern period would be pursued through government bodies rather than directly between College and parliament.[62]

## The coming of the NHS

The first few decades of the twentieth century saw a change in the direction of national as well as College politics. Of prime concern was now the health of the population as opposed to regulation of the medical profession. Following the introduction of National Insurance in 1911, and in the light of ongoing attempts to improve the health of the Scots, it was perhaps inevitable that proposals for some sort of inclusive medical service would be made. In the period leading up to the construction of the NHS legislation, the College was invited, along with many other institutions, to give its opinion on proposals for the reform of health services in Scotland. In the early 1930s it was requested by the Department of Health for Scotland's Committee on Scottish Health Services to comment on, *inter alia*, the Statutory Medical Services, Hospitals, Public (Voluntary) Medical Services, Consultation Services, Nursing Homes, Medical Teaching and General Policy.[63] The College's views were submitted in 1935, and oral evidence given by College representatives, in which strong support was voiced for the proposed key function of the general practitioner. The subsequent report, known as the Cathcart Report, appeared in 1936.[64] Though its recommendations were not implemented, the Cathcart proposals did stimulate debate and shape opinion on these matters.[65] In May 1942 the College was invited to give evidence to a committee chaired by Hector Hetherington on post-war hospital problems including EMS and voluntary hospitals.[66]

By 1943, and with a continuing eye to post-war needs and in the context of the Beveridge Report, the College participated in discussions with the other Scottish medical corporations and the Royal College of Obstetricians and Gynaecologists concerning the role of consultants after the war. The report of these proceedings, minuted on 20 October 1943, outlined in considerable detail what would be required, including approved hospital training, the possession of a higher degree or diploma and a recognised hospital appointment. It was also stated very firmly that 'consultants must not engage in general practice'. In the new scheme of things it was quite clear that the consultant would be at the apex of the hospital pyramid and this may be seen as the final separation of the hospital doctor and the general practitioner. Until almost the last minute, though, the profession remained largely unconvinced of the merits of the proposed national provision. There were considerable reservations regarding the salaried nature of the service, and threats to the autonomy of consultants within the hospital setting, but doubters were eventually convinced, and the National Health Service (Scotland) Act reached the statute book in 1947.[67]

The implementation of the Act from 1948 had considerable implications for the College. In addition to its being represented on a plethora of boards and committees, the new structures effectively ended undergraduate teaching in the medical colleges and confirmed them as major providers of postgraduate training. As all hospital consultants were henceforth required to have a higher qualification, this placed the College in a pivotal position. (The sections in this chapter on training and examinations will illustrate the major changes in the period between the Medical Act and the NHS.) The political activities of the College were thus moulded by the context, and by 1945 this was primarily focused on the politics of national health care provision and the requirements of surgical training.

## THE COLLEGE AND SURGICAL TRAINING

For much of the period covered by this chapter, apprentices continued to take out indentures with College Fellows, though their training, especially from the latter part of the eighteenth century, was very different. As discussed, one group which did disappear was the servants, and by the end of the nineteenth century the apprentices themselves were very much in the minority.

After the Medical Act came into force, the GMC made considerable efforts to regulate and standardise medical and surgical training, and the College was in regular contact, commenting at length on various proposals and refinements to proposals. In November 1863 the College questioned exactly what the GMC considered to be a medical school, and also the precise number of winter and summer sessions that would be required before qualification. The GMC also encouraged the formation of joint examining bodies, so that students would not have to sit multiple similar examinations. All of this can be seen as part of the continued drive towards standardisation, and this may have hastened the end of the apprenticeship system as much as the expanding curriculum.

Ongoing tensions between the College and Edinburgh University can be illustrated by the complaint in March 1864 that new regulations proposed by the University would restore the monopoly of the University professors in medical teaching. This problem continued, as in July 1869 a strongly worded memorial was sent to the Home Secretary advising that the next holder of the Edinburgh University Chair of Clinical Surgery should not have a monopoly, and that 'all the wards of a recognised hospital' should be made available for the instruction of students.[68] There were also problems about the University's awarding of medical and surgical degrees, which the colleges considered inadequate as licences to practise. Medical schools in cities which did not house a medical corporation perhaps had fewer difficulties to overcome, or at least the problems were rather different.[69]

Extra-mural teaching in the nineteenth century was significant. As the University Medical School declined in reputation, so the extra-mural teachers gained in popularity, and it is arguable that for much of the nineteenth century, students who acquired their surgical training outside the walls of the University were better equipped for practice than their contemporaries who had received their instruction from the University professors. Extra-mural teachers, particularly of anatomy, were able to offer a system of teaching which was much more 'modern' in terms of its approach, methods and relationship to surgery and comparative anatomy.[70] Once their classes were recognised as acceptable for University curricular requirements in the period following the Medical Act, their importance in the sphere of medical training was confirmed, and not just in Edinburgh.

### School of Medicine of the Royal Colleges

As the numbers of extra-mural lecturers in Edinburgh grew, and there was a 'virtual' extra-mural school in operation, it was inevitable that they would wish to have a more coherent organisation, and in 1883 they proposed that they be constituted into a school of medicine, under the auspices of the College and the RCPEd. Signatories to this proposal included Joseph Bell and Charles Cathcart, and the School of Medicine of the Royal Colleges came into operation in 1895. This School was not unique; there were other extra-mural schools in Scotland, notably Queen's College and Anderson's Institute in Glasgow, but once it had been established, it attracted large numbers of students. In the winter session 1899–1900, for example, over 1,000 students were registered, and in summer 1900 the number was 1,109, with 42 lecturers to cover the various courses.[71] The School continued to be well patronised by students and lecturers, many of whom were Fellows of the College, although there was a natural drop in numbers during the First World War – in 1917–18 there were only 275 students and 20 lecturers.[72]

By the end of the Second World War, though, the role of the School of Medicine was diminishing. It was eclipsed by the universities, which had become the major entry portal for the basic medical qualification – a role which they had long sought and which had long been opposed by the Colleges. By the middle of the twentieth century it was probably inevitable that this would be the case. The relationship between the College and the University had always been a little tense – very tense on occasion – though Fellows occupied surgical chairs and participated in the academic side of surgery and surgical education. The School closed its doors in 1949, and, from that point, although the TQ examination was still available, the College for practical purposes gradually ceased to provide initial medical qualifications. It had done this in various forms for some 450 years, but was forced to accept that its future lay in higher training, especially after the publication of the Goodenough Report.

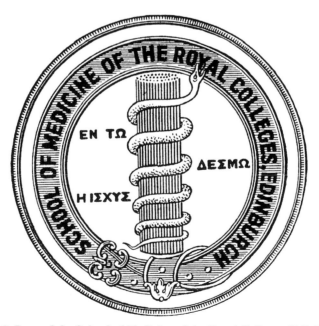

*FIG. 5.3* *Logo of the School of Medicine of the Royal Colleges, Edinburgh.*

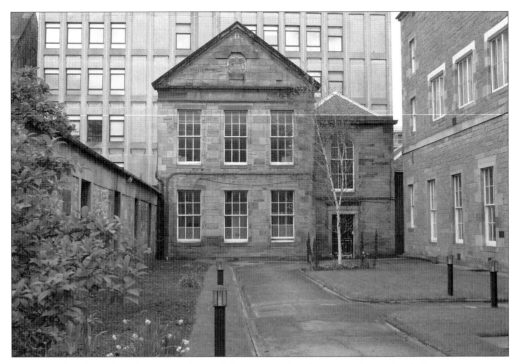

**FIG. 5.4** *Building which housed the Extra-Mural School of the Royal Colleges.*

The extra-mural schools in Glasgow were amalgamated with the University in 1947, after pressure from the University, it seems partly because of resentment at the high numbers of Jewish American students taking the TQ examinations (this does not seem to have been such a concern in Edinburgh).[73]

## The Polish Medical School

Though not directly organised or run by the College, the College did have connections with this unique institution, which was established in 1940 under the aegis of Edinburgh University. As a result of the war in Europe, a large number of Polish medical personnel had arrived in Scotland, and in an attempt to maintain their medical skills had been allowed to visit some Scottish hospitals, despite the considerable language difficulties. They were also able to gain some clinical training and experience within the military hospital at Edinburgh Castle, and following further discussion and negotiation with the University, the Polish Medical School opened its doors on 4 March 1940.[74] Most of the teaching staff were Polish, but the College was represented by, among others, Sir James Learmonth, who taught surgery between 1947 and 1949 and also acted as an examiner.

The role of the College here was indirect, but none the less important, not least in affording support for the enterprise as well as supplying teaching staff. The College minutes note on 22 July 1941, for example, that permission had been granted to the members of the Polish Faculty of Medicine to use the College

Library, and in May 1942 it was decided to award an Honorary Fellowship to Professor Antoni Jurasz, Dean of the Polish Faculty of Medicine (who had been Professor of Surgery at Poznan University before being exiled to Scotland). Further possible connection with the College is noted on 1 October 1945, when permission was granted to two graduates of the Polish Medical School to appear for the Fellowship examination, but neither appears to have been successful.

By the end of the war some 330 students had passed through the School, of whom 227 graduated.[75] Some students, presumably those who had acquired the necessary language skills, transferred as undergraduates to British universities, including Edinburgh, and so would have contact with College Fellows who were involved in university teaching. Many graduates of the School chose to remain in Scotland after the war. The School closed in 1949, having served its purpose, but many of its graduates pursued their surgical careers in Britain.

In summary, the teaching activities of the College in the century after 1858 were largely channelled through its individual Fellows who were university professors, or taught extra-murally, or assisted with the Polish School. The earlier cornerstone of surgical training, the apprenticeship, had largely gone by the turn of the twentieth century, when basic training was taken according to a prescribed curriculum for the Licentiateship diploma, most of the elements of which were acquired in academic classes and hospital wards.

The College may have introduced more and more detailed and prescriptive regulations on training, as did the University, but the experience of individuals could still be interesting. One example comes from the memoirs of College Fellow, President and surgical pioneer Sir Harold Stiles, who described his training in the late-nineteenth century. Of dubious ethical provenance, he noted that he had fallen 'heir to a dissected arm, leg and head and neck specimens which belonged to my grandfather – he got them for £5 from a resurrectionist in London'.[76] Stiles, though, was training during a key period for both College and surgery. He studied physiology, which was essential 'because surgery has now become as much of a science as an art', and acted as spray clerk to John Chiene in the early days of antisepsis, as well as spending some in America, at the Mayo clinic, but stated that 'in many ways my greatest teacher has been the war'.[77]

## Postgraduate training

Continued study has been encouraged by the College since the start, and by the early years of the twentieth century the context was such that formal organisation was necessary. Wherever physicians and surgeons achieved the initial qualification which entitled them to a licence to practise, it was agreed that this was no longer adequate, and that further training would have to be undertaken. The College was closely involved in early moves, and efforts were made even before the outbreak of the 1914–18 war.

When the first serious efforts were made to formalise further training, it was claimed that this was the first occasion on which the Faculty of Medicine and School of Medicine of the Royal Colleges 'combined forces for the common good'.[78] There was something of an eye to commerce here, though, as in the light of the fact that some of the English provincial medical schools, such as Birmingham and Leeds, had gained university status, it was feared that fewer students would be attracted to Edinburgh. There was also the aim of keeping Edinburgh graduates in touch with their Alma Mater. Eventually a joint committee was set up between the Faculty and School of Medicine, of which Andrew Logan Turner was a member. It was decided in the first instance to extend the scope of the vacation courses which had been offered previously, and in 1905 a three-week course for general practitioners was run, with seventy-one graduates taking part. Courses in summer were offered subsequently on general practice, surgery and internal medicine; by 1911 children's diseases and urology were covered, and by 1913, urology had its own course. There was an enforced break during the war years – it was advertised in 1914, for example, that 'owing to the war, the Committee of the Edinburgh Postgraduate Course were reluctantly compelled to cancel all arrangements for post graduate teaching during August and September'.[79] After the war the emphasis was laid more strongly on increasingly specialised courses, though some of these did not attract sufficient students to render them viable.[80]

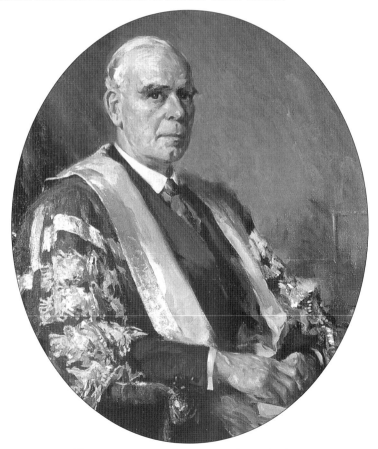

*FIG. 5.5* *Portrait of James Methuen Graham.*

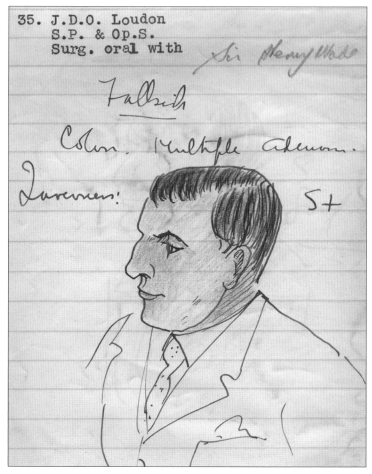

35. J.D.O. Loudon
    S.P. & Op.S.
    Surg. oral with

**FIG. 5.6** *Caricature of Dr J. D. O. Loudon by his examiner,*
*James Methuen Graham.*

The natural consequence was to extend teaching from the vacation period into the academic terms themselves, and in 1926 the surgical staff in the Royal Hospital for Sick Children introduced daily postgraduate clinical lecture/demonstrations. Harold Stiles offered a six-week course in clinical surgery, including orthopaedics and neurosurgery, and by 1937–8 similar courses were attended by some 220 postgraduate students.

Following a further enforced break in postgraduate teaching during the Second World War, and in view of the recommendation of the Goodenough Committee that each university outside London should appoint a Dean of Postgraduate Medical Education, a General Purposes Board was set up, Chaired by Sir John Fraser. This Board included representatives from the University, the College and the RCPEd and at its first formal meeting in October 1944, the College was represented by Robert Johnstone, James Methuen Graham[81] and Keith Paterson Brown. Johnstone was appointed Chairman in 1945, and Graham in 1949, thus bringing the College, through its representatives, to the core of new developments in postgraduate training.

Academic closeness became physical closeness when in 1949 the Board moved to accommodation within Surgeons' Hall.

In the early post-war years, the immediate priority was to train demobilised officers from the forces, and courses were mounted for those who had been general practitioners, officers recruited to arms within a year of graduation, and individuals already acting as specialists in various fields of medicine and surgery. There were also considerable numbers of graduates who had still to complete periods of higher diploma training which had been interrupted during the conflict. Fifty-three individuals attended the ten-week surgical course run by the College in 1946, and from then the demand grew, boosted by increasing interest from overseas graduates. Participants in these courses were given clinical attachments in the RIE, they attended specialist units where clinical lecture/demonstrations were given, and pathological demonstrations were mounted in the College Museum. The numerical bulge caused by the war declined by the early 1950s, and this was not just because the initial complement of ex-military had passed through the system. Considerable numbers had finished their periods of higher surgical training, the impact of the NHS was being felt on academic structures, and with the introduction of the Primary FRCSEd Examination (see below), most surgeons in training did not participate in courses run by the Postgraduate Board until they had completed the basic science stage of their training. All of these factors served to push both Board and College in new directions, not always of their own desire or choosing. It was proposed that the Postgraduate Dean be made *ex officio* a member of key University committees, and that the Board itself would be a committee of the University, thus strengthening the links with the University.

The emphasis on basic science training spawned courses on anatomy, physiology and pathology, all of which required laboratory facilities and lecturers from University departments. Inexorably, therefore, the stage was being reached where a formal structure and purpose-built accommodation were necessary. The aim initially was to set up such a body in Surgeons' Hall, with links to a number of University departments, but much delay was caused by financial difficulties, and the fact that access to any funding from the University Grants Commission would need formal connections with the University (buildings were not constructed until the 1960s).

## EXAMINATIONS

### Regulations

From 1858 the College was constrained by the requirements of the Medical Act and GMC, and was involved in frequent correspondence in response to requests to provide examination statistics and information. In April 1860 the College was asked to submit to the House of Commons the number of qualifications granted without examination since 1858. The rather righteous reply was that the College had 'never at any time either before or since the passing of the Medical Act granted any qualifications to practise medicine or surgery without examination. Nor is anyone eligible for the Fellowship of the College who is not already a Licentiate in Surgery'.[82] The College was quick to claim that its regulations were equal to, or in advance of, those stipulated by national bodies. Any perceived slight was taken very seriously, particularly if it happened to come from the University, as witnessed by the heated reaction to 'certain remarks made by Professor Bennet on the 1st instant in his address to the graduates in medicine at the Edinburgh University wherein every effort was made to disparage the Medical Corporations and hold them up to public odium'.[83] A robust reply was dispatched forthwith, 'in order to prevent the public from being misled'. Shortly thereafter it was agreed that courses taken at provincial medical schools could henceforth be counted towards the required curriculum, on the same basis as those from 'metropolitan schools'. These would, of course, require to be validated in the usual way.

Self-righteousness did bring some problems, though, as the College in 1863 complained bitterly to the GMC that it had fully implemented GMC directives regarding the necessity to pass preliminary examinations before commencing training, and that the full period of professional study should commence with beginning of period of study at medical school. The problem was that other centres had not implemented these rules and so it was possible for students to qualify elsewhere in a shorter period of time, with inevitable economic consequences for the College.[84] The College was forced to suspend its regulations until the GMC enforced them more generally.

This whole situation is interesting. This period was one of considerable flux in a number of areas. The universities, after several centuries of relative difficulties, were able to offer legitimate and – mostly – comprehensive medical training. In the past the Colleges had been able to complain that the universities were not providing graduates with the skills and knowledge to *practise* medicine and surgery as opposed to abstract conceptual knowledge and expertise. Hospitals were a good thing for the universities just as they had been for the development of medicine as a whole. Hospitals could be used by the universities as centres of clinical training just as by the Colleges. So in effect the medical and surgical colleges, which had long prided themselves on the practical as well as the academic aspects of the training and qualifications they offered, were by now in competition with bodies which were very different, but which were increasingly able to offer and demand a curriculum with residence and practical requirements which were very similar.

In the wake of the Medical Act and its subsequent periodic revisions, the Scottish Colleges faced considerable dangers, not the least of which was pressure to set up conjoint examination boards, which would have given the universities too much (in the view of the medical corporations) power. As with the original Medical Act, a number of measures were proposed and submitted to parliament, but most met with considerable opposition and delay. The minutes of the Senatus of the University of Edinburgh illustrate the tensions which existed between the University and the medical corporations. It was noted in December 1871 that the Medical Faculty had received a request from the medical colleges for a meeting to discuss proposals to establish a conjoint examining board – following the resolution of the

GMC that arrangements to institute these boards should be undertaken without delay. The Faculty, though, took the view that 'the changes recently introduced into the examinations of the various medical and surgical Boards in Scotland, under the direction of a Royal Commission and of the General Medical Council, have already provided the means of effecting all that is required in the way of improvement, and that there is no necessity of revolutionising the whole system of examination in the United Kingdom'.[85] The Medical Faculty did, though, make a number of tentative suggestions, including the introduction of an examination to test clinical competence, which would have to be passed before any candidate could be licensed to practise. Further, it was considered at a special meeting in 1872 that a single entry portal via a conjoint board would be detrimental because of fears that 'academical honours will be neglected, that students will be content with a lower amount of medical and surgical acquirement, and that the universities will be discouraged and impeded in their efforts to elevate the standard of medical teaching and examination'.[86]

By this time, of course, the Colleges were not fully independent or free to implement regulations as they wished. The GMC had a role to play if standardisation were to be established and maintained across the country. It required that examination candidates had studied vaccination 'under a competent and recognised teacher', and that 'observations with the microscope should form part of the examinations of Candidates for a Licence'.[87] The Colleges themselves were agreed from the start that 'in examinations in Anatomy, Candidates should understand that they may be called upon to perform actual dissections, and Candidates in Examinations in Surgery should understand that they may be called upon to perform one or more operations on the dead subject'. In summary, the consequences of the Medical Act for examining were that the College was not, and would not be, independent. The consequences for the medical profession as a whole seemed to be to end one long chapter by standardising qualifications, but it may also have heightened divisions in terms of the growing separation of hospital doctors from general practitioners, though the medicalisation of hospitals was perhaps more important here.[88]

## Fellowship

As mentioned, the Fellowship rules were altered in 1822, and further amendments came in 1838, when it was agreed that henceforth candidates must possess the Licentiateship diploma, and that the only other formal examination would be conducted in private, on the topic of the probationary essay, but with the scope to question the candidate on any aspect of the required curriculum.[89] This continued until 1850, when one of the apparently less prudent moves taken by the College was to discontinue the separate examination for Fellowship candidates, requiring them only to have the Licentiateship and then petition for election by vote of Fellows. A remark made in 1863 hints at a perhaps less than intellectually sound reason for instituting the move. It was noted that:

the new Charter has removed another obstacle to the increase of the College, by abolishing the old system of examination at admission to our Fellowship; a practice found to be not merely useless for the purposes for which it had been instituted, but injurious to us, by deterring some of the very best and fittest men from becoming candidates for that distinction. Since its abolition a great number of new Fellows, as you are well aware, have been added to our list, many of them men of the highest rank and character in our profession . . . the Fellowship of our College will in future be more and more sought after, as one of the highest of professional distinction.[90]

A further admission, a few years later, again does not set the College in a good light, it being stated that the old Fellowship examinations 'were never very extensive nor stringent, considerably less so, in fact, than the examinations for the Licence of the College'.[91] So much for diligent observance of the Seal of Cause.

Eventually, though, in the light of growing criticism of the apparently less than rigorous admission procedures for College Fellows, a separate Fellowship examination was reinstated in October 1885. Henceforth entrant Fellows would undertake examinations in Clinical and Operative Surgery and an optional subject from:

- Surgery in any one of its Ophthalmic, Aural, Laryngeal or other special branches
- Advanced Anatomy and Physiology
- Pathology and Morbid Anatomy
- Midwifery and Gynaecological Medicine and Surgery
- Medical Jurisprudence and Hygiene
- Practice of Medicine and Therapeutics[92]

The College Letterbooks give useful information on the examinations that is not found elsewhere in the records. For example, the scope of the practical side is hinted at in the statement that 'in operative surgery operations on the dead body are not usually given owing to a want of subjects for the purpose, but the candidate is usually required to trace out on the living body the method of operation'.[93]

The scope of the ophthalmology option can be seen in the questions set in September 1899:

1. What is meant by sclerectasia posterior? What is its cause? How is it recognised? What are its complications? How should it be treated?
2. Describe the operation of enucleation and mention the circumstances that may demand its performance.
3. Describe the so-called pulsating tumour of the orbit, its symptoms and treatment.[94]

In a reply to a candidate in 1895, James Robertson wrote that the 'examiners expect something more than mere book knowledge for the Fellowship, and candidates

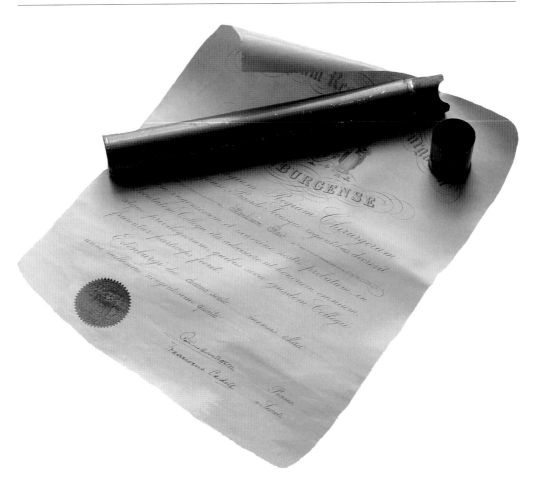

**FIG. 5.7** *Fellowship Diploma awarded to Stanley Raw (1905).*

should be able to state reasons for adopting particular lines. A good knowledge of clinical work and of use of surgical apparatus is also required.'[95] Among the books recommended were Joseph Bell's *Operative Surgery*, and works by Erichsen, Holmes, Spence and Bryant.[96]

The Fellowship remained largely unaltered thereafter until 1948, when a Primary examination was instituted in recognition of the growing importance of laboratory and basic sciences.[97] In terms of success or failure, the available statistics for the 1930s show a 36 per cent pass rate out of 314 candidates; and in 1947 a 32 per cent pass rate from 752 candidates (a post-war bulge). There was a fair degree of consistency in the pass rates against a sharp rise in numbers of candidates, and also against increasing prescription and supervision of surgical training.[98]

A hint of ongoing suspicions about the RCSEng appeared in a reply to a query at that time as to whether the correct designation of College Fellows was FRCSEd or merely FRCS. The reply was that the 'Ed' was not strictly necessary but that it was better to put it in as the English College Fellows usually called themselves FRCS 'on the presumption that their College is the only one'.[99]

### The Double and Triple Qualifications – unprecedented intercollegiate bonding

Though the College's own Licentiateship examination was popular, it was realised fairly quickly that intercollegiate co-operation would be needed if the medical corporations were to survive as examining bodies.[100]

Almost before the ink of the Medical Act had dried, the Edinburgh Colleges took steps towards co-operation in terms of negotiations for the establishment of a Double Qualification award. Each College initially undertook separate, unsuccessful negotiations with Edinburgh University with a view to a Triple Qualification. In the event, a Triple Qualification did appear, but one of a rather different nature. Agreement between the two Colleges was reached relatively swiftly, and in August 1859 proposals were approved by the GMC, bringing in the first intercollegiate examinations.[101] Candidates who were successful in these examinations would be deemed qualified in both medicine and surgery, in effect confirming the standard 'general practitioner' of the time. The College records indicate that cadavers might not be available for surgical examinations, but the RCPEd records declare that in the medical part of the DQ students would be obliged to undertake 'actual examination of persons labouring under disease'.[102] The numbers of individuals obtaining this qualification were relatively low at the start, with only around ten qualifying by 1863, but this situation did improve, and in July 1867 alone some forty-four successful candidates were recorded. The RCPEd also had a DQ in combination with the FPSG, but numbers here were much smaller.

The next move was stimulated by the continued threat of the enforcement of conjoint boards by the GMC, consequent on the report of the 1881 Royal Commission Appointed to Inquire into the Medical Acts. This report had recommended that conjoint boards be set up and that a double medical and surgical qualification should be required for registration. Such a system was implemented in England, but the Scottish corporations chose to set aside any lingering hostilities and offer a Triple Qualification, which would obviate the need for a Scottish conjoint board and, therefore, prevent further encroachment by the universities. The Triple Qualification Examination, which brought the FPSG into play, with the aim of strengthening the Scottish Colleges as a group, was established in 1884.[103] This decision was of considerable importance for the College in a number of ways, and so justifies full coverage. Articles of Agreement were drawn up as follows:

**ARTICLES OF AGREEMENT** between the Royal College of Physicians of Edinburgh, of the First Part; The Royal College of Surgeons of Edinburgh, of the Second Part; and the Faculty of Physicians and Surgeons of Glasgow, of the Third Part, being the three Medical Corporations of Scotland, otherwise called Medical Authorities entered into under their respective Corporate Seals, for uniting or co-operating in conducting the Examinations required for qualifications to be registered under Section 19 of the 'Medical Act' 21st and 22nd Vict. Cap. 90.

1. That each of the said three Medical Corporations of Scotland – namely, the Royal College of Physicians of Edinburgh, the Royal College of Surgeons of Edinburgh, and the Faculty of Physicians and Surgeons of Glasgow, while reserving to itself liberty to confer its Higher Qualifications as it may deem proper, resolves, That on and after the 1st day of October 1884, it shall abstain from the exercise of its power of granting its Licence separately and independently, except only in the cases herein provided for: That is to say, the Royal College of Physicians of Edinburgh may, notwithstanding this Agreement, grant its Licence to Candidates already possessed of one or other of the Surgical Qualifications mentioned in Schedule A of the Medical Act 1858 and the Royal College of Surgeons of Edinburgh and the Faculty of Physicians and Surgeons of Glasgow may each grant its licence to candidates already registered Licentiates of one of the Colleges of Physicians of the United Kingdom or graduates in medicine or [sic] a British or Irish University mentioned in Schedule A of the Medical Act.

2. That the three medical authorities above mentioned shall co-operate to form an examining Board to conduct their examinations in combination and that from the date to be fixed for the commencement of this scheme, the Agreement or Convention at present subsisting between the Royal College of Physicians of Edinburgh and the Royal College of Surgeons of Edinburgh, by which, under Section 19 of the Medical Act 1858, these two Colleges conduct examinations in combination, and the similar agreement or convention at present subsisting between the Royal College of Physicians of Edinburgh and the Faculty of Physicians and Surgeons of Glasgow by which, these two bodies conduct examinations in combination, shall cease and terminate and the provisions of this present Agreement, in respect to combined examinations shall alone be valid.

3. That each of the co-operating Medical Authorities shall elect two Members of a Committee, herein called the Committee of Management. Of this Committee of six members, three members shall retire annually, that is to say one elected by each of the Authorities but they shall be eligible for re-election, but shall not at the same time hold office as examiners. To the members of this Committee, reasonable remuneration shall be paid for attendance at the meetings.

4. That the duties of the Committee of management shall be:
   (a) To elect annually a Chairman who shall also be Convener and have both a deliberative and casting vote.
   (b) To fix the period and places of examination, in accordance with the provisions of this scheme.
   (c) To convene the Examiners, and to apportion their work at the different periods and places of examination, in accordance with the provisions of this scheme.

(d)  To appoint a general Treasurer and any other executive officers they may consider necessary.

(e)  To determine the fees to be paid to the Examiners and other officers.

(f)  To arrange for the visitation of Examinations.

(g)  To act generally as a Committee of Superintendents and reference under the provisions of this Scheme, and also in all matters concerning the examinations which are not specially provided for in this scheme.

5.  That each of the co-operating Medical Authorities shall elect its own Examiners to examine on special or allied subjects, each of these Authorities determining the number to be elected on each subject and the period for which they shall hold office; and notification of the names of the Examiners, with the subject for which they are appointed, shall be duly made to the Committee of Management.

6.  That the Examination on the Principles and Practice of Medicine (including Clinical Medicine) and in Therapeutics, and except only so far as is provided otherwise in the note appended to this Article, shall be conducted wholly by the Examiners in these subjects appointed by the Royal College of Physicians of Edinburgh; that the Examination on the Principles and Practice of Surgery (including Clinical Surgery) and on Surgical Anatomy, shall be conducted wholly by the Examiners on these subjects appointed by the Royal College of Surgeons of Edinburgh, and by the Faculty of Physicians and Surgeons of Glasgow, and that in all the other subjects the Examinations shall, subject to the provisions of Article 7, be conducted by the Examiner of the three co-operating Authorities.

> Note: At the Examinations to be held in Glasgow, the Examination in Clinical Medicine shall be conducted by Examiners of the Faculty of Physicians and Surgeons of Glasgow, being Hospital Physicians, and by the Examiners of the Royal College of Physicians of Edinburgh.

7.  In arranging for the Examinations at the different periods and places the Committee of Management shall apportion the Examiners in the different subjects of the three co-operating Authorities, on the plan provided for in the Schedule appended to this Agreement, which plan may from time to time be modified, with the consent of the three co-operating authorities.

8.  The Examinations shall be held in Edinburgh and in Glasgow, it being arranged that at every third period they shall be held in Glasgow, and at the other periods in Edinburgh.

It was agreed that a Committee of Management would be set up, that every third examination diet would be held in Glasgow, and that there would be three Professional Examinations – at the end of the first and second years, and at the end of the full period of study. The favoured curriculum was set out as:

First Professional      Chemistry, Practical Chemistry, Anatomy/Histology

Second Professional    Anatomy, Physiology, Material Medica, Pharmacy

Third Professional      Principles and practice of medicine (including Thera-peutics, Medical Anatomy, Pathology), principles and practice of surgery (including Surgical Anatomy, Operative Surgery, Pathology), Clinical Surgery, Midwifery and Diseases of Women; Medical Juris-prudence and Hygiene

Candidates with passes from two of the Colleges were granted the Triple Licence. The printed regulations outline the scope of what appeared to be a comprehensive examination and one which was very similar in most respects to the University MD curriculum.

Despite the apparent view nowadays that it is no longer necessary or even advantageous for students to dissect as part of the undergraduate curriculum, it certainly still was thought to be imperative even in the dark days of the Second World War. On 6 April 1943 a letter was sent from the TQ Management Committee to all anatomy lecturers in Glasgow and Edinburgh, which stated: 'The committee have been informed that certain omissions have been occurring in the curriculum, such as the dissection of the whole body by each candidate ... The Triple Quali-fication Committee is creditably informed that all students have not, in fact, done this, although so certified'. The current lack of bodies was noted, and lecturers asked to inform the Board of problems in advance of the imminent visit of the Goodenough Committee.

When the Triple Qualification Examination was instituted in 1884, restrictions were placed on candidates for the single College licence (which gradually came to an end), and holders of the Licentiateship of the Society of Apothecaries of London were excluded, but by 1896 holders of the latter were allowed to proceed directly to the final TQ Examination. In the early days a number of candidates who were about to complete the 'wrong' curriculum were given dispensation to sit the exam-ination 'sine curriculo', but the last opportunity to do this was in 1888. This was very much in line with the need to allow candidates to finish one set of regulations and phase in the next, a situation which continues with each new recasting of College Fellowship and other examinations. (The TQ became part of the United Education Board in the 1980s and, though the last diet was held in 1990, it is still technically available.)[104]

The TQ Examination was open to women, and the first recorded female recip-ient was Emma Littlewood, in November 1886. The numbers of female TQ candidates remained small but did increase gradually, so that in October 1888 five out of sixty-five successful candidates were female, and in August 1895 there were thirteen women among the sixty-eight successful candidates. Around this time Sophia Jex-Blake appears in the records as validator of courses of study undertaken by female students (see the section on women below). Jean Robertson, who qualified in 1892, had her entire curriculum signed by Jex-Blake's bold signature, though her tutors

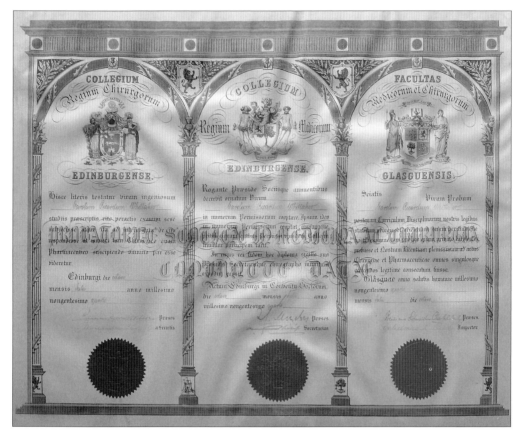

**FIG. 5.8** *Triple Qualification Diploma awarded to Charles Whittaker (1904).*

had also included Charles Cathcart (one of the founders of the School of Medicine of the Royal Colleges) and Henry Littlejohn (first MOH in Edinburgh). One female Licentiate who studied both in Edinburgh and London, Janet Gray, divided her studies between the two cities, and her work at the Royal Free Hospital in London was confirmed by the signature of Elizabeth Garrett Anderson.

The TQ rapidly became a popular qualification, and in its first 15 years some 3,020 candidates were successful. What is also interesting about the schedules submitted by the candidates to prove that they had fulfilled all the requirements is that they give useful insight into the wide medical market place. They also show that the extra-mural schools were being well used.

Further evidence about the TQ examinations comes from the College Letterbooks. The long-serving James Robertson (who by February 1885 found himself appointed Inspector and Treasurer of the Triple Qualification Examination in addition to his other duties as Secretary to the College and registrar of the local branch of the GMC) complained about his workload in this regard, which prevented him from taking a holiday. (He did manage a short trip to Bridge of Allan in the summer of 1885 and felt 'very much the benefit of the water there'.)[105] He demonstrates at times a little impatience as well as an acerbic wit. On one occasion, when he had received a query too many about TQ Examination regulations, he replied: 'It is clear as noon day that one only and any one of the three optional subjects can be selected'.[106] A few years later he wrote, in a letter to Joseph Bell concerning a possible case of impersonation of a deceased Licentiate, that 'if the careful gentleman who is writing from appointment in Ireland, found the College ready to grant him a duplicate diploma, he would at once slip off with it and perhaps kill no end of Yankees!'[107]

Some insight into the practicalities of the diploma examinations comes from a letter dated 22 October 1888, which mentions 'a lady to be up for the single examination'. This indicated that 'the answers [to the written examination] will be taken to the President who will examine them. For the oral two tables will be enough and you can summon as examiners the president, Dr Watson, Dr Argyll Robertson and Dr Underhill. The questions will be sent around on the morning of the examination day. The hour of examination is 11 o'clock'.

Perusal of a sample of the schedules for successful TQ candidates gives good indication of their path to qualification. The surviving schedules start at 1887, and the first of these was John Rogerson, from Lochrutton, Kirkcudbrightshire. He had achieved his curriculum by means of five winter sessions and one spring session at Glasgow University, together with a summer at Anderson's College and a winter at Glasgow Royal Infirmary. He gained his main hospital experience at Dumfries and Galloway Royal Infirmary, and dispensing practice at the Andersonian Dispensary. This was a fairly typical 'cafeteria' pattern. Another interesting individual that year was Frederick Primrose. Born in Nova Scotia, he acquired his preliminary qualification from the Nova Scotia Medical Board, then undertook hospital experience in Philadelphia before travelling to Scotland, where he spent periods at the Edinburgh Maternity Hospital, RIE, The Royal College of Surgeons and Minto House school[108] – a truly eclectic experience. Adam Merson, who finally qualified in 1892 after three failed attempts, studied at the universities of Aberdeen and Edinburgh, as well as Surgeons' Hall, the RIE, the New Town Dispensary and a pharmacy and vaccination station in Yorkshire. The schedules also hint at the workload of examiners, as in most cases eight or nine examiners are listed on each schedule. One of the farthest-travelled candidates in 1892 was George Rose, from Port of Spain, Trinidad, who undertook his entire curriculum in Edinburgh, combining periods at the University and Surgeons' Hall.

Elsie Inglis' training schedule shows her route to the set curriculum. She gained the preliminary examination of the Educational Institute of Scotland, then studied at the Edinburgh School of Medicine for Women, the Medical College for Women, Edinburgh, and at Leith Hospital, Glasgow Royal Infirmary and the Glasgow Royal Infirmary Dispensary. Her entry on the register of Licentiates is countersigned by her examiner, Charles Thatcher.[109]

By 1900 the patterns were well established and demonstrate the continuing importance of extra-mural education. Of the two hundred successful candidates that year, thirty-four had trained solely in Edinburgh, thirty-one in Glasgow and seventeen in London, while forty-eight candidates offered a combination of sources for their qualifications. Of the single-source candidates from outwith Scotland, twenty had attended English centres, with eighteen from Ireland, eleven from Canada, fourteen from India and one from Argentina. Around 9 per cent of the total were female.[110]

Ten years later, a relatively lean year with fewer than one hundred successful candidates, one candidate had taken thirteen attempts to pass the final part of the examination, while two candidates with the same surname, place of birth and training programmes in the USA were either husband and wife or brother and sister.[111] The statistics for 1910 show that of the ninety-two successful entrants, five were female, seventeen trained wholly in Edinburgh, six in Glasgow and one in London, with twenty-two showing combination training. The remainder received their education in Ireland, England, Canada, Australia, the USA and New Zealand.

One of the most noteworthy TQ candidates was Benjamin Alexandrowitsch Belilovsky. Qualified in medicine at the University of Kiev, he had been, among other things, liaison officer between the British and Russian staffs during the occupation of Archangel and Chief Medical Officer of Health for North Russia. There are possible connections with the College here, given that Elsie Inglis was closely involved with the Scottish Women's Hospital Movement in Archangel, and, further, one of the validation letters for Belilovsky's application to sit the TQ was signed by J. D. Comrie, who would write the first full history of medicine in Scotland, published in 1932.[112]

These schedules are extremely useful in illustrating a number of aspects of the medical market place at the turn of the last century and the important role of College Fellows in extra-mural teaching as well as examining. It may have been a very different market place from that which characterised the seventeenth or eighteenth century, but it was, none the less, a market place, however restricted by the constraints of the Medical Act or pronouncements of the GMC. It also shows clearly the extent to which not only the College, but also many individual Fellows, were involved in the delivery and validation of surgical training in Edinburgh at this time.

There are also intriguing insights into Empire and non-transferability of qualifications. George Green, a candidate for the TQ in 1920, already possessed the MD of the Medical College, Richmond, USA, and had practised for many years as a medical missionary in Nigeria, but found that 'in the course of progress in the British Colony of Nigeria British laws regulating the practice of Medicine and Surgery are very wisely being applied to Nigeria, but sad to relate from my point of view American Degrees not being registerable in Great Britain are not registerable in Nigeria'.[113]

The records for the 1940s show also a significant number of candidates from the USA who also completed their entire period of medical education in Scotland. This was also a time when candidates tended to gain their whole curriculum either intra-murally or extra-murally, but by the 1950s the eclecticism had returned. The general situation in Europe in the 1940s is illustrated by the twenty-nine candidates whose birthplaces were in Europe, mainly Austria, Hungary, Romania, Lithuania and Poland, and also by the number of name changes, from the obviously Jewish to something more neutral in appearance. Most of these candidates had trained almost entirely in their home country but completed hospital experience in London, Edinburgh or Glasgow. Among the College Fellows who had taught many of these individuals were Sir John Fraser, Sir David Wilkie, and Mr Pirie Watson, while two noted historians of Scottish medicine, J. D. Comrie and Douglas Guthrie, pursued surgical practice and taught extra-murally as well as gathering information for their historical publications. Table 5.2 illustrates the pattern of curricular origins of TQ candidates.

**Table 5.2 Triple Qualification schedules, 1890–1990: sources of curricular requirements.** (Source: TQ Registers)

|       | Edin. | Glas. | Lond. | UK/Ire. | Foreign | Combined | (Female) | Total |
|-------|-------|-------|-------|---------|---------|----------|----------|-------|
| 1890  | 41    | 16    | 14    | 54      | 21      | 39       | 9        | 185   |
| 1900  | 36    | 31    | 16    | 37      | 32      | 43       | 19       | 195   |
| 1910  | 17    | 6     | 1     | 17      | 30      | 22       | 5        | 93    |
| 1920  | 22    | 15    | –     | 8       | 5       | 12       | 9        | 62    |
| 1930  | 25    | 8     | –     | 5       | 38      | 23       | 6        | 99    |
| 1940  | 87    | 81    | –     | 10      | 14      | 19       | 8        | 211   |
| 1950  | 68    | 47    | –     | 5       | 2       | 8        | 32       | 130   |
| 1960  | 6     | 1     | –     | 5       | 17      | 3        | 6        | 32    |
| 1970  | –     | –     | –     | –       | 7       | –        | 2        | 7     |
| 1980  | –     | 1     | –     | 1       | 38      | –        | 4        | 40    |
| 1990  | –     | –     | –     | –       | –       | –        | –        | –     |
| Total | 302   | 206   | 31    | 142     | 204     | 169      | 100      | 1054  |

It is sometimes imagined that medical practitioners could never be lawbreakers, but the medical profession has always had its share of fraudsters and charlatans. By the middle of the nineteenth century the problem for the College was no longer that of dealing with the outrageous claims of quacks or mountebanks, but rather the difficulties of ensuring that fraudulent claims of ownership of qualifications from the College were detected and dealt with. It appears that before 1875 the College had not had the power to strike off individuals who claimed fraudulent qualifications or were convicted of criminal offences, but in a letter to Joseph Bell on 20 November 1882, the Secretary indicated that he had taken legal opinion at that time, and had constructed a bye-law which 'catches all such fish in its net'. The specific case referred to at this point was of an 'Australian felon'.

Licentiates or Fellows who were caught advertising were dealt with severely (though advertising had been a normal part of medical life for centuries in the past). In February 1888 a letter was sent to Thomas Ritchie in Bristol, a dental Licentiate, noting that he had apparently been advertising in the *British and Colonial Druggist*. He was reminded strongly of 'the declaration signed by you previous to your admission and that you would refrain from advertising or employing any other unbecoming modes of attracting business . . . in the event of the commission of any offence by any Licentiate the College may recall his diploma and declare the same to be void.'[114] There was a steady trickle of similar cases, including forged TQ certificates, and the language of the ensuing debate confirms the particular sensitivities of the College to outside perceptions of its status as a fully professional and learned organisation, which had the highest ethical standards. It did not matter that these ethical standards changed with the times. By the late-Victorian period this sort of advertising was deemed highly unsuitable for a medical professional – it had been acceptable previously, but that was not the point.

## WOMEN AND THE COLLEGE

By the second half of the nineteenth century, against the background of a society which was changing rapidly but which still held to older notions and the currently popular 'separate spheres' argument regarding the role of respectable women in respectable society (advocating separate roles for women based on arguments relating to biological and emotional differences),[115] the question of women and their rights and suitability to enter the medical profession as doctors became more pressing. The College became embroiled in the controversy in 1870, when a formal protest was received from extra-mural students. It was signed by sixty-five students who complained that:

> several of the lecturers at the Royal College of Surgeons have admitted women into their classes without the least endeavour to ascertain the opinion of the male students, and, as now appears, directly contrary to their desire . . . That the presence of women at the classes of anatomy and Surgery, and in the dissecting room of the College, gives rise to various feelings which tend to distract the attention of the Students from important subjects of study . . . that as the institution of mixed classes had not been determined upon when many of the present students attached themselves to this school of medicine, we are of opinion that those gentlemen who commenced their studies under the old system have suffered a certain breach of Contract; inasmuch as a new element has been introduced which would have demanded consideration in their choice of classes.[116]

The reply was a classic example of 'not our fault'. The College stated that it was 'not a teaching body, and though it recognises, and is interested in the success of all the extra academical classes it has no direct control over them, and is not responsible for the decisions of the lecturers'. It was stressed that the extra-mural lecturers were only tenants of the College, and that the students should direct their grievances to them, not to the College. Patrick Heron Watson was one prominent College Fellow who taught mixed extra-mural classes.[117]

Many women were forced to travel to Europe, where medical training was open to women at some centres, such as Paris, Zurich or Bern.[118] The famous case of

Sophia Jex-Blake and her lengthy, unsuccessful battles with the University of Edinburgh has been well documented elsewhere.[119] The attention of the College was not drawn directly to the issue again until 1885, when it received an application from a female who wished to take the Dental Examinations. The reply sent by the College Secretary stated:

> Dear Madam, I have to acknowledge receipt of your letter of 9th ulto. In answer I have to state that yours is the first application that has been received from a person of the female sex to be admitted to any professional examination at this College. The question of such admission has therefore never been considered.[120]

The College Secretary referred her to the Registrar of the GMC for further advice regarding registration and examinations. Matters were helped along the way a little by the 1876 Act to Remove Restrictions on the Granting of Qualifications for Registration under the Medical Act on the Ground of Sex (Russell Gurney Enabling Act), and the TQ Regulations stated that 'Female Candidates are admitted to the Examinations for this Qualification equally with male candidates; and throughout these Regulations the masculine pronoun is to be read as standing for Candidates irrespective of sex.'[121] The 1889 Universities (Scotland) Act allowed degrees in medicine to be conferred on women, but it was not till 1894 that Edinburgh University allowed women to graduate in medicine, and it took until 1916 for women to be admitted to all University classes under similar conditions to their male counterparts. By 1889 the College was receiving applications from women for Licentiateship examinations without comment, but Robertson stated in a terse reply to Miss E. E. Ward that 'Ladies are not admitted to the Fellowship of this College'.[122]

The University Senatus minutes noted in 1894 that courses given by the Edinburgh School of Medicine for Women in Surgeons' Square, and the Medical College for Women in Chambers Street, would be acceptable for graduation, provided that they conformed to the University Ordinances.[123] It would, though, be some time before the College admitted its first female Fellow. In a letter to the Secretary of the FPSG in 1896, it was stated that when women were admitted to the Licence of the College they were not admitted to the Fellowship: 'As regards the right to refuse admission I think the College would be protected by the decision in the case of Jex-Blake v. the University of Edinburgh. I have had only one or two applications for admission, but when the applicants were informed of the regulation on the subject I heard no more from them'.[124]

Glasgow University was the first in Scotland to allow females to graduate on equal terms with men – the shadows of Jex-Blake and the 'battle of Edinburgh' lingered in the east. Much of the debate about female higher education in general as well as medical education in particular centred around the 'separate spheres' issues about the social role and identity of women, and as claims of intellectual inferiority were dismissed, these were replaced with concerns about unsuitability in general – in medicine one of the problems was the examination of men by female practitioners.[125] All of this was bound up, as was the College, in the prevailing social ethos of the late nineteenth century. Viewed from a distance the College seems reactionary and unwilling to 'move with the times'. However, that is precisely the point – it reacted to its times, and once legislation was introduced to allow women to take medical qualifications, the TQ was immediately opened to them. The question of College Fellowship was quite another matter, as it was the historic core of the College's functions.

Other areas of professional society were equally difficult for women to penetrate. The College was also nudged along the path by the passing of the Sex Disqualification (Removal) Bill in 1919, though it did not act until it had taken legal advice. The opinion of Counsel was that the Act applied to all such bodies, whether public or private, and that henceforth women should be admitted to the Fellowship on the same terms as men, and with identical privileges as Fellows once admitted. The College had tried to argue that the 1851 Charter – and, indeed, its precursors – had been intended to cover male surgeons, by implication, and that it was therefore *ultra vires* that it should be compelled to admit women under its terms. Many attempted justifications are made on semantic grounds, and this was no less so here.

The College eventually admitted its first female Fellow, Alice Headwards (later Headwards Hunter), in 1920.[126] (Miss Caroline Doig, first Female member of the College Council, has endowed a Hunter Doig Medal, to be awarded in recognition of significant contributions to surgery by female surgeons.) Headwards did not go on to follow a surgical career in Scotland, but a few months later Gertrude Herzfeld gained her Fellowship and became the first practising female surgeon·in Scotland, specialising in paediatrics and disorders of women. This is one area where the FPSG was a little ahead, as its first female Fellow, Yamani Sen, was admitted as a surgical Fellow in 1912, while Eleanor Davies-Colley achieved similar status in the RCSEng in 1911.[127]

Gertrude Herzfeld spent her professional life in Edinburgh, and her surgical career was spent mainly in paediatric and gynaecological surgery, starting out as House Surgeon to Harold Stiles at the RHSC. By 1925 she was full surgeon to the RHSC and served there for twenty years. From 1920 to 1955 she was also surgeon to the Bruntsfield Hospital for women and children.[128] During her long career she published widely, on such diverse topics as rupture of the intestine, uterine prolapse, hernia, congenital talipes (club foot), and malformations of the newborn.[129] The first female dental 'Fellow' appears to have been Dr Dorothy Johnston, who held the TQ qualification and passed the HDD RCSEd, the precursor of the FDS RCSEd, in 1948.

The way was now clearly open, but relatively few females took up the challenge, with only thirty-five female Fellows elected in the ten years after 1920 (as compared with some 995 male Fellows entering during this period). The numbers who took the TQ examination were consistently higher. The reasons for this were probably partly domestic, partly social and partly economic, since before the NHS, hospital work had to be subsidised from private practice. The activities of female medical practitioners during the campaigns of the First World War have been well documented,[130] but it does not seem that this vital contribution to the war effort on the European Front was to help women enter formal hospital surgical training in numbers in the post-war period. This of course was true of many occupations undertaken by women during this time – once the conflict was over they were expected mostly to return to the domestic sphere from which they had come. All was not entirely lost, though, and women increasingly gained a foothold in a number of branches of medicine, mainly in public health, gynaecology and paediatrics. Besides admitting female Fellows, the College itself did not at that point feel the need to take any active measures to assist women onto the surgical ladder. Indeed, one female consultant surgeon admitted that as a medical student, she felt that her apparent role as a 'diffident, loyal nurturer' seemed at the time to be 'not a very terrible thing'.[131] So it is important to remember that not all women felt frustrated by their apparent lack of progress in the male-dominated surgical world. The College was probably no more (or less) mysogynistic than any other institution at the time.

## THE COLLEGE AND THE ROYAL INFIRMARY

One of the major threads running through the history of the College since 1729 is its often difficult relationship with hospital surgery and, in particular, the RIE.[132] Masters of the Incorporation and Fellows of the College have served the RIE (and, eventually, hospitals in all parts of Britain and the world) since its foundation, and by the 1830s a more stable surgical service was in operation. In a report covering the years 1854–92, Joseph Bell gives a good survey of arrangements in the surgical side of the RIE. In 1854 the visiting surgeons comprised James Miller (Professor of Systematic Surgery), James Syme (seventy-two beds), two ordinary surgeons (approximately sixty beds), two assistant surgeons and one 'specialist' (William Walker, pioneer ophthalmologist). By 1881 there were two professors, three acting surgeons, six assistant surgeons and six specialists.[133] Because his own contemporaries had by that time 'gone over to the majority', Bell felt able to give brief sketches of their surgical lives, and indicates, *inter alia*, that Syme had 'a very little veiled voice, and no eloquence' and 'his hands were too small, and his whole physique too dapper to allow him to be brilliant or rapid with the amputating knife at a thigh or a hip joint'; that it was a 'treat' to watch Miller performing lateral lithotomy; that James Spence's idea of surgical 'bliss' was 'a vast amphitheatre where the souls of the blessed were continually cutting the souls of the lost for stone'; and that William Walker, the 'only pure ophthalmic surgeon in Edinburgh', 'lectured to those few men who were wise enough to think it important to know something about eyes'.[134] In terms of good surgical practice, Bell cautioned against too much time being spent in the primary surgery of severe accident cases, in order to prevent shock, it being better to 'get the patient off the table as soon as possible, even though only a few stitches approximate the flaps'.[135]

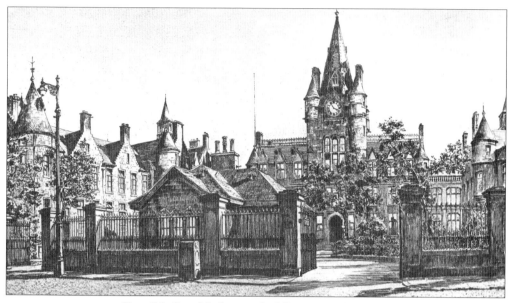

**FIG. 5.9** *Royal Infirmary building, opened in 1879.*
(Book of the Old Edinburgh Club, *15 (1927), facing p. 134.*)

The College as a corporate body gave its opinion routinely on proposed changes to RIE arrangements, and expressed its strong opposition to the amalgamation of the maternity hospital with the main hospital, as proximity would mean that maternity patients would be at considerable risk from erysipelas, fevers and other infectious diseases 'to which puerperal patients are particularly susceptible.'[136]

The close links between the College and the RIE have been important since the establishment of the hospital, and continued with the move to the Lauriston Place building in 1879. The proverbial tonsillectomy performed on the kitchen table may still have featured, but as the nineteenth century wore on and both surgery and technology became more and more complex, it was no longer possible to do heroic surgical deeds on kitchen tables, although more recent episodes, such as that when a life was saved by a College Fellow using bits of coathanger and in-flight brandy on a long-haul flight, continue to hit the headlines on occasion.[137]

The general arrangements for the surgical department of the RIE continued to expand, and by the 1930s it comprised seven 'units', each headed by a 'chief' – David Wilkie and John Fraser (both University professors), together with George Chiene, James Graham (who made significant contributions to the fields of blood transfusion and thyroid surgery), John Struthers, William 'Pussy' Stuart, and Henry Wade (pioneer of urological surgery).[138] At that point surgical services were still general in nature, though several of the surgical chiefs focused their attention on what would become specialties. In addition, and importantly, the outer circles of laboratory sciences, radiology and the paramedical disciplines were becoming more fully established. The separation of the surgical wards into more specialised units went in parallel, but slightly behind the emergence of the specialties themselves.

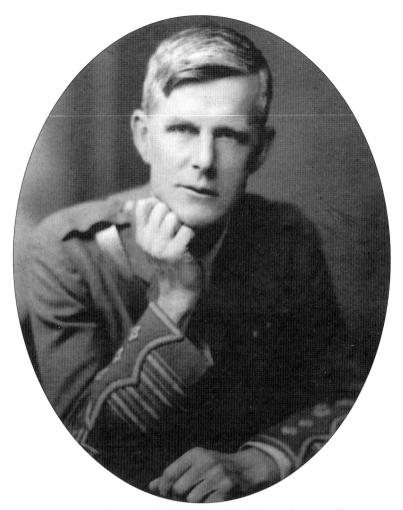

***FIG. 5.10*** *Photograph of Sir Henry Wade in military uniform.*

It would not be until after the NHS altered hospital staffing arrangements as well as all other aspects of health care that the legacy of Wade, for example, would be seen in the setting apart of two wards exclusively for urology. In the same way, wards for cardiothoracic and vascular surgery were established. The role of the College in the RIE was therefore multifaceted. Many Fellows acted as consultants and carried out adventurous surgical procedures as well as routine operations; many were involved in clinical teaching as well as management and a variety of boards and committees.[139] By the end of the 1940s the staffing and organisation of NHS hospitals would present new challenges for College Fellows.

## THE COLLEGE AND SURGICAL DEVELOPMENTS

By the middle of the nineteenth century, when anaesthetics and antiseptics made their hesitant entrance into the surgical world, hospitals were still insanitary, unhealthy places, but the situation improved gradually, helped by the advent of nursing training, so that College Fellows by the turn of the twentieth century were able to develop their techniques to the extent that the beginnings of surgical specialisation were evident. However, the skilled general surgeon was still very much to the fore.

Arguably the most famous College Fellow of the mid-nineteenth century was Joseph Lister, son-in-law of Syme and the first and only individual to be both Fellow and Honorary Fellow of the College. As well as his antiseptic fame,[140] Lister made significant contributions to the debate on the nature of inflammation and to research on the eye and skin, publishing widely on these and other topics, as well as teaching extra-murally and operating at the RIE. Also notable in this era was Thomas Annandale, renowned for his work on knee surgery.[141] Thomas Keith, a keen photographer as well as surgeon, was apprenticed to J. Y. Simpson and may have been the last surgical apprentice in Edinburgh.[142] 'Specialising' in obstetrics,

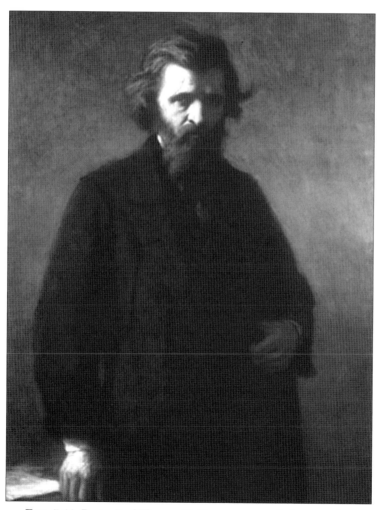

*FIG. 5.11* *Portrait of Thomas Keith, surgeon and photographer.*

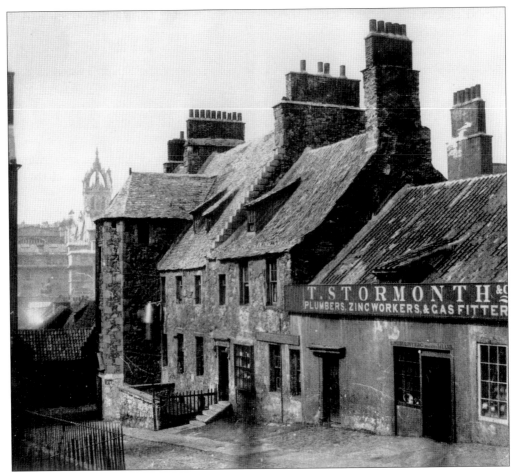

*FIG. 5.12* *Photograph of Brown Square, taken by Thomas Keith.*

he performed his first ovariotomy in 1862, and went on to undertake around 136 of these operations, with over 80 per cent survival recorded. He was also proficient at hysterectomy, recording thirty-three cases and losing only three patients.[143] Patrick Heron Watson (College President in 1878 and 1905) saw surgical service at Balaclava during the Crimean War, and by 1875 had performed excision of the larynx and thyroidectomy as well as splenectomy and nephrectomy. His transitional status in terms of the threshold of surgical specialisation is confirmed, though, by his expertise in ophthalmology and venereal disease, not to mention general medicine.[144]

This was the beginning of 'scientific surgery', the more measured approach rendered possible by the luxury of operating time. Speed was no longer the essence; technical care and innovation were. The next step, though, was to link surgical advance to progress in the laboratory sciences, and John Chiene provided such a link, establishing the first teaching bacteriological laboratory in Britain, and publishing important papers on major blood vessels. Among Chiene's more memorable remarks was the comment that 'surgery is nothing but applied anatomy with a little bacteriology'.[145]

As confirmation of the continuing general organisation of surgery, a handwritten survey of operations carried out in two surgical wards of the RIE in 1929 and 1935 gives good illustration of the scope of general surgery, and, therefore, the activities of College Fellows. In these two wards (one male, one female) in 1929 were undertaken some 414 surgical procedures, among which there were 86 appendicectomies, 6 perforated ulcers among 165 gastrointestinal procedures, 20 hernias, 12 breast cancer procedures, 25 operations for tuberculosis and 104 orthopaedic cases. Among the twenty-seven operations classified as miscellaneous there was one 'cut throat' and one 'vicious circle'.[146]

In 1935, some 987 surgical procedures were recorded, of which 732 were general cases and 255 orthopaedic. Of these, there were: 178 appendicectomies; 23 cholecystectomies; 89 procedures were undertaken on genito-urinary tract problems, including 13 prostatectomies; 24 neurological operations; 3 thoracotomies for lung cancer; 42 operations for tuberculosis in various sites; 22 cases of breast cancer; 38 insertions of radium needles; and 26 laparotomies. On the orthopaedic side there were eighty cases of fracture, four bone tumours and sixteen amputations, while the group labelled 'miscellaneous' included everything from semimembranosus bursa, to hammer toe, hallux valgus and ingrowing toenail.[147] It is clear that here was almost the whole range of what would become surgical specialties.

During the first half of the twentieth century the Fellows produced by the College were true general surgeons, turning their hand to all sorts of conditions. Till that point the FRCSEd had been adequate to prepare surgeons for just this sort of career – and indeed to a career in large part private in nature. The advent of the NHS would alter the latter, and the emergence of the specialties as well as rapid advances in laboratory sciences would force the College to consider modifications to its longstanding examinations (see below).

### Early specialisation

In the period following the First World War, the surgical specialties began to emerge more rapidly, and a number of enabling factors can be recognised. The experience of wartime surgery and the extra hospital space provided by the EMS and wartime hospitals before, during and after the Second World War were key factors, as these institutions survived for a considerable time in the post-war period and were used in some instances as specialist units. It was not just the surgical stimulus of war which brought about these changes, though. The scourge of epidemic disease was no less potent than it had been for centuries, and the pressures of many cases of poliomyelitis, tuberculosis and other crippling conditions ensured that progress would be made in orthopaedics, thoracic surgery and the paramedical areas of radiography, physiotherapy and occupational therapy.

The specific role of the College in bringing about surgical specialisms was both direct and indirect – indirect insofar as Fellows pioneered these surgical subdivisions during their individual careers, and more directly in its role as examiners of these Fellows and validators of their surgical skills. Once it became evident that the future of surgery lay in specialist areas, the College was forced to amend its examinations, beginning with the introduction of a Primary Examination for the FRCSEd (see below).

It may be claimed with some justification that the first of the College specialties was dentistry, and this is covered in a separate section below. What follows here is a brief survey, *not* a comprehensive review, in order to illustrate the range of specialisation and, particularly and primarily, the role and influence of the College through its Fellows and, eventually, its examination systems. Specialties not covered are included by implication in the general conclusions on major contextual influences and links.

Ophthalmology was one of the first areas to specialise. Peter Lowe had described cataract surgery in his surgical textbook, first published in 1599, and following the contributions of James Wardrop, Benjamin Bell and others in the late-eighteenth and early-nineteenth centuries, the Edinburgh Eye Infirmary was in operation by the 1830s,[148] and William Walker (College President 1871–3 and Ophthalmic Surgeon to Queen Victoria) was appointed as the first specialist ophthalmological surgeon at the RIE in 1885. John Argyll Robertson, extra-mural lecturer, specialised

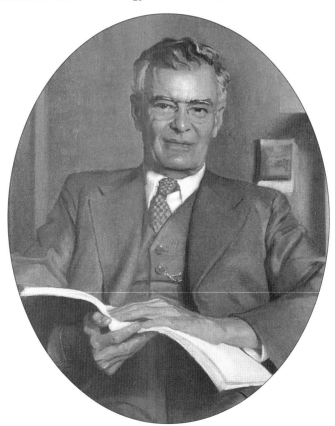

**FIG. 5.13** *Portrait of Norman Dott.*

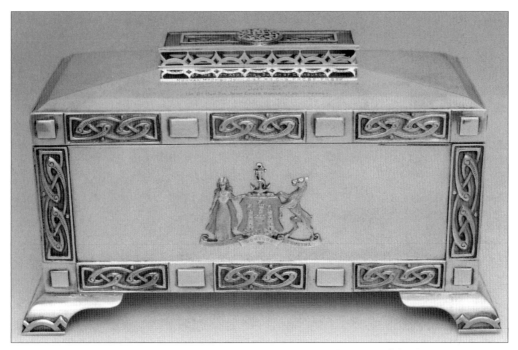

**FIG. 5.14**  *Casket presented to Norman Dott as Freeman of the City of Edinburgh, July 1962.*

early in this area, and his son Douglas Argyll Robertson (President 1886–8) continued the family interest.[149] The latter's combination of scientific research, extensive surgical practice and teaching activities epitomised the contributions of College Fellows in this period, and well reflected the increasingly scientific contemporary context.

Plastic surgery was one area which owed much to wartime. John Shaw, a College Fellow who had worked in this area with Sir Harold Gillies, pioneer of plastic surgery, was appointed assistant surgeon at the RIE in 1924, as well as undertaking duties for Craigleith Hospital.[150] The Second World War brought renewed need for this sort of service, and another College Fellow trained by Gillies, A. B. Wallace, was appointed to organise plastic surgery services at the Bangour EMS hospital. After 1945 these services were maintained and expanded – a clear example of the needs of war utilised to cater for very different peacetime requirements. Orthopaedics was similarly influenced by the necessities of war (see Chapter 6) as well as by the major contributions of Fellows such as Sir Robert Jones, whose main influence was south of the border.

In the field of neurosurgery, the pioneering work of Norman Dott was crucial. Appointed first Professor of Surgical Neurology in 1947, he founded University departments dealing with brain and spinal injuries.[151] A future College President, John Gillingham, who succeeded Dott, was renowned for his work in neurosurgery during the Second World War, in England, the Middle East and Italy. This expertise was translated to peacetime and continued the development of the specialty.

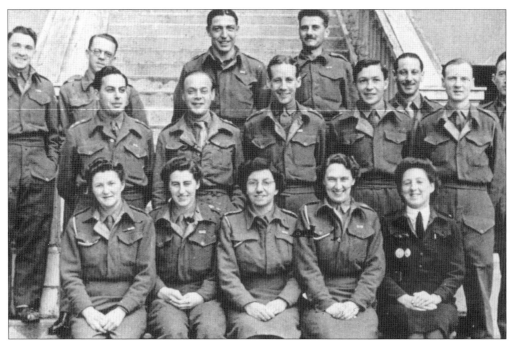

**FIG. 5.15a** *No. 4 Mobile Surgical Unit, Italy 1944. John Gillingham second from right, middle row. The unit operated on 1,556 brain and spinal injuries in 56 days. (F. J. Gillingham.)*

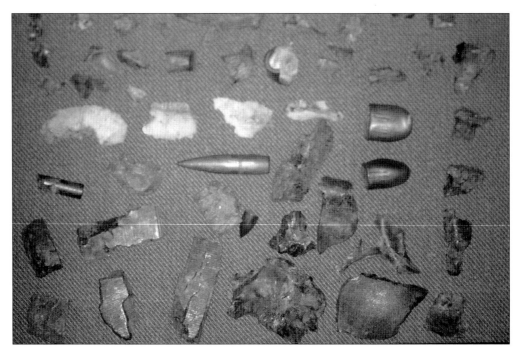

**FIG. 5.15b** *Shrapnel and bullets removed from patients treated in Gillingham's unit.*

Gillingham later pioneered stereotactic surgery, and progress in that area required the further, crucial, factor of technology, both surgical and radiological.

Other specialties required rather different contextual encouragements, which owed more to general conditions than to war. Paediatric surgery, for example, required not only medical expertise, but also some general improvement in the survival and nutrition of young children. The RHSC opened in Edinburgh in 1860, and James Miller, Professor of Systematic Surgery, and James Spence were appointed consulting surgeons.[152] Joseph Bell, Thomas Annandale, Harold Stiles and Gertrude Herzfeld were among the College Fellows who served the institution and not only contributed to surgical techniques, but also pioneered the notion that paediatric surgery could be a full-time occupation and not merely added on to adult surgical practice.

In an account by Joseph Bell of surgical procedures carried out in the RHSC from 1887 to 1892, it was claimed that it was not the urgent cases which found their way to the RHSC initially, but rather the 'deformities of childhood' (cleft palate, spina bifida, club foot, 'late manifestations of spinal and hip disease').[153] Bell claimed that no patient of his had died within three months of surgery, which

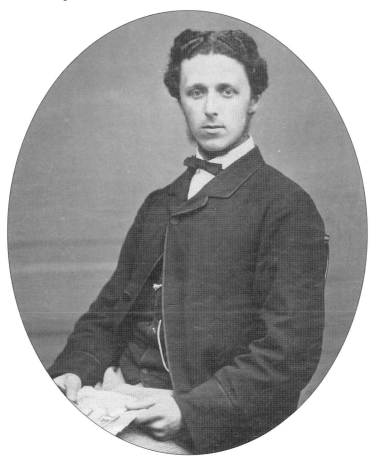

**FIG. 5.16** *Photograph of Joseph Bell from College Presidents' album.*

is a little surprising given the heroic nature of some of the procedures described, including one case where a child had undergone 'excision of the malar bone and lower jawbone, excision of left wrist followed by amputation of forearm, tracheotomy, above knee amputation of leg and scraping of elbow joint'.[154] It is clear that paediatric surgery at this time was largely concerned with the consequences of social deprivation, disease and congenital malformation. (In addition to his full surgical career, Bell gave systematic instruction to nurses, and served as editor of the *EMJ* from 1873 to 1896).

Harold Stiles served the RHSC for over twenty years and assisted the advance in paediatric abdominal surgery, using asepsis rather than the antiseptic approach.[155] During the 1914–18 war, Stiles was consultant to the forces in orthopaedics (developing an interest in peripheral nerve injuries), and was eventually appointed to the Chair of Clinical Surgery at Edinburgh University, but retained his deep interest in paediatric surgery, with major contributions in the general field of urology and transplantation of the ureter.

The paediatric specialty fairly quickly spawned 'system specialties', initially in orthopaedics, not surprisingly in view of the general conditions of the time, when nutritional deficiencies consequent on poverty resulted in rickets,[156] and other conditions such as congenital dislocation of the hip were not detected early enough to be dealt with by conservative means. College Fellows provided specialist services to the RHCS in orthopaedics (Robert Stirling), neurosurgery (Dott) and plastic surgery (Wallace), while outwith Edinburgh, Fellows such as Edward Barrington Ward were developing the specialty in their own areas.

The major surgical features of this period, then, were the possibilities afforded by anaesthetics and antiseptics, as well as expansion of the hospitals and the emergence of the hospital doctor as separate from the general practitioners. New surgical techniques, influenced by war and epidemic disease, began to emerge, given the luxury of operating time and the increasing likelihood that patients would not die of shock or infection. All of these factors shaped College policy and actions, particularly in the lengthy process of refocusing and amending training requirements and examinations. This process would accelerate markedly in the post-1945 period, and will be considered in the next chapter.

## THE COLLEGE AND DENTISTRY

During the Victorian period a number of College Fellows began to consider dentistry as a significant but increasingly separate part of their activities. This almost spontaneous specialisation, combined with legislation aimed at standardisation in the same manner as the Medical Act of 1858, was the origin of the Dental Faculty of the College, though it would be well into the twentieth century before such a Faculty came into being. Before the more formal organisation of dental education, a number of College Fellows had shown an interest in this branch of medicine, and indeed the connection can be traced from the very origins of the College, as James IV was an enthusiastic amateur dentist.

Up to this point dentistry had remained largely 'amateur' and almost completely unregulated, with all sorts of individuals offering to pull teeth or advise on cures for toothache or gumboils. By the turn of the nineteenth century there were as yet few real attempts to organise or improve dentistry on the same lines as medicine. There was no separate qualification for dentistry and it was not perceived as a reputable profession, being unordered and rather chaotic. A few College Fellows had made inroads during the second half of the eighteenth century, but still within the context of surgery in general. It would take considerable efforts to persuade both the medical profession and the public that dentistry had its place alongside medicine, surgery and pharmacy within the spectrum of the increasingly organised and regulated medical profession. Gradually, though, more and more adherents of the College began to practise dentistry alongside surgery and once this process began, *pace* postmodernists, the logical consequence was to offer specialised teaching in this area.

The first real evidence comes from the middle decades of the eighteenth century, when James Rae, grandson of George II's barber, instituted teaching specifically related to dental disease and treatment (see Chapter 3). During the early part of the nineteenth century, James Syme and Robert Liston, more famous in other areas of surgery, included in their publications descriptions of surgical procedures related to the maxillo-facial area, and in 1825 Robert Naysmith (or Nasmith) 'co-operated with Liston in the splinting of mobile mandibular fragments following resection of part of the jaw for neoplasm'.[157] (Naysmith's brother Alexander gave his name to the eponymous membrane which covers the enamel surface of newly erupted teeth.) Other notable individuals who influenced the legitimate practice of dentistry included Francis Brodie Imlach, Licentiate, Fellow and President of the College, who spent the major part of his practice on dentistry, was an acquaintance of J. Y. Simpson, and, perhaps not surprisingly, had a keen interest in anaesthesia. Imlach served as President in 1879 and 1880–1, one of only two dentists to do so, the other being John Smith, in 1883–4. Given his friendship with Simpson, it is not surprising that Imlach performed the first extraction of a tooth under chloroform, in 1847, only a few days after Simpson had tried chloroform in an obstetric case. Keeping things in the family, Smith's son-in-law, William Guy, served as Dean of the Edinburgh Dental Hospital and School in the early years of the twentieth century, and was prominent in the treatment of facial injuries sustained by casualties of the Great War, who were treated at the Second Scottish General Hospital at Craigleith. Given the accepted need for clinical instruction in any area of medicine by this time, it was significant that in 1863 Smith was formally appointed to the RIE in order to provide dental services.

Perhaps the most important stimulus to College dentistry in the third quarter of the nineteenth century came from Smith, who did a great deal to further both dental education and the provision of dental treatment in the form of the Edinburgh Dental Dispensary in Drummond Street in 1860, in the establishment of which he was a prime mover (having resigned from his post as Surgeon Dentist to the Royal Public Dispensary, in order to promote an independent centre managed by dentists).

In 1856 he had instituted a comprehensive course of lectures on diseases of the teeth, and pushed for dental practitioners to be subject to a licensing process in the same way as medical practitioners, in an attempt to prevent the worst excesses of the amateur teeth-pullers. Smith described the situation well in the introduction to his lectures: 'I am entering on an experiment as yet untried in this place; I therefore do so with less confidence since not having the advantage of a predecessor in the same province . . . I am left very much to my own resources in the arrangement and manner of conducting the course'.[158] Meanwhile, the work of the Dental Dispensary appears to have gained repute quickly, as by 1865, RCSEng accepted attendance there as counting towards its required dental curriculum.[159] Progress towards professionalisation was further enabled by the passing of the first Dentists Act in 1878, and in 1879 by the establishment by the College of the LDS RCSEd diploma (in 1895 Lilian Lindsay became the first woman in the United Kingdom to graduate in dentistry, with the Edinburgh LDS).[160] The topic of professionalisation is controversial, but whatever the case it does seem clear that in any branch of medicine, or indeed any other profession, formalised validation must be a feature.

By 1878 the Scottish Dental Education Committee was in operation, and in the same year the Dentists Act reached the statute book,[161] establishing supervisory and registration frameworks along the same lines as those instituted by the 1858 Medical Act. Once the British Dental Association was set up shortly thereafter, both Smith and Imlach served as its President, confirming the key role played by College Fellows in the politics of early dental organisation. The first Dental Hospital and School were located in Brown Square, before moving via Lauriston Place to Chambers Street, in 1894.[162]

In the medical world, publications and societies were becoming increasingly important, and Smith made an unsuccessful attempt to set up a dental society in 1865, with the purpose of encouraging its members to practise 'ethical dentistry'. Though this initial move failed, two years later the Odonto-Chirurgical Society of Scotland was founded. The contemporary perception of dentists was that they were largely unprincipled and poorly educated, and the Society aimed to alter this image by enforcing what it considered to be ethical standards on the part of its members. Advertising was banned, on pain of expulsion from the Society, and in keeping with the notion that learned societies benefited from the awarding of honorary memberships to notable individuals in the wider world, the first honorary member of the Society was Charles James Fox, elected in 1869.[163]

The Society held regular meetings, considered scientific presentations, and subscribed to the available journals. Its lecture programme contained a wide range of topics, including 'conservative dentistry of exposed pulp' and 'case of sarcoma of the lower jaw', and in March 1890 one of the prominent members, W. Bowman Macleod, spoke on the very Scottish topic of 'the effects of bagpipe playing on the teeth'. The Society demonstrated a keen interest in the latest science and its application, hearing papers on 'nitrous oxide gas' (1868), 'inhalation of gas and ether' (1898) and 'micro-organisms of the mouth and their relationship with disease'

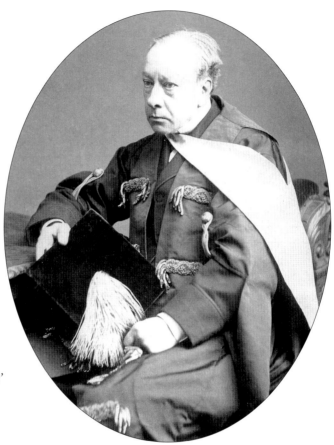

*FIG. 5.17 Photograph of John Smith, dentist and College President, 1883–5.*

*FIG. 5.18 Map showing Surgeons' Square, Old Surgeons' Hall, Argyle Square and Brown Square, 1850. (Edinburgh Medical Journal, 27 (1882), facing p. 780.)*

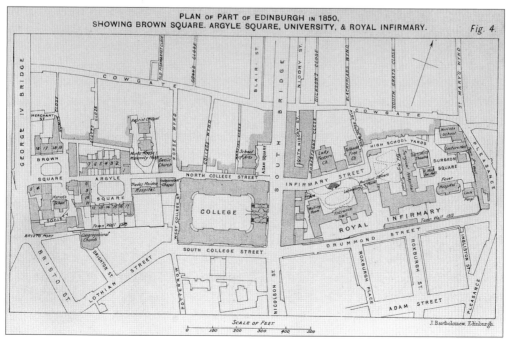

(1883) – laboratory sciences were by this point becoming key to progress in most areas of medicine and the same was the case with dentistry.[164]

By the turn of the twentieth century there was a need for some sort of higher examination, given the combination of an increasing cohort of qualified dentists, the development of maxillo-facial surgery and the growing – however slowly – technology of dentistry. In 1920 the Higher Dental Diploma (HDD RCSEd) was established, drawing in fair numbers of candidates, particularly those aiming for a career in hospital rather than community dentistry, albeit part-time before the NHS. This examination was superseded by the FDS RCSEd in 1949, but during its lifetime it allowed the College to offer qualifications which recognised competence at a higher level than the basic LDS RCSEd (The RFPSG had a similar qualification). In time, as with medicine in general, dentists would gain their initial qualification at a university, but for the moment the dental side of the College, pioneered by a few determined individuals, offered further evidence that the College was 'famous and flourishing'. It may be argued of course that these things came about only because of the immediate stimulus of the Dentists Act, but it is clear that from the time of James Rae, whether of its own volition or not, the College made a significant contribution to the cause of removing dentistry from its background of quackery or a mere sideline for a surgeon or other practitioner.

There was also the other key factor of hospital facilities and the beginnings of the specialty of oral and maxillo-facial surgery (OMS). Dental staff had been appointed to the RIE since 1863 and there was still a close connection between dentistry and anaesthetics, with several anaesthetists in the inter-war period also having a dental qualification and running dental practices in addition to their duties as anaesthetists. These included John Gibbs, who served in the RIE from 1903 to 1929, and was considered to be the 'father of oral surgery in Edinburgh'.[165] Despite this label, he also worked as an anaesthetist within the ENT department of the RIE. David Middleton also combined dental and anaesthetic practices before leading a field ambulance unit in France at the start of the Second World War.[166] After the war he and a colleague, Frederick Gibbs, established the Oral Surgery Department in the RIE, and he was one of only two Fellows to be elected to both College and Dental Councils (the other being J. F. Gould).

In terms of dental organisation, the College made a detailed and comprehensive report to the Inter-Departmental Committee on Dentistry in 1943, in which it recommended the establishment of a General Dental Council on the same lines as the GMC, and made the point strongly that adequate funding would be required before substantial scientific research could be undertaken.[167] The GDC was eventually established in 1956 following a further Dentists Act.

The role of the College at this time in relation to dentistry was characterised by several factors, including the general socio-economic and political context, advances in knowledge, requirements of legislation, necessities of war, and the enthusiasm of individuals who wished to change the negative image in which their calling was portrayed and help to establish it as a medical profession in its own right, not just an occasional function of surgeons or a sideline for unqualified amateurs. As with surgery in general, the College was both proactive and reactive according to the complexities of the medical spheres in which it operated.

## THE COLLEGE AND PUBLIC HEALTH

The College had always taken an interest in matters of public health, and was involved in several areas from the 1830s. A number of measures were proposed, some of which were enacted, to try to improve general health and, in particular, to prevent or at least lessen the devastating effects of endemic and epidemic diseases.

In 1831 the College was involved with the Board of Health, set up by the Edinburgh Town Council in anticipation of an outbreak of cholera, and in June 1840 it was consulted by Edwin Chadwick, who asked for assistance in preparing his ground-breaking sanitary report.[168] Fellows were also in favour of the recording of vital statistics, and petitioned parliament to that effect in 1845 (the statutory recording of this information came later in Scotland than in England), and support was given to various initiatives on removal of nuisances.

The question of compulsory vaccination occupied the College for much of the first half of the nineteenth century.[169] Inoculation against smallpox had been available since the early decades of the eighteenth century, but at the start it took the form of after-dinner entertainment for the upper levels of society rather than a measure to combat the disease for all. Moves to make it widely available had met with a degree of opposition which was not remarkable in its day but perhaps rather surprising to modern observers. Objections to compulsory inoculation or, later, vaccination were based on two elements: firstly, the religious objection to artificial interference with the will of God and, secondly, the degree of compulsion involved. While wholeheartedly in favour of vaccination, some Fellows had severe reservations about compulsion and penalties for non-compliance, and were concerned about the practicalities of any legally enforced programme of vaccination, importantly on the question of whether specialist vaccinators should be appointed or whether the procedure could be carried out by any qualified general practitioner. Legislation was passed for England in 1853, but it took another decade before similar measures could be put in place for Scotland.

For much of the earlier period in its history, inoculation was administered by a variety of mostly unqualified individuals who, with greater or lesser skills, undertook to carry out the task. As with many things, though, particularly things of a practical nature, repeated performance of a procedure generates skills, not necessarily requiring detailed theoretical knowledge to carry them out efficiently. Given also the pivotal role of the parish minister in Scottish society, it was frequently he who performed inoculations as well as offering general medical and legal advice and caring for the spiritual needs of his parishioners.

By the 1850s the College was rather more concerned with its rights and privileges than the compulsion factor, and was opposed to the creation of specialist vaccinators. Its views were expressed thus:

The College do not require to be reminded of the notorious fact that Vaccination has to a very lamentable extent been neglected in Scotland, that the result of this is that small-pox has shown itself in Scotland extensively and fatally, especially of late years, – and that an Epidemic of this disease is at the present moment prevalent throughout the country. In this respect Scotland stands in striking and unfavourable contrast to other European countries, which enjoy a comparatively large immunity from small-pox, traceable to the wise and stringent measures which they have adopted and enforced for promoting the universal practice of vaccination. The Vaccination Act, of which England has for several years enjoyed the advantages, has, so far as it is operative, produced good results ... The College Council believe that the College will agree with them in holding that there is no reason why Scotland should not enjoy the advantages of a Vaccination Act, rendered effective by the supplying of those omissions which have interfered with the successful operation of the act for England.[170]

The view was expressed that public vaccinators should have certificates of competence, but also that Licentiate candidates should possess a certificate of having 'witnessed the progress of six successful cases' under the supervision of a registered medical practitioner. The competency certificates would obviate the 'invidious distinction' of specialist vaccinators. The College was generally in favour of the introduction in Scotland of measures similar to those which had been enacted south of the border, as the Vaccination Act applied to England had 'so far as it is operative produced good results', though the penalty clauses posed considerable problems.[171]

Individual Fellows objected, and one of the most vociferous was William Brown, who was opposed 'because the efforts of the College may be more beneficially exerted in bringing the important subject of vaccination before its Fellows and Licentiates, before the Ministers of Religion, before the Parochial Boards, before the Educational and Charitable Institutions throughout the Country, and thus securing a large and intelligent moral influence on those people who chiefly need it.'[172] The background to this of course was the whole debate on poverty, charity and the responsibilities of government in areas of public health and preventative medicine. Historians are divided on the question of whether legislation in this period was to enforce or enable change at local level – whatever the case, it is clear that government had a significant part to play.[173]

Debate continued until 1863, when final drafts of the legislation were being put together and commented on by the College at each stage. The main objections were that vaccination on the one hand, however compulsory, could not be expected to wholly eradicate the disease and also that in England it had not been fully successful owing to problems with the administration of the programme. On the other hand, though, it was pointed out in May 1863 that:

is it not discreditable to Great Britain, the native country of Jenner, that

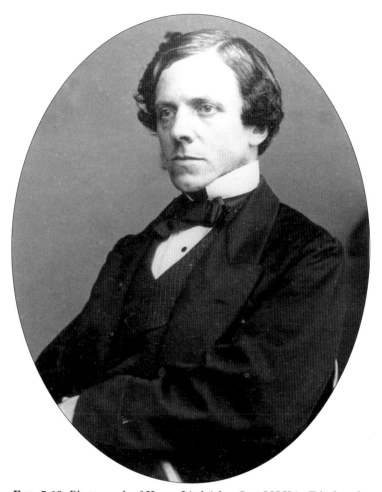

**FIG. 5.19** *Photograph of Henry Littlejohn, first MOH in Edinburgh.*

because of a certain squeamishness in applying compulsion, the mortality among us from Small-pox is 1 in 1,700 whilst in Austria it is only 1 in 4,800, in France 1 in 11,000, in Sweden 1 in 27,000 and in Denmark (we are sorry we cannot give the exact figures), in a still smaller ratio. Shall we not, ought we not to do what these countries have done in order to reap similar benefits? Why should we then scruple to enact them [legislation] when the health, beauty and life of the community are at stake in deference to the ignorance of indolence or prejudice of a small minority of the population (a large part of that minority not indigenous) who by their neglect whether wilful or otherwise keep up a continuous supply of victims of a loathsome and dangerous disease?

Even after the belated addition of the Scottish Vaccination Act to the Statute Book, there were still grumblings. In August 1863 the College complained to the Town Council that reports in the press had inferred that the College had not been as active as had the physicians and other bodies in discussions prior to the passing of the Act. Any perceived insult was greatly resented.[174]

In terms of individual College contributions to public health, Sir Henry Littlejohn, President 1875–6, Professor of Forensic Medicine and Edinburgh's first MOH, epitomised the multiple influences which institutions could bring to bear through the work of individual Fellows. Littlejohn produced the highly influential *Report on the Sanitary Condition of the City of Edinburgh* in 1865, two years before the Public Health Act (Scotland) reached the statute book. He was appointed MOH in 1862, recommended by the RCSEd and RCPEd in view of his expertise in the area and the fact that he was already a police surgeon.[175] (By that point the Police Commissioners had been subsumed into the Edinburgh Town Council.) Though faced with considerable opposition from the medical establishment, Littlejohn was the prime instigator of disease notification, which would have considerable influence on epidemiology and the control of public nuisance.[176] Unlike James Burn Russell,[177] who served full-time as MOH in Glasgow, Littlejohn worked at this aspect of his career part-time, in conjunction with his other offices, but was, none the less, a significant force. This was very much in the period of the 'sanitation' approach to public health, at a time when there was not, as yet, agreement as to whether disease transfer took place by contagion or miasma.[178]

In terms of College action, in addition to giving its views on public health measures proposed by the Town Council, moves were made to introduce a Diploma in Public Health in the late 1880s, and the scope of this examination illustrates what were perceived to be the main priorities. Subjects to be examined included: 'chemistry, physics, topographical atmospherics and climatic influences in their relations to disease', together with 'epidemic and endemic diseases, contagion, drainage, water supply and conservancy, construction of public buildings, barracks, hospitals, schools, factories and dwelling houses, establishments connected with food supplies, cemeteries, sanitary science in general and sanitary laws, laws related to the duties of an officer of health in all its departments including vital statistics'.[179] There would also be a practical examination in which students would be required to demonstrate procedures concerning 'examination of water, air, foods, beverages, condiments, sewage, soils, disinfectants and deodorisers, building materials, clothing, bacteriology and examination of water, bread, milk and tea'. This apparently wide-ranging qualification would seem to anticipate the duties of modern Health, Safety and Food Standards authorities. The DPH was finally offered conjointly by the three Scottish Colleges in 1892. A similar diploma was instituted by the RCSEng in 1887.[180]

By the early decades of the twentieth century, the language of 'public health' was changing slightly, as seen, for example, in the nomination of a Fellow to serve on the Edinburgh Council of Social Service in July 1922. The emphasis was by that time on schemes for health insurance and for the welfare of mothers and children, not to mention the problem of dealing with the scourge of tuberculosis and, later, poliomyelitis – the latter of which would stimulate significant developments in orthopaedic surgery.

## MUSEUM AND LIBRARY

### Museum

From the start the College Museum had contained an eclectic mixture of the patho-logically significant and the frankly curious, and this was a continuing feature of the period covered in this chapter, despite the much stronger organisation and acquisition of pathological specimens which had taken place during the earlier part of the nineteenth century.

The middle part of the nineteenth century was, though, a period of relative stagnation. It is noted, for example, that during William Sanders' tenure as Conservator from 1853 to 1869, not a single entry was made in the Museum Catalogue, though apparently Sanders did deliver some teaching to medical students. The situation of intertia continued throughout the conservatorships of James Pettigrew and Robert Cunynghame between 1869 and 1887, so that, in effect, there had been almost no development for almost half a century. Some curiosities did appear, including 'two casts from the head of a homicidal maniac' (12 November 1862) and a collection of serpents (12 November 1868), while the more medical donations included 'a portion of Collier's lung' (3 February 1872).

It is difficult to account for this prolonged period of inactivity, given the rapid development in surgery, anatomy, hospital surgery and extra-mural teaching. One reason which has been given is that Council had imposed stringent economic limits on such activities[181] – this is plausible (and would not be the only time), but was also rather going against the general aims of the College in terms of improving its status and teaching abilities. However, the next Conservator, Charles Cathcart, who held the post from 1887 to 1900, was much more active and energetic. Under his patronage a new catalogue was prepared, and new methods of pathological classi-fication were described, though these were not introduced until 1929. Cathcart claimed that 'the canons of logical division can be applied to the working out of any system of classification in pathology', and his justification for his system was firmly embedded in the classical principles of logic.[182] Cathcart's activities and general developments in laboratory techniques combined to bring about an accom-modation crisis, which was not resolved until the major reconstruction of the Playfair Building undertaken by Balfour Paul in 1908–9. Cathcart's interest in histopathology was also a feature of this period, reflecting the growing importance of the laboratory sciences in medicine. Cathcart resigned as Conservator in 1900, but continued to wield influence as Chairman of the Curators, and indeed was involved in the committee appointed to organise the Balfour Paul renovations. In addition to Cathcart's own energies there was the important factor of the requirements of the School of Medicine of the Royal Colleges for anatomical and pathological teaching, and also a diagnostic service was made available as a possible alternative to the RCSEd Laboratory. This was perhaps the zenith of the Museum in terms of its teaching functions. The Museum was opened to the public annually, but restrictions had to be imposed in 1913 as a result of suffragette activities.

Following the reconstruction of the Museum premises in 1908, there was of necessity a lull in activity during the First World War, which disrupted the Conservatorship of Henry Wade, who during his term of office promoted the pathological sciences, particularly histopathology and bacteriology, as well as improving conservation of specimens. Following Wade's resignation in 1920, David Greig became the first full-time incumbent of the post.[183] On accepting this offer, Greig donated a large part of his extensive pathological collection to the Museum. He implemented Cathcart's classification plans, and acquisitions included collections of gynaecological, ENT and dental specimens, reflecting the emerging specialties. This period was also notable for the emphasis placed by Greig and his successors on scientific research based on the collections as well as publication of this work. Scientific research as part of the life of the active surgeon would be encouraged strongly in the future. A precursor of the Menzies Campbell dental collection came on 4 February 1931, when the report of the Museum Committee noted that Dr J. H. Gibbs had presented a collection of specimens illustrating dental pathology to the College.

The Second World War period saw the Conservatorship of John Struthers. The specimens were removed to the basement between 1930 and 1943, at which point it was deemed safe for them to be brought into use again. At the end of hostilities, attention was again given to teaching (which had been carried out privately before the war), though the consequences of the Goodenough Report (1944) were that henceforth the main focus of the activities of the College and its Museum would be on postgraduate matters. During the century or so covered here, the Museum underwent a combination of periods of stagnation and of significant change according to changing context, College policy, economics and the individual interests of conservators. The next half-century would see more rapid progress, with developments in radiological and dental collections in particular, though there would be considerable political and economic tensions.

### Library

As mentioned, the library collection was lost to Edinburgh University in 1763, and there was increasing friction between the College and University over such matters as numbers of surgeons borrowing books. Complaints were made to the University Commissioners, and the agreement with the University was terminated finally in 1887. Meanwhile, once the Playfair Hall opened its doors, a priority for the 'famous and flourishing' society was to resurrect its own library collections. It was noted by January 1834 that the Library contained some 150 volumes, and the collection was enhanced substantially by the donation of over 1,000 volumes by the Misses Abercrombie in 1845, these books having belonged to their father, Dr John Abercrombie. From that point the College continued the process of rebuilding its library stock as well as amassing a number of non-medical but important antiquarian books and artefacts. This was also a time when medical periodicals proliferated, and subscriptions were made to, among other things, the *BMJ*, *EMJ* and *Lancet*. This, naturally, resulted in an increasing need for library space, which was again part of the impetus for the Balfour Paul alterations (see Chapter 7). Over the years, Fellows and others have donated sizeable collections to the Library, and a significant number of rare books, medical and non-medical, have been acquired, including a copy of Cranmer's Bible, which belonged to James Haig Ferguson, Fellow, President and pioneer in the field of obstetrics. In recent times attempts have been made to retrieve the books lost to the University, but these have so far been unsuccessful.

## CONCLUSION

This period was of considerable importance for the College in a number of ways. The spheres of influence and threat with which it had to contend were themselves shaped by the restructuring of society as a whole. The extension of the franchise and the determined drive by successive governments towards medical reform, enforcing or enabling measures to improve public health, the heyday of Empire, the dislocation of world wars and the coming of the NHS all combined to provide a changing background discourse and a very different medical market place by 1948. The College started the period covered by this chapter in a brand new and very impressive building and continued to develop its 'campus' thereafter. It started this

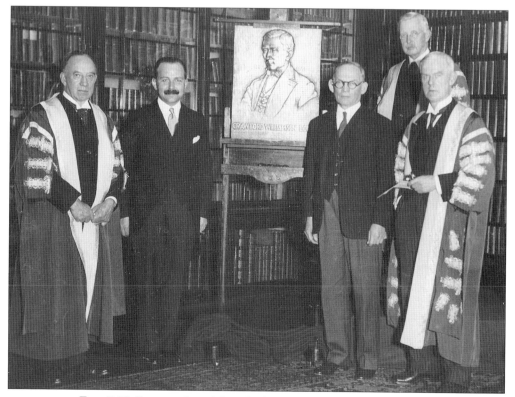

*FIG. 5.20* *Presentation of Crawford Long Memorial, 30 March 1937.*
*Long was an American physician who excised a neck tumour using ether in 1842,*
*although this was not publicised until after the demonstration by*
*Dr W. T. G. Morton in Boston, 1846.*

period as a provider of basic surgical qualification – it ended it still with this right, but accepting the inevitable and changing its focus towards the provision of higher education. It survived economic threat and the many failed medical Bills which would have had much more limiting effects on the College than the one which eventually reached the statute book in 1858. It saw a period of unprecedented co-operation between and among the British and Irish colleges; the dental wing of the College was in an embryonic stage; and by 1948 the College was relatively stable within a changing environment. This situation would not last too long, as more, greater and very different challenges were ahead. The Victorian social and medical spheres were complex, and the influences which shaped the College at this time were equally complicated. Overseas connections and courtesies were maintained and would be developed much further in the second half of the twentieth century. The next chapter will consider the College's most recent past and the different challenges which it faced, in a much more global context.

## NOTES

1. Letter from the College to promoters of Mr Warburton's Medical Reform Bill, 12 December 1840.
2. Bynum, W. F., *Science and the Practice of Medicine in the Nineteenth Century* (Cambridge, 1995), p. 219.
3. Jenkinson, J. L. M., *Scotland's Health 1919–1948* (Bern, 2002), pp. 153–270.
4. Sturdy, S., 'Alternative publics. The development of government policy on personal health care 1905–11', in S. Sturdy (ed.), *Medicine, Health and the Public Sphere*, p. 253. See also McLachlan, G. (ed.), *Improving the Common Weal. Aspects of Scottish Health Services, 1900–1984* (Edinburgh, 1995).
5. *Report of the Committee on Social Insurance and Allied Services* (HMSO, 1942) (Cmnd. 6404) [The Beveridge Report].
6. College Minutes, 12 November and 20 December 1861.
7. College Minutes, 20 December 1861. Further addresses were sent on the coming of age of the Prince of Wales in 1861 and the attempt on the life of the Duke of Edinburgh in 1868.
8. Ibid., 3 February 1862. There was concern, though, over whether the College had the right to give a corporate opinion, given its separation from the Town Council. Support was expressed for business to be rated for this as well as householders.
9. Ibid., 16 May 1862. The Lunacy Act was passed in 1857, enforcing the certification of the insane.
10. Smith, J., *The Origin, Progress and Present Position of the Royal College of Surgeons of Edinburgh 1505–1905* (Edinburgh, 1905), p. 29.
11. The College in 1929 incurred considerable expense – over £680 – in dealing with the College Clerk, who 'had allowed his habits to interfere not only with his health, but also with the punctual and efficient performance of his duties'. The College had 'sent him, along with his wife, to the Canary Islands' for a long holiday, but this had not improved the situation. An independent audit revealed discrepancies in the accounts, and on 28 December 1928 the Clerk was suspended and his appointment subsequently terminated. The Assistant Clerk was promoted though he was eventually dismissed also.
12. College Minutes, 27 July and 18 October 1911.
13. Ibid., 16 May 1911.
14. See the more detailed account in Hull and Geyer-Kordesch, *The Shaping of the Medical Profession*, pp. 66–8.

15. College Minutes, 12 December 1912; Hull and Geyer-Kordesch, *Shaping of the Medical Profession*, pp. 70–4. By 1913 most doctors had signed up to the scheme. In December 1912 a manifesto was issued with the aim of helping the profession 'to maintain its independence' – in other words, to maintain the hierarchy with consultants at its apex.

16. College Minutes, 14 May 1912.

17. Ibid., 25 July and 12 December 1912.

18. Ibid., 3 February 1870.

19. Ibid., 12 October 1863.

20. *Report on the State of the Widows' Fund of the Royal College of Surgeons of Edinburgh as at Lammas 1868* (Edinburgh, 1868), pp. 4–5.

21. Though by 1868 the list included non-resident Fellows.

22. The Victoria Cross is awarded for 'most conspicuous bravery, or pre-eminent act of valour or self-sacrifice or extreme devotion to duty in the presence of the enemy', though between 1858 and 1881 an amendment allowed for awards 'under circumstances of extreme danger'.

23. College Minutes, 16 December 1914.

24. Ibid., 9 May 1915. It was considered that the circular had had good effects in speeding up recruitment to the RAMC. For a history of the RAMC see Blair, J. S. G., *The Royal Army Medical Corps 1898–1998. Reflections of One Hundred Years of Service* (Royal Army Medical Corps, 1998).

25. College Minutes, 29 July 1940. It was decided not to contribute to the Lord Provost's appeal for subscriptions towards a fighter aircraft, the investment option being considered more appropriate.

26. Ibid., 22 July 1941.

27. RCSEng, Council Minutes, 4 June 1833.

28. Ibid., 2 June 1838.

29. Ibid., 15 October 1840.

30. Ibid., 7 February 1840.

31. Ibid., 11 February 1841.

32. Ibid., 31 January 1842. Graham kept in close touch with the RCSEng and provided assistance in its acquisition of a new charter. He was at that point Home Secretary in Sir Robert Peel's government, 'which had no leanings to radicalism but was in earnest about social reform'.

33. RCSEng, Council Minutes, 4 November 1852. There is no explanation given as to how this conclusion was reached.

34. Lawrence, C., *Medicine in the Making of Modern Britain*, pp. 27–8.

35. RCSEng, Council Minutes, 10 June 1857.

36. Geyer-Kordesch and Macdonald, *Physicians and Surgeons in Glasgow*, pp. 368–96.

37. RCSI, Minutes, 27 February 1838. See also Widdess, J. D. H., *The Royal College of Surgeons in Ireland and its Medical School 1784–1984*, third edn (Dublin, 1984).

38. RCSI, Minutes, 7 May 1638. The sum of £30 was paid for the specimen.

39. Ibid., 5 February 1841.

40. Ibid., 12 May 1854.

41. Geyer-Kordesch and Macdonald, *Physicians and Surgeons in Glasgow*, p. 370. For example, the Passenger Vessels Act of 1803, designed to regulate the flow of emigration, stipulated that a surgeon had to be on board every vessel with more than fifty passengers, but those qualified to undertake this task did not include Licentiates of the FPSG. Similarly, the Bill for Regulating the Practice of Surgery throughout the United Kingdom of Great Britain and Ireland, mooted in 1816, made no mention of the FPSG.

42. RCPSG, Minutes, 26 March 1833.

43. Ibid., 25 April 1838.

44. Ibid., 17 December 1838.

45. Geyer-Kordesch and Macdonald, *Physicians and Surgeons in Glasgow*, p. 378.

46. RCPEd, Minutes, 11 March 1853. Part of the problem was that, at that point, the FPSG

was in favour of the universities having a representative on any proposed board of supervision, but the other corporations were not.

47. RCPSG, Minutes, 25 March 1853.
48. Craig, *Royal College of Physicians*, p. 238.
49. The RCPEd co-operated even to the extent of agreeing in 1831 that members of the RCSEd should in future be invited to the President's breakfast on the morning of his election. RCPEd, Minutes, 1 November 1831.
50. Ibid., 4 February 1817.
51. At this point the RCPEd also voiced its opposition to Glasgow's call for a Royal Charter.
52. The licensing powers of the universities would continue to be a problem for the medical corporations after the passing of the Medical Act.
53. There is a useful narrative account of the various Bills and college activities in Craig, *Royal College of Physicians*, pp. 251–83.
54. RCPEd, Minutes, 7 February 1854.
55. The first telegraphic message by morse code had been sent on 24 May 1844.
56. Clark, C., *A History of the Royal College of Physicians of London*, vol. 2 (London, 1966), p. 680.
57. For a history of the GMC, see Stacey, M., *Regulating British Medicine. The General Medical Council* (Chichester, 1992).
58. College Minutes, 13 December 1859.
59. Ibid., 3 February 1860.
60. Hull and Geyer-Kordesch, *Shaping of the Medical Profession*, pp. 6–47.
61. See the detailed account of the struggle for legislation in Hull and Geyer-Kordesch, *Shaping of the Medical Profession*, pp. 20–47.
62. Cooter, R., 'The rise and decline of the medical member: doctors and parliament in Edwardian and inter-war Britain', *Bull. Hist. Med.*, 78 (1) (2004), p. 97.
63. College Minutes, 5 March 1934. Further discussion took place on 19 December 1934.
64. Department of Health for Scotland, *Committee on the Scottish Health Services Report* (HMSO, 1936) (Cmnd. 5204) [The Cathcart Report]. See Jenkinson, *Scotland's Health*, pp. 144–9.
65. Jenkinson, *Scotland's Health*, pp. 142–8.
66. College Minutes, 25 May 1942. Hetherington was one of the prime movers for reform of medical training in Glasgow, giving an enhanced role to the universities. Hull and Geyer-Kordesch, *Shaping of the Medical Profession*, pp. 105–7.
67. For an assessment of the NHS in Scotland, see Nottingham, C., *The NHS in Scotland. The Legacy of the Past and the Prospect of the Future* (Aldershot, 2000); Webster, C., *The National Health Service. A Political History* (Oxford, 1998).
68. College Minutes, 27 July 1869.
69. In Aberdeen the major problem was rivalry between the two University Colleges, while the lack of hospital facilities was difficult for St Andrews. See Pennington, C., *The Modernisation of Medical Teaching in Aberdeen in the Nineteenth Century* (Aberdeen, 1994); Blair, J. S. G., *History of Medicine at the University of St Andrews* (Edinburgh, 1987).
70. See Struthers, J., *Historical Sketch of the Edinburgh Anatomical School* (Edinburgh, 1867).
71. RCPEd, Minutes, 7 August 1900.
72. Financial details show that income from this source from 1862 to 1935 amounted to the not inconsiderable total of £149,221. From a fairly modest £132 in 1862, by 1935 the figure was £5,125; and, following an expected dip between 1914 and 1918, from the 1920s income was relatively steady at £4,000–£6,000 each year.
73. Hull and Geyer-Kordesch, *Shaping of the Medical Profession*, pp. 88, 92; Collins, K. E., 'American Jewish medical students in Scotland 1925–40', in D. Dow (ed.), *The Influence of Scottish Medicine* (London, 1986), pp. 143–58.

74. Wojcik, W. A., 'Time in context – the Polish School of Medicine and Paderewski Polish Hospital in Edinburgh 1941 to 1949', *Proc. Roy. Coll. Phys. Ed.*, 31 (2001), pp. 69–76. See also Rostowski, J., *History of the Polish School of Medicine at the University of Edinburgh* (London, 1955).

75. Catford, E. F., *The Royal Infirmary of Edinburgh 1929–1979* (Edinburgh, 1984) p. 227.

76. Stiles, H. J., *Reminiscences of a Surgical Training* (Edinburgh, 1919), p. 17.

77. Ibid., pp. 27, 31.

78. Bramwell, E., 'Postgraduate medical students and teaching in Edinburgh – the past, the present and the future', *University of Edinburgh Journal*, 9 (1937–8), p. 118.

79. 'Editorial Notes', *EMJ*, 8 (1914), p. 292.

80. There is a full account of these developments in LHSA, 'History of the Edinburgh Post-graduate Board for Medicine 1905–50' [no author noted].

81. Graham was an accomplished artist, and drew caricatures of the candidates he examined for the FRCSEd.

82. College Minutes, 27 April 1860.

83. Ibid., 2 August 1860.

84. Ibid., 16 May 1863.

85. EUL, Minutes of Senatus, 16 December 1871 and 24 February 1872.

86. Ibid., 14 June 1872.

87. RCPEd, Minutes, 26 December 1884.

88. There is a full discussion of this in Loudon, I., 'Medical Education and Medical Reform', in N. Nutton and R. Porter (eds), *The History of Medical Education in Britain* (Amsterdam, 1995), pp. 241–5.

89. College Minutes, 6 July and 9 August 1830.

90. Ibid., 16 May 1863.

91. Ibid., 16 May 1877.

92. *Laws of the Royal College of Surgeons of Edinburgh* (Edinburgh, 1885), 20–1.

93. RCSEd, Letterbooks, 19 December 1888.

94. Ibid., September 1889.

95. Ibid., 23 January 1895.

96. These were works such as: Bryant, T., *A Manual for the Practice of Surgery* (London, 1879); Erichsen, J. E., *The Science and Art of Surgery; Being a Treatise on Surgical Injuries, Diseases and Operations* (London, 1853); Holmes, T., *Treatise on Surgery* (London, 1875); Spence, J., *Lectures on Surgery* (Edinburgh, 1864). Several of these works ran to many subsequent editions.

97. A committee was set up as early as 1943 to consider modifications to the Fellowship Examination, and by 16 May 1946 these had been agreed, the new regulations to come into force on 1 January 1948.

98. In 1957, 39 per cent of 491 candidates passed; in 1967 the figure was 37 per cent of 1,217 candidates (a dramatic rise in candidate numbers over the decade); and in 1977, 32 per cent of 1,012 candidates were successful.

99. RCSEd, Letterbooks, 22 May 1896.

100. In December 1859, Dr Andrew Wood referred to the unusually large number of students who had offered themselves for the preliminary examination for the single Diploma as an evidence of the good reputation of that qualification, and of the need for the College to continue to offer it, notwithstanding the introduction of the Double Qualification.

101. Craig, *Royal College of Physicians*, pp. 306–8.

102. RCPEd, Minutes, 13 August 1861.

103. College Minutes; see also Craig, *Royal College of Physicians*, pp. 308–11.

104. If such an examination were held at the present time, the TQ qualification would still be awarded in Scotland.

105. College Minutes, 24 August 1885.

106. RCSEd, Letterbooks, 1 November 1882.

107. Ibid., 6 January 1883.

108. Kaufman, *Medical Teaching in Edinburgh*, pp. 125–7.

109. Inglis also listed additional experience at the Cowgate Dispensary, the Edinburgh Maternity and Sick Children's Hospitals and St Mungo's College, and she was taught by, among others, Henry Littlejohn. Inglis' close colleague Jessie MacGregor qualified a few months earlier. She too gained preliminary entry via the Educational Institute of Scotland. Her medical training was undertaken at the School of Medicine for Women in Edinburgh, Leith Hospital, Glasgow Maternity Hospital, Edinburgh Dispensary for Women and Children and the Richmond Street vaccination station. Her additional experience included a course of lectures on mental diseases by Thomas Clouston, together with attendance at the Eye Dispensary in Leith and the Extracting Room of the Dental Hospital. Within the context of the period this was a comprehensive and rounded training.

110. As an example of 'mixed sources', James Gray studied at the University of Aberdeen for three years, then undertook medical courses at Minto House and Surgeons' Hall, hospital experience at the Aberdeen and Edinburgh Infirmaries, dispensing at the Cowgate Dispensary and vaccination at the Royal Dispensary.

111. RCSEd, TQ Schedules 1910, nos 4685 and 4701.

112. Confirmation by the Russian Consulate in London is complete with a photograph of Belilovsky and a colourful postage stamp for 1 rouble 50 kopeks.

113. RCSEd, TQ Schedules, letter dated 2 July 1920. He asked for an early time for his oral, 'so as not to be unduly rushed to make my steamer at Southampton'.

114. Ibid., 7 February 1888.

115. Vickery, A., 'Golden age to separate spheres. A review of the categories and chronology of English women's history', in R. Schoemaker and J, Vincent (eds), *Gender and History in Western Europe* (London, 1988), pp. 197–228.

116. College Minutes, 12 December 1870.

117. Turner, A. L., *Story of a Great Hospital*, p. 247.

118. Bonner, T. N., 'Medical women abroad: a new dimension of women's push for opportunity in medicine 1850–1914', *Bull. Hist. Med.*, 62 (1998), p. 64. See also Bonner, T. N., *To the Ends of the Earth. Women's Search for Education in Medicine* (Massachusetts, 1992); Dyhouse, C., *No Distinction of Sex? Women in British Universities 1870–1939* (London, 1995).

119. Roberts, S., *Sophia Jex-Blake: A Woman Pioneer in Nineteenth Century Medical Reform* (London, 1993). Jex-Blake's own views are covered in Jex-Blake, S., *Medical Women. Two Essays. I. Medicine as a Profession for Women. II. Medical Education of Women* (Edinburgh, 1872); Jex-Blake, S., *Medical Women. A Thesis and a History. I. Medicine as a Profession for Women. II. The Medical Education of Women. I. The Battle in Edinburgh. II. The Victory Won* (Edinburgh, 1886). Sophia Jex-Blake eventually set up her own medical school for women in Edinburgh.

120. RCSEd, Letterbooks, 27 June 1885.

121. *Regulations to be Observed by Candidates for the Qualifications in Medicine and Surgery Conferred Conjointly by the Royal College of Physicians of Edinburgh, the Royal College of Surgeons of Edinburgh and the Faculty of Physicians and Surgeons of Glasgow* (Edinburgh, 1887 and subsequent editions).

122. RCSEd, Letterbooks, 30 July 1889.

123. EUL, Senatus Minutes, 20 October 1894.

124. RCSEd, Letterbooks, 12 December 1896.

125. Geyer-Kordesch, J. and Ferguson, R., *Blue Stockings, Black Gowns, White Coats. A Brief History of Women Entering Higher Education and the Medical Profession in Scotland, in Celebration of One Hundred Years of Women Graduates at the University of Glasgow* (Glasgow, 1994), pp. 14–18.

126. Admitted on 20 October 1920, Alice Headwards Hunter practised medicine in India for

many years and was awarded the Kaiser-I-Hind silver medal by the Indian Government in 1945.

127. Hull and Geyer-Kordesch, *Shaping of the Medical Profession*, p. 82.

128. Herzfeld chaired the Edinburgh branch of the BMA from 1960 to 1962 and served as the National President of the Medical Women's Federation from 1948 to 1950.

129. Examples of Herzfeld's publications are: 'Traumatic rupture of intestine without external injury', *Lancet*, 1 (1920), p. 377; 'Treatment of burns and scalds by tannic acid', *Practitioner*, 122 (1929), pp. 106–11; 'Injuries and malformations of the newborn', *Practitioner*, 164 (1950), pp. 52–60.

130. Crofton, E., *The Women of Royaumont. A Scottish Women's Hospital on the Western Front* (East Linton, 1997); Leneman, L., *In the Service of Life. The Story of Elsie Inglis and the Scottish Women's Hospitals* (Edinburgh, 1994).

131. Wilson, J., 'Training women for surgical leadership', *J. Roy. Coll. Surg. Edinb.*, 41 (1996), p. 212.

132. For an account of a similar period in Glasgow, see Jenkinson, J. L. M., Moss, M. and Russell, I., *The Royal. The History of the Glasgow Royal Infirmary 1794–1994* (Glasgow, 1994).

133. Bell, J., 'The surgical side of the Royal Infirmary of Edinburgh 1854–1892. The progress of a generation', *Edinburgh Hospital Reports*, 1 (1893), p. 5.

134. Ibid., pp. 6–10.

135. Ibid., p. 16. Bell was careful to emphasise that this referred to serious accident cases, and that appropriate time should be allowed in cases of, for example, operations for tubercular joints, where 'time is well spent in scraping cavities and giving the part a chance of union by first intention'.

136. College Minutes, 5 May 1868.

137. Wallace, W. A., 'Fortnightly Review: managing in-flight emergencies', *BMJ*, 311 (1995), pp. 374–5, describes the author's experience in treating a patient with tension pneumothorax during a long-haul flight from Hong Kong.

138. Gardner, D. L., 'Early twentieth century surgical urology: the 1909–1939 experience of Henry Wade', *The Surgeon*, 1 (3) (2003), pp. 166–76, gives a detailed account of Wade's work in this period on developing the field.

139. For a full account of the more recent past, see Catford, *Royal Infirmary*.

140. Lister's carbolic technique, however, was not approved by all. There is coverage of the debate in, for example, Granshaw, L., '"Upon this principle I have based a practice": the development and reception of antisepsis in Britain 1867–1900', in J. V. Pickstone (ed.), *Medical Innovations in Historical Perspective* (Basingstoke, 1992), pp. 17–46.

141. For more detail on Annandale and the other individuals mentioned here, see Ross, J. A., *The Edinburgh School of Surgery after Lister* (Edinburgh, 1978).

142. Comrie, *History*, ii, pp. 606–7.

143. Keith published a series of articles on his cases, including Keith, T., 'Cases of ovariotomy', *EMJ*, 12 (1866–7), pp. 493–509.

144. It is claimed that this plethora of interests was a factor in Watson's failure to gain the Chair of Surgery at the University. Ross, *Edinburgh School of Surgery after Lister*, p. 13.

145. Ibid., p. 19. Chiene was the first President of the Scottish Rugby Union, for the season 1877–8.

146. RCSEd, GD15/23/48, Sir John Bruce papers.

147. RCSEd, GH15/23/49, Sir John Bruce papers.

148. First annual report in Watson, A., 'Report of the Edinburgh Eye Infirmary by Alexander Watson Esq., Fellow of the Royal College of Surgeons and Surgeon to the Institution', *EMJ*, 43 (1835), pp. 126–36.

149. Of note also is the fact that he delivered the first practical physiology class at the University. Ross, *Edinburgh School of Surgery After Lister*, p. 197.

150. I am grateful to Miss A. B. Sutherland for notes on the emergence of plastic surgery as a specialty, and the role of College Fellows in this area.

151. Dott instituted the Department of Surgical Neurology in Edinburgh, and was awarded the Freedom of the City of Edinburgh in 1962. Lister had been the last surgeon to receive the honour previously.

152. I am grateful to the late Professor James Lister for information on the development of paediatric surgery.

153. Bell, J., 'Five years' surgery in the Royal Hospital for Sick Children', *Edinburgh Hospital Reports*, 1 (1893), p. 3.

154. Ibid., p. 9.

155. Stiles is credited with introducing the first steam steriliser in Scotland in the RHSC.

156. Nutrition was a key political topic in the 1930s, when debate centred on whether children suffered from undernutrition or malnutrition. See discussion in Jenkinson, *Scotland's Health*, pp. 252–63.

157. I am grateful to Mr L. D. Finch, Dr J. F. Gould and the late Professor Dorothy Geddes for providing me with detailed notes on this topic.

158. Quoted in *Centenary Brochure of the Edinburgh Dental School and Royal College of Surgeons Licence in Dental Surgery* (Edinburgh, 1979), p. 1.

159. Menzies Campbell, J., *Dentistry Then and Now* (privately printed, 1981), p. 303.

160. Lilian Lindsay faced the same sort of problems as did female medical students – being informed by Henry Littlejohn that she was 'taking the bread out of some poor fellow's mouth'. Cohen, R. A., 'Lilian Lindsay 1871–1960', *British Dental Journal*, 131 (3) (1971), p. 122.

161. Antecedents of the Dentists Act are covered in Forbes, E. G., 'The professionalization of dentistry in the United Kingdom', *Med. Hist.*, 29 (1985), pp. 169–76.

162. Kaufman, *Medical Teaching*, pp. 143–5.

163. Ibid., pp. 128–44.

164. Geissler, P. R., *The Royal Odonto-Chirurgical Society of Scotland* (Edinburgh, 1997), p. 29; Jenkinson, J. L. M., *Scottish Medical Societies 1731–1939* (Edinburgh, 1993), pp. 185–6.

165. Gould, J. F., manuscript notes on development of oral surgery in Edinburgh, 2.

166. Middleton was a prisoner of war with Sir Michael Woodruff in Chengi.

167. College Minutes, 24 March 1944.

168. Ibid., 20 June 1840. The report was eventually published in 1842 as Chadwick, E., *Report on the Sanitary Condition of the Labouring Population of Great Britain 1842* (Edinburgh, 1965).

169. College Minutes, 11 November 1806; 28 March 1809; 18 December 1810; 2 February 1811; 15 May 1812; 5 December 1813.

170. Ibid., 3 December 1860.

171. Ibid., 3 February 1860.

172. Ibid., 17 March 1860.

173. There is a discussion on the 'enabling or enforcing' question in Finlayson, G., *Citizen, State and Social Welfare in Britain 1839–1990* (Oxford, 1994).

174. There is an account of the controversy in Brunton, D., 'Practitioners versus legislators: the shaping of the Scottish Vaccination Act', *Proc. Roy. Coll. Phys. Ed.*, 23 (1993), pp. 193–201. The Glasgow situation is covered in Macdonald, F., 'Vaccination policy of the Faculty of Physicians and Surgeons of Glasgow, 1801–1863', *Med. Hist.*, 41 (1997), pp. 291–321.

175. Circumstances of the appointment are outlined in Tait, H. P., *A Doctor and Two Policemen. The History of Edinburgh Health Department 1862–1974* (Edinburgh, 1974), pp. 17–18.

176. Ibid., pp. 29–30.

177. For a biographical account of Russell, see Robertson, E., *Glasgow's Doctor. James Burn Russell 1837–1904* (East Linton, 1998).

178. Dingwall, *History of Scottish Medicine*, pp. 167–74, discusses the sanitation approach to public health. See also Crowther, M. A., 'Poverty, health and welfare', in W. H. Fraser, (ed.), *People and Society in Scotland Vol II, 1830–1914* (Edinburgh, 1990), pp. 265–87.
179. RCSEd, Letterbooks, 21 February 1890.
180. Hull and Geyer-Kordesch, *Shaping of the Medical Profession*, p. 52; Cope, Z., *The Royal College of Surgeons of England. A History* (London, 1959), p. 155.
181. Tansey, V. and Mekie, D. E. C., *The Museum of the Royal College of Surgeons of Edinburgh* (Edinburgh, 1982), p. 24..
182. The system was outlined in considerable detail in Cathcart, C. W., 'Classification in Pathology', *EMJ*, 42 (1896), pp. 37–46; 141–8.
183. Greig also acted as College Librarian. At this point the designation of Curator appears to have ceased, thenceforth reference in the records is to the Museum Committee.

# 6

# Five hundred years on — technology, global communication and new horizons, 1948–2005

Without Fellows, we are nothing.[1]

## INTRODUCTION

The last half-century of the first 500 years of the life of the College has seen considerable change in the nation itself as well as in the College's own development. The political countenance of Scotland in the 1930s and early 1940s had been very similar to that of the United Kingdom as a whole and during the early part of the century, a number of government functions were devolved to Scotland, so that there was some semblance of independent government, if not in reality. The landslide Labour victory in the 1945 general election ushered in significant change, and by the early 1960s the political orientation of Scotland was markedly different. From that point the Labour party has been the dominant force in Scottish politics, despite the determined efforts of the Scottish National Party to acquire that role.[2] The coming of devolution and the – as yet – uncertain impact of the revived Scottish parliament have yet to be fully assessed. Many of the difficulties and problems in modern Britain are reflected in modern Scotland, whether these are tackled by Holyrood or Westminster. Scots have been involved in the many armed conflicts of recent times, from Korea, through Suez, to the Falklands and Iraq; Scottish politicians use the politics of healthcare provision as a political end in itself (though postgraduate standards of medical education and training are reserved to Westminster); Scotland is affected by the endless plethora of European directives just as much as elsewhere; the Scottish economy is shaped by the vagaries of the global economy; and Scots suffer from the same health problems as in other parts of Britain, though in some areas much more seriously. The Scottish Executive has declared war on the ill-health of the Scots, setting ambitious targets for improving the statistics on such areas as heart disease, cancer and mental illness – whether these can be met remains to be seen. It is also difficult to assess the Scottish national identity at this point.[3] Many of the factors which currently shape the nation are British and international rather than local, and historiographical

213

analysis of devolved Scotland must wait until a decent interval has passed. What is also clear, though, is that the last fifty-five years of the College's history have been influenced to a much greater extent than in earlier periods by global communication, technology and surgical advances.

At the end of the Second World War, and in anticipation of a new future, the College turned its mind to the directions in which it should – or could – now go, in view of the imminent arrival of the NHS, which altered permanently the role of both surgeon and College, particularly in the organisation and staffing of hospitals, and in restrictions placed on surgeons in terms of private practice. A former President, James Ross, described the resentment felt by some surgeons, who had built up substantial private surgical practices, at the perceived opposition to hard work and individual enterprise which the new arrangements would bring in, as well as the loss of individual freedom which would come with a salaried service.[4] The NHS was clearly the end of an era, but it was also the beginning of a new one.

The second half of the twentieth century was something of a paradox. The College remained fairly independent within the sphere of surgical education, but at the same time was constrained increasingly by the prescriptive nature of training regulations, government reports and attempts to ensure reciprocity of standards and qualifications, while also trying to develop a more modern administrative structure, plan new training courses and build up the candidate base in the UK, Europe and worldwide as far as possible. As medicine and surgery and the peripheral disciplines developed, each of them evolved an administrative structure, and the College sent representatives to sit on an increasing number of boards and committees concerned with all aspects of surgery, hospital organisation, NHS operation and surgical research and development.[5] The political influence of the College has perhaps become rather more diffuse in recent times, and channelled through representation on other bodies, rather than directly on its own account as a corporate body.

This chapter will assess the College in the short period from 1948, looking at the impact of the NHS, the role of the College in education and the pioneering of new courses and qualifications, adaptation to the needs of specialist surgical training and validation, the opportunities afforded by technological advances, the problems of modern management and business priorities, and continued overseas outreach and expansion.

GENERAL COLLEGE AFFAIRS

**Social**

In the aftermath of the Second World War it was perhaps not surprising that the College would turn its attention to more social and domestic matters, in addition to the more serious concerns of the NHS and higher surgical training. It considered designs for a College tie, and the minutes of 13 April 1955 note gloomily that 'the design submitted met with rather a lukewarm reception, and it was decided that a further design should be obtained'. In March 1978, discussions opened on the important question of the laying down of a College wine cellar, and, with an eye to good food, a request was placed in the *Newsletter* in November 1983 for suggestions for a College pudding, which should be 'delightful, light and tasty, to be served at dinners both large and small' (it is not clear whether it 'large or small' referred to the pudding or the dinners). Turning to sporting matters, on 7 June 1985 the minutes recorded mournfully that 'Council noted with despondency that the Royal College of Surgeons' curlers had failed to regain the Chiene Curling Cup, having lost to the Royal College of Physicians by 20 to 11'. This was the case, unfortunately, on a number of occasions, although occasional victories were recorded. Fishing and golf competitions were also organised. More recently the College has acquired its own tartan, in suitably restrained hues, as well as developing a range of merchandise, while on 19 April 1991 came the inaugural meeting of the Senior Fellows' Club, which combines academic and social activities for retired Fellows. Some of these things may appear rather trivial in the grand scheme of College affairs, but they illustrate the wide spectrum of functions of such institutions.

## National

Ever mindful of the need to commemorate national events, the College suspended business on 6 February 1952 on the death of the King, and the President stated:

> We meet today under the shadow of a great national loss – none the less heavy for not being entirely unexpected. The gallant soul of King George the Sixth has passed to an eternal home . . . We thank God that his end, after an illness borne with a fortitude which aroused the admiration of all, and most of all those in closest touch with him, was calm and peaceful.

The College had a long tradition of submitting loyal addresses and messages of congratulation or sympathy to the royal family, and these links would be strengthened by the acceptance of the role of Patron by the Duke of Edinburgh in 1955. In the past, royal patronage was less symbolic and much more practical, but ceremonial links have just as much significance now as they did several centuries ago.

The College had always taken an interest in external affairs and had, for example, supported vaccination, though voicing strong opposition at times to compulsion. It supported the government of the day, mostly, but was not afraid to oppose measures it considered to be ill-judged (any relationship between the College and the current Scottish parliament is too immature as yet to allow proper comment). With an eye to publicity, politics and promotion, Council occasionally invited newspaper editors to lunch, though no specific reasons are given for these invitations.

On the important question of impending devolution, the College took an uncompromisingly negative stance, giving reasons of fear for the future of the health services. In commenting on the White Paper *Devolution to Scotland*,[6] it was stated that:

We could not accept any form of contract from a Scottish Assembly which was in any way restrictive of professional freedom . . . The White Paper appears to be completely lacking in an appreciation of the value of independence of professions . . . We agree with the comment made by the Royal College of Physicians of Edinburgh; as the health services are presently organised, the collaboration between the Scottish Home and Health Department, the Area Health Boards and the Medical Schools, and the three independent Scottish Royal Colleges ensures that the people of Scotland are provided with a higher standard of national medical care than elsewhere in the United Kingdom. We urge the Government to devolve no powers to a Scottish Assembly, the exercise of which might jeopardise the continuation of this satisfactory state of affairs.[7]

Maintenance of professional independence was clearly the crucial concern. On the equally important question of reform of the NHS, the College voiced strong opposition to the Consultative Document prepared by the Scottish Home and Health Department in 1976, *The Health Services. The Way Ahead*. Council expressed concern that 'in the immediate future acute medicine, including all branches of Surgery, was going to be starved of resources for development in favour of geriatrics and provisions for the care of the mentally disordered and physically handicapped.'[8] The document was considered to be 'in the nature of a political tract rather than a reasoned presentation of medical priorities', and Council resolved to express its opposition in the strongest terms.

One event which was initially a College rather than a general political matter, but which had considerable ramifications later, was the donation to the College of some £350,000 by Dr Hastings Banda, College Licentiate, Church of Scotland elder and dictator of Malawi, in 1977. This donation, 'the largest ever received by the College, was greeted by Council with astonishment and delight'.[9] Dr Banda was subsequently awarded Honorary Fellowship of the College on 6 September 1979, and on 6 October 1982 he performed the inauguration ceremony for the new postgraduate residences adjacent to the College (see Chapter 7). By the early 1990s, though, there was increasing pressure on both the College and the Church of Scotland to return donations made by Dr Banda, with headlines such as 'Hastings Banda the Malawi dictator, is welcomed to the palatial home of the Royal College of Surgeons in Edinburgh', which appeared in the *Sunday Times* on 9 February 2003. The College's response was that surgeons from Malawi were currently training in Edinburgh and that Edinburgh surgeons provided expertise to the College of Surgeons of East, Central and Southern Africa, thus making a return contribution. This was one delicate area in an age when all sorts of actions are open to more and more public scrutiny. Large financial donations can become heavy political millstones.

In the more recent past, general support was expressed during the campaign for the compulsory use of seat belts, while the late 1980s saw concern voiced about the burgeoning problems of HIV and AIDS. It was also resolved on 7 October 1993 to ban smoking in the main hall (the next meeting voted to ban smoking in all

College buildings – renewing a ban which had been imposed in the seventeenth century).

### Patron, chaplain and regents

In line with its wish to maintain the sort of high-level connections perceived to be part of the trappings of the learned institution, in 1954 HRH the Duke of Edinburgh was invited to become Patron of the College, and to accept an Honorary Fellowship.[10] This of course was very much in line with the tradition dating from the middle of the seventeenth century, whereby the College had appointed many individuals of public note as Honorary Fellows. At that time these individuals were expected to act on behalf of the College in terms of political patronage and influence. By the middle of the twentieth century, this patronage was perhaps rather less practical but none the less significant. At the present time similar honours are given, mostly, but not exclusively, to medical persons of note. At a special meeting on 3 December 1954, discussion centred on the arrangements for the celebration of the 450th anniversary of the College, but these could not be finalised until the Duke of Edinburgh indicated when he would be able to attend the College in order to receive his Honorary Fellowship.

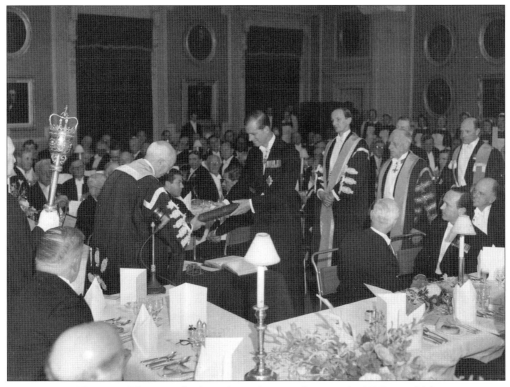

**FIG. 6.1** *Photograph of 450th anniversary banquet in 1955, at which HRH Prince Philip, Duke of Edinburgh, was awarded Honorary Fellowship of the College and installed as its patron.*

One perhaps less predictable but no less historically appropriate appointment came in October 1952, when Dr Charles Warr, the minister of St Giles', was appointed *ex officio* as Chaplain to the College, 'in view of the long association of the College with the Kirk of St Giles'. In the early days, meetings and examinations had occasionally been held in the 'Ile' of St Giles', and even before then, the craft had maintained an altar dedicated to St Mungo. The Reformation changed many things, but the historic link remained and the Fellows wished to emphasise and sustain it. The current Chaplain, the Very Reverend Gilleasbuig Macmillan, was recently awarded Honorary Fellowship of the College, marking twenty-five years' service in this office. The long connection with St Giles' is symbolised in the stained-glass window in the clerestory of the Cathedral.

In line with the College's practice of fostering close contacts with influential individuals from outside the surgical world, it was resolved in 1979 to set up a Court of Regents, consisting of 'persons of distinction who have an interest in and a concern for the Royal College of Surgeons of Edinburgh'.[11] Suitable individuals would be appointed by Council on the advice of the Nominations Committee (which advised on the award of Honorary Fellowships), and Regents would be entitled to wear a special gown. The intention was that the Regents would provide expertise and experience in areas otherwise outwith that of the College. The Regents also assisted with the College appeal during the 1980s, and their activities lapsed following the end of that initiative. It was decided in 1990, though, to reactivate this group, which would henceforth comprise fifteen members, including the three previous Presidents. The Regents provide valuable advisory and 'networking' services, particularly during periods when active financial appeals are underway, offering a very different kind of patronage, but patronage none the less.

## Management, laws and possible mergers

One of the major proposals in the early post-war period was that there should be a combined College to cover the whole of Scotland, and this proposal engendered considerable and at times acrimonious debate. On 19 July 1950, a report was submitted to the College by Mr Keith Paterson Brown, which noted that in the early stages of debate, the College had not been involved directly, but only with the status of observer. The initial proposal had been put forward by the RFPSG for a National College 'on the Glasgow model'. This, not surprisingly, proved unacceptable, and the next move considered was the setting up of separate National Colleges in medicine and surgery, which would, of course, create problems for the Glasgow College, given its binary nature. There were also financial concerns, in terms of the funding of the Glasgow 'sub-college' if it ceased to operate as an examining body, and of the Edinburgh College, which would have expanded responsibilities but no concomitant increase in finances. The College was eventually involved more directly in the negotiations, but the main problem remained finance and the role of Glasgow. In the event, it was reported to the College that 'it is with deep regret that the Committee, after prolonged negotiation, have formed the opinion that it is impracticable at present to form a National College of Surgeons in Scotland. In these circumstances it is felt that the Committee can no longer serve any useful purpose and should be discharged'.[12] This subject may arise again in the future, and was indeed raised during the presidency of Professor Arnold Maran in the late 1990s.

In parallel with this question of merger, in January 1949 John Struthers produced a document entitled 'Some comments on the future prospects of the College prompted by the recent closure of the School of Medicine in Surgeons' Hall and the coming into force of the National Health Service Act 1948'. In his introductory remarks, Struthers expressed the view that the College 'seems at the moment to have lost direction and purpose', emphasised by the closure of the School of Medicine of the Royal Colleges. The College had not itself been directly responsible for organising the teaching in the School, but its physical proximity to the College as well as the participation of many Fellows as lecturers confirmed the close links. Lack of finance had in large part prompted its closure, linked to the dominance of the University as the major initial port of entry to basic medical qualification. The School's inability to provide modern laboratory and other teaching facilities had created in some quarters a detrimental view of the College itself, despite the fact that it did not run the School. The extra-mural schools in Glasgow also closed around this time,[13] and it was considered that the TQ examination would rapidly cease to attract candidates (though in fact it survived till the 1990s as a means of registration for individuals with foreign qualifications who wished to practise in the UK, until these rules were also altered; the last diet took place in November 1993).[14] The Goodenough Report of 1944 was also an important factor here, as it recommended that universities should be the prime centres for medical education.[15] Dental teaching was also available at the University, thus drawing away a further source of student recruitment, and it was considered that the Public Health Diploma would also not survive the short-term future.

Among the suggestions proffered to remedy the situation were proposals that the College should become a centre for the dissemination of the results of research; that the Library could be expanded; that the social activities of the College be developed; and, most importantly, that the College might 'acquire for itself a worthy place in the medical field by undertaking the teaching of graduates in surgery and the allied subjects *on its own responsibility*.' This last suggestion would indeed be the key to the future. It was around this point that the RFPSG went through something of a crisis of redefinition as, according to the recent history of that body, in the period before the Second World War, it had 'signally failed to appreciate the magnitude of the change that was imminent in medical education and practice'.[16] The College may not have failed so signally, as it had been involved in postgraduate education for several decades, but it would have to adapt quite considerably to major changes in medical education.

At an extraordinary meeting of the College in November 1952, a range of proposals concerning the future structure and activities of the College was discussed. These included recognition of the increasingly specialised nature of surgical practice, by means of the establishment of sectional committees to advise on matters pertaining to these areas, with provision to add further committees where necessary, in line with future advances and divisions into new surgical specialties. It was also agreed that a priority should be the establishment of an 'active' School of Graduate Surgery in association with the EPGBM, and that this should not be confined to the Basic Sciences courses, but should also include intensive courses in a range of surgical areas, including vascular, thoracic and plastic surgery. The office-bearing structure of the College was altered, so that there would henceforth be two vice-presidents, elected by postal vote of the Fellows, and also separate posts of Treasurer and Secretary. Further committees were set up to cover Finance, Fabric and Medical Education.

A major external management review was undertaken in the mid-1960s, by which time much executive responsibility had passed to the College Council, allowing for closer control and better planning, but more radical change would require alteration of the laws. By June 1969, concern was expressed about delays in the activities of the *ad hoc* Laws Committee, which had not met for over a year, but progress was eventually made. There were some problems with the Privy Council concerning powers of investment of funds and maximum rates of fees, and the view was also taken that much of the domestic detail currently in the College Laws should be transferred into regulations.[17] The College Law Agent felt that this was important as the terms of the proposed new Royal Charter were such that any future change in the laws would require Privy Council approval. If many of the routine matters were redesignated as coming under Regulations rather than Laws, these could be altered much more easily, without recourse to successive new Charters. An extraordinary meeting of the College was held on 18 October 1977 to ratify the new laws and regulations, and the Supplementary Royal Charter was passed in 1979. Annual College Meetings are still held at which alterations to Laws and Regulations are ratified, but full executive power lies with the College Council.

As a further step towards setting the College on a more businesslike footing, it was decided in February 1987 to appoint a business manager to oversee computerisation in the first instance and then assume responsibility for the management of general College affairs. At this time also the role of the College Clerk was undertaken for the first time by individuals who were not lawyers, including Mrs Wilma Thomson and Miss Margaret Bean, who was the last to hold that office, which has now disappeared into the modernised management structure of the College. In order to streamline operations further, in October 1993 the administrative structure of the College was altered to comprise four Boards covering Education, Examinations and Training, Finance, and Developments.

In July 1997 the College Council approved a document entitled 'RCSEd Business Plan'. This title is, surely, of some significance in indicating the thinking of the College on its activities and its future. The difficulty with institutions of this sort is that they wish to retain their original ideals and activities, but have to do so in a world of business plans, networking, opposition from other 'businesses', local and national government intervention and economic uncertainty. For an institution whose major income comes from examination fees and Fellows' subscriptions, the problems are clear, whether or not the institution achieves charitable status, which in itself results in constraints. There is a trend, increasingly, among large companies to desert their imposing city centre premises and decant to impersonal, but cheaper, 'business parks', in order to reduce some of their spiralling costs. The problem for historic, professional institutions, as opposed to strictly commercial enterprises, is that central urban location and the symbolism of grand buildings are still of importance. Visual symbolism may not be so important as it was in medieval times, where sight and sound took precedence over other means of communication, yet ancient institutions generally still wish to appear 'ancient'. None of the British Colleges has yet given up the symbolic city centre presence of an imposing building. This of course has implications for finance, management and physical distribution of departments within a restricted and unwieldy space (see the further discussion on buildings in Chapter 7).

In the 1997 document, produced as the result of a very modern 'away-day' for College staff, the purpose of the College was enunciated thus: 'The Royal College of Surgeons of Edinburgh is concerned with the education and training for medical and surgical practice and for the maintenance of high standards of professional competence and conduct'. The College motto is *Hinc Sanitas* – from here, health. At this meeting a Fellow made a telling remark, which may indeed be a more appropriate motto for 2005 – 'Without Fellows, we are nothing' (*Sine Societate Nihil*). The document went on to outline a new administrative structure for the College, with power and responsibility devolved to a network of directorates and committees. The strategic objectives noted were: 'to recruit and retain Fellows; to meet the educational and training needs of surgeons at all stages; to achieve financial stability; to improve external relations'. Apart from the last of these, the sentiments are, in modern language, precisely those articulated by the earliest recorded masters of the Incorporation. The implications, though, are very different and much more complex and difficult to achieve. The details of the plan, which included particular attention to IT and electronic media, were peppered with business language, such as 'line management', 'projected costs', 'roles and goals' and sponsorship. This could be any modern business, and herein lies one of the major problems of retaining the particular identity of a historic academic body in a changed, management- and government-dominated world. Perhaps even more important and recognisably businesslike were the decisions to develop a corporate house style and 'improve media and lobbying skills' – the latter had been well honed in the 1850s but now required to be adapted to the modern political scene. There was even a SWOT analysis – strengths, weaknesses, opportunities and threats. The major threat to continuing survival, if not prosperity, was loss of markets relating to overseas candidates, together with devolution and the effects of the European Union on postgraduate qualifications.

Over the last ten or so years in particular, the College has seen a number of radical changes made to its organisational structure. Following the advice of a further external management review in the late 1990s, the managerial structure is now headed by a Chief Executive, who has overall responsibility to the President and Council for the operation of the College. In addition to Council as a body, individual Fellows serve as Directors of Standards, Training, Education, Communication, and as Examinations Convener.[18] Recently the entire gamut of education, training and examinations has come within the remit of the newly formed Careers Department, located in a separate building, the Adamson Centre. This will allow easier access for candidates in all aspects of their surgical training and examinations, from first tentative enquiry to presentation of the Fellowship Diploma.

The practical infrastructure of the College now has separate sections dealing with Professional Business, Careers, Property and Facilities, and Support Services, together with administrators for the faculties contained within the College. Any organisation that wishes to survive in the modern world must have this sort of professional infrastructure, and what has been set up recently would seem to have the potential to see the College through the medium-term future. What this future has in store may be problematic.

As the College enters its second 500-year span, it is no longer possible for such an institution to be run by surgeons devoting part of their time to the College. Individuals who are highly trained surgeons but who are mostly not trained at all in matters of management, finance or forward economic planning are no longer sufficient to ensure the sound future of the College. All that the office-bearers in earlier times had to concern themselves with was that the surgeons conducted themselves in a professional manner, that unauthorised practice was policed and that dues were collected. Matters are very different nowadays. College Fellows are scattered worldwide; the financial and administrative structures are complex; and all of this requires a permanent staff to ensure its operation. Of course the main office-bearers who lead the College and plan its future are still and should still be surgeons. The time has long gone when President, Secretary and Treasurer, changing every three years, could manage all the affairs of the College, but it is right and, indeed, essential that these office-bearers should continue to serve the College in the way that they have done for the past five centuries. The major potential problem with the regular change at the top is that the vision of the College's future may also change radically every three years. In the modern world this is not always practicable.

## Publications

College Fellows had published individually from the middle of the eighteenth century, producing many surgical books and contributing to the growing number of medical journals on offer. This would, of course, continue in the modern period, but it was decided, partly on the initiative of Sir John Bruce, to institute a College journal, and the first edition of the *Journal of the Royal College of Surgeons of Edinburgh* appeared under his editorship in 1955. Most of the medical corporations publish a journal, and such publications offer a further opportunity for Fellows and others to make contributions to the literature on their specialties. The *Journal* operated independently until 2002, when it was amalgamated with the equivalent publication of the RCSI, and is now entitled *The Surgeon*.

In addition to the formal journal, the College has for a number of years issued a regular *Newsletter* to staff, Fellows and members, containing items of news, information on examinations and training, and matters of general interest. In the very recent past this has been superseded by a much more wide-ranging publication, *Surgeonsnews*, which contains short scientific papers and 'second-opinion' responses to published articles, as well as the general-interest items on matters concerning the College.

As well as the formal *Journal* and more informal *Surgeonsnews*, the College has published, or supported the publication of, a series of books on a variety of topics, including books on the College's portraits, furniture and other artefacts, as well as military surgery, Audubon's links with the College, a volume of biographies of surgeons, a history of the College Museum and one of the Royal Odonto-Chirurgical Society.[19]

This eclectic range of publications reflects several of the main functions of the College: to publish surgical papers, to highlight notable individuals with College connections, to describe the College's possessions and to support publications on specific aspects of surgical or dental history. All of this reflects the wish to support surgical science and provide a forum for dissemination and discussion.

## TRAINING – IMPLEMENTATION OF THE CONTINUUM?

Since 1948 the College's role in education has broadened out of all recognition, but at the core is still, in many ways, the surgical apprenticeship.[20] The candidate may no longer live in the house of the master, or be directly under the control of one individual surgeon, but what he or she does in the way of training still owes something to the past. Higher surgical training nowadays follows a pattern of academic education combined with strictly defined and supervised hospital rotations (a very different sort of apprenticeship) in validated posts to cover basic surgical skills and procedures, followed by a period of concentrated and closely supervised experience in the specialty of choice. Candidates are assessed annually and are required to maintain logbooks of the procedures they have undertaken; these are scrutinised during the examination diets in order to ensure the sufficiency of practical experience. Continuous assessment is very much part of the wider educational world these days.

### Postgraduate Board

In addition to its own training functions, the College has been closely involved in the activities of the EPGBM, in conjunction with the RCPEd and Edinburgh University, since its inception in the early part of last century, although relations have not always been perfect. Within the report of the Postgraduate Board for Medicine dated 20 December 1950, there is mention of moves being made towards the establishment of a postgraduate school in Surgeons' Hall, and that negotiations were continuing with the Town Council Planning Authorities, the Lister Memorial Trustees and the University in this regard. A year later it was noted that the architect's plans were under discussion, but by June 1957 matters had not been resolved, and there remained difficulties with the University as well as with buildings. It was agreed that the Lister Trust Scheme should be adopted rather than wait for lecturers to be appointed by the University, which was not likely to happen within the next few years at least. Ultimately, in May 1965, the Pfizer Building was opened, giving better facilities for postgraduate training. The Lister Building opened its doors in 1967, finally signalling the fruition of plans made on the death of Lister. These facilities are adjacent to the College, and ensure close involvement with all aspects of postgraduate training.

Relations among the constituent parts of the Board were not always cordial. In 1966 the College expressed its disappointment when the University made an appointment to the Chair of the EPGBM without consulting the Royal Colleges.[21] This in part stimulated the College to make independent provision, and in the early 1970s it appointed Sir John Bruce as Adviser in Postgraduate Studies, and arranged a series of clinical meetings, all with the earnest wish that the 'health of the College will be nurtured and ensured'.[22] The JCHST, established in 1969 and comprising the Colleges, Specialty Associations and University Professors, was also a focus of College activity, as was the JCHTD for dental training and examinations.[23]

The SCPGME was set up in 1970, and the central British Postgraduate Committee disbanded following the establishment of the three individual Councils for Scotland, England and Ireland. There were close links between the College and the EPGBM during Sir James Fraser's term of office as Dean, which coincided with his period as College President.[24] The establishment of the SCPGME did not alleviate the great concern about the status of the College as an awarding body in the light of the increasing role of the universities in postgraduate education and about the influence of the GMC in all of this:

> It may be accepted that in contemporary postgraduate training the Universities play an increasing part and that as a corollary the Colleges might be unacceptable as the sole recommending body. It was not our impression, however, that the Universities would raise any objection to the Colleges retaining their present role of a recommending body. Furthermore, no case had been made against the continuation of the Colleges in this role and for the interposition of the Specialty Boards. Council felt that the introduction of Specialty Boards 'constituted an irrelevancy' and that the 'Colleges should continue to be the examining body where relevant and the Colleges, through their Specialist Advisory Committees, should act as the recommending body'.[25]

It is clear that the medical corporations felt threatened by a complex of influences exerted by the universities and the GMC, as well as the emergent surgical specialties, and the institution of American-style Specialty Boards would have diluted the corporations' influence further. This was, therefore, a time of some danger for the ancient medical corporations, competing as they had to do in an atmosphere much changed from the climate in which they were born.

## College training

The second half of the twentieth century was a period of intense change and new directions for the College in the area of surgical training, but a strong link to the past came in 1970 when 'it was agreed that the College should appoint a Prosector in Anatomy every six months to make an anatomy of one body per annum for use during the Primary FRCSEd Examination, and that this prosector be called the Monro Prosector in Anatomy of the Royal College of Surgeons'.[26] Even the terminology – 'make an anatomy' – is redolent of sixteenth-century language.

More than ever, though, the focus was forced by outside circumstances (outlined in the previous chapter). It was essential, therefore, that effective communication and co-operation were established with the hospitals and other agencies involved, as it was there where the trainee surgeons would receive the practical training necessary for accreditation as surgeons. It was essential that any approved hospital could provide adequate access to expertise in the full range of basic and advanced surgical procedures, and that the most up-to-date methods were being used and passed on. The College was closely involved in the visitation and validation of hospital posts for this purpose.

On its own account, the College provided representatives to the specialist sub-committees of the JCHST (which was financed by the Colleges and the Nuffield Foundation). Whatever the reality of the situation in regard to collegiate training initiatives, the sense of the College documentation is that suspicion of encroachment by the London College was still very real, and in August 1971 the President, Donald Douglas, stated that Council was 'determined to resist the southward drift and to preserve our ancient right to instruct and examine young surgeons'.

Building on its earlier training provision, the courses and other educational activities run by the College have diversified into many areas. Starting with Basic Surgical Skills courses to support the Primary FRCSEd examination, introduced in 1948, the College's offerings now include many courses or workshops aimed at developing general and specific surgical skills. Training is available in such areas as vascular and gastrointestinal anastomotic techniques, early trauma and critical care, and, more recently, Highlights of Basic Surgery (which is geared specifically towards the MRCS examinations – see below). The Scottish Intercollegiate Board for Standards and Training in Surgery (SIBSATS), under the auspices of the College and the RCPSG, now has oversight of the recognition and inspection of Senior House Officer posts. This body aims to liaise with the JCHST and other agencies to streamline the process of hospital visits and to oversee the work of the

Scottish Royal Colleges Board for the Recognition of Surgical Posts – one body at least which does not easily lend itself to an identifying acronym.

The College also arranges and participates in surgical masterclasses in a variety of topics, and an important area in which it was an active participant was the MATTUS project (Minimal Access Therapy Training Unit, in conjunction with the University of Dundee), which offered training in the techniques of minimal access, or 'keyhole', surgery. It is important that trainee surgeons are trained in the most up-to-date techniques available, and it is also important that examining bodies are aware of new developments and take steps to offer training themselves or participate in corporate training, in order to ensure that surgeons who become Fellows are trained to the highest standards possible in the most modern 'cutting edge' areas of their specialties. In 1993 the College appointed a small group of Fellows to advise on the drawing-up of guidelines for the practice of minimal access surgery, recognising that this was a rapidly developing area which would require close supervision and control, if disasters were to be avoided. The group was led by Professor Sir Alfred Cuschieri.[27] Although the MATTUS project has come to an end, it served its purpose when required – very much in the mould of the temporary College Professors and Professors of Military Surgery in the early nineteenth century.

Further innovations in training in the recent past have included the introduction of distance learning programmes for surgical and dental trainees and the Surgical Skills area of the College website. BASIC, SELECT and PASS courses are all designed to lead the trainee through the core curriculum. They are not meant to take the place of attendance at 'real' courses, but are an important addition to the training armoury of the College. The College Surgical Skills website contains a large variety of interactive learning aids and is widely used and expanding, and the College Library maintains a collection of educational videos and CDs which can be used by candidates as part of their study programmes.

### Virtual reality, the internet and modern surgical education

At the beginning of the twenty-first century, the great new tool for everyone, not just surgeons, is the technology of virtual reality and the internet. It seems, though, that those in charge of surgical training and also, perhaps surprisingly, young surgeons undergoing training, are reluctant to embrace these possibilities too enthusiastically. A recent analysis by a postgraduate student, assessing attitudes to the use of virtual reality training in a group of English hospitals, showed that in general there was reluctance to embrace this technology because, in the words of one trainee, it seemed to be 'Nintendo surgery', and was not widely used or accepted by the surgical world – perhaps in part because it was not a formal requirement of surgical training as yet.[28] The author of the study made the very obvious point that 'cadavers are in short supply and are not reusable',[29] but that is one thing – convincing surgeons that practice on anything other than patients or bodies is useful may be quite another. In the area of minimal access surgery, while training boxes for practice with the instruments are common, the next step towards virtual training may take some effort. There is also the question, if this sort of training method is to be employed, of creating an assessment method to measure the skills acquired by virtual reality practice.[30]

Another recent research project has assessed the value of web-based surgical training, focusing on the field of interventional radiology. This study covered the use of multimedia tool-text, images and videos in order to simulate the clinical situation and these are claimed to be more effective in both training and evaluation than virtual reality.[31] As with most technological approaches to training, this is dependent on current technical possibilities, and the future will depend just as much on technical progress as on the willingness of surgical trainers and trainees to embrace these methods and for appropriate assessment techniques to be worked out. The College itself was involved in the development of a training simulator – the Stirling Simulator – used in multidisciplinary training in resuscitation, and it assisted with the funding of research projects in this area.

In 1999 the College was represented at a conference which considered these matters, and there seemed to be general agreement on the need for improved training and validation to suit the requirements and technical complexities of modern surgery. Papers were given at this event by individuals from a number of non-surgical areas, including a representative from the NASA Space Flight Training Division, who gave a paper on proficiency training for astronauts – the methodology rather than the end product being of interest, in relation to the use of simulators, methods of evaluation and refresher courses.[32] In his general introduction to the published reports of this conference, Sir Barry Jackson, President of the RCSEng, stated eloquently that 'it is no good being able to handle tissue with great delicacy or to make beautiful sutures if you are not sure when and where to do it; equally, it is not much use knowing what needs to be done if it cannot be done skilfully.'[33] One of the major concerns facing all groups and institutions connected with surgical training is the view that clear and objective structures must be put in place for reliable systems of validation during surgical training and subsequent revalidation, whether by peer review or other means. As early as 1982, a candidate who had taken the new Specialty Fellowship in Neurosurgery stated that he was 'reinforced in my opinion that we should all have to requalify from time to time'.[34]

These matters have been aired very recently in *Surgeonsnews*, and the comment of one surgeon in training that 'simulation in surgery is only just taking off – enjoy the ride'[35] perhaps indicates that the tide is beginning to turn in favour of these kinds of training methods.

## Research

Connected to all of this is the essential sphere of independent scientific research as a key part of surgical training. In the 1980s the College established the Lister Professorships, which gave recognition to original research carried out by younger surgeons as part of their training. The first lecture in the series was given by Mr I. H. Thomas, on 12 November 1982, who spoke on 'Caisson disease of bone' (funding had been secured from Johnson and Johnson Ltd to support this scheme). This was carrying on a tradition from at least the 1930s. On 3 February 1932, the minutes note approval of a grant of £100 to a College Fellow to assist him in research on 'metabolic changes in patients suffering from burns and septic infections'. Closer links with medical industry were forged when in 1969 a donation of £15,000 was made to the College for the establishment of an Ethicon Foundation Fund for the 'purpose of promoting international good will in medicine and surgery by means of grants to assist the overseas travel of surgeons and others, or for such other purposes as Council might from time to time determine on the unanimous recommendation of the Advisory Board'. Nowadays the College supports a range of research, including small grants, pump-priming awards, the King James IV Professorships, travel grants and joint Fellowships with the Medical Research Council.

College lectures, colloquia and symposia also contribute to the general exchange of knowledge and opinion and the presentation of research, and a nice illustration of the combination of old and the new can be seen in the titles of two College lectures in 1975, when Mr Philip Caves lectured on 'Cardiac Transplantation today', while Mr M. H. Irving discussed Syme's Amputation.[36]

### Government actions on surgical training

Parallel to all of this, the College was involved not only with implementing the recommendations of government-appointed bodies, but also in giving evidence or participating on commissions through its Fellows. The Royal Commission on Medical Education 1965–8 produced the Todd Report, which concluded that all doctors should be 'specialists in particular aspects of medicine', and that there should be an agreed pattern of training for all specialties.[37] The College was not represented on the Commission but gave evidence. It was shortly thereafter that the medical and surgical colleges began to consider specialist training more closely. It did have a representative on the body which produced the Merrison Report in 1979, which, *inter alia*, emphasised that the career structure for hospital doctors required to be recast in view of its 'obvious defects',[38] and several College Fellows were involved in the enquiry which produced the Shaw Report in 1987 – these included Sir James Fraser, John Cook and Malcolm Macnicol. Among its recommendations were that the Colleges should advise on criteria for SHO posts and on the nature and length of training periods and should co-operate with the regional postgraduate committees.[39] The Calman Report was, of course, of crucial importance to the directions taken by the College and its Fellows, and in 1991 it was again involved, in an enquiry chaired by Dr Kenneth Calman, ahead of the main Calman Report published in 1993. This report concluded that significant changes should be made to the structure and organisation of postgraduate medical and dental education in Scotland, and that a new Scottish Council should be set up.[40] This was followed in 1997 by the Specialist Medical Order, which founded the

Specialist Training Authority (STA) and enforced the keeping of a register of specialists – though this would last only a few years until the imposition of the next acronym. All of this has meant that College training (as with the other surgical colleges) has had to adapt to deal with increasingly prescriptive legislation and recurrent government initiatives, as well as the complexities of modern surgery. A direct link between Calman and the College comes in the person of Professor Sir John Temple, past President, who was closely involved in the politics of reform of surgical training and was appointed by Calman in 1995 'as his special adviser on implementation of the changes to specialist medical training'.[41]

### The future after Calman – the age of the acronym?

The Calman Report recommended sweeping changes to the ways in which surgeons were trained, particularly with regard to the structure of registrar grades, in anticipation of the implementation of the EWTD, and the aim was that better structured and more streamlined training programmes would compensate for the necessary reduction in the time available.[42] 'Calmanisation' is in its relatively early stages, and was part of the background leading to the introduction of the latest acronym. The PMETB was established by the government with a view to standardising the operation of the fourteen medical Royal Colleges. It will now oversee most aspects of postgraduate surgical training, taking over the responsibilities formerly held by the Joint Committee on Postgraduate Training for General Practice (JCPTGP) and the Specialist Training Authority. The College is a constituent member of the STA, which has six representatives from the medical and surgical Colleges, but they must make their voice heard in order to continue to have some influence on the future shape of surgical training. The aims of the PMETB are to improve standards and ensure the quality of postgraduate medical education and training for the modern NHS:[43]

> Through its committees, the Board will draw on the medical Royal Colleges for their knowledge, experience and expertise in setting standards. It will look to the medical Royal Colleges to provide professional members of its visiting panels . . . The Royal Colleges will support the Board by working within the framework and standards which its [sic] has set.[44]

There are clearly challenging times ahead for all of the medical Royal Colleges. The PMETB will have a medical majority, at least at the start, but the six representatives of the Colleges on the twenty-five-strong Board are very much a minority. Though the Board will be influenced by the Colleges, the future of surgical training is, effectively, outwith their direct control. This body and others, such as JCHST, together with the Intercollegiate Boards and Senate of Surgery of Great Britain and Ireland, will shape surgical training, though the restrictions of the EWTD will make it difficult for trainee surgeons to have adequate training time unless some flexibility can be introduced. A very recent concern has been aired in the press, with the claim that surgical training will be reduced drastically, from 30,000 to a mere 6,000 hours. Press reports are often less than reliable, but there does seem to be a concern that this will be too little, unless it is extremely well organised, 'quality' training for the whole of the period in question. In an editorial in the *BMJ* on 21 February 2004, the authors claim that 'to become a competent surgeon in one fifth of the time once needed either requires genius, intensive practice or lower standards'.[45] It was also stated that in a recent survey of consultant surgeons, 'two-thirds would not wish to be operated on by a Calman trained consultant colleague'. This is clearly a time of considerable flux in terms both of national organisation and the recasting of the College's training and examinations.

In the broadest sense, then, the most fundamental activity of the College has continued in various, increasingly complex, forms for five centuries. Given the ways of modern science it is likely that training courses in future will be concerned with computers, robots and other 'inert objects'. It is difficult, though, to envisage a stage at which human surgeons will be rendered obsolete. As technology takes over, though, it will probably be increasingly the case that computer programmers and experts in robotics will take part in the delivery of training as well as surgeons and teachers of anatomy, physiology and pathology. Although no system and no institution is perfect, and although there may be ongoing problems with intercollegiate medical and surgical politics, it may be claimed with some degree of justification that the College is endeavouring to fulfil the exhortations of the Seal of Cause in its most modern form. The days are now past when 'see one, do one, teach one' was the norm. The College is preparing for this, and with the acquisition and adaptation of the Forbes Laboratory (see Chapter 7) to provide more extensive training facilities, should be able to compete on equal terms with similar courses of instruction offered by other Colleges and surgical training centres.

It is historically noteworthy that in a recent article outlining 'the way forward' for surgical training, the College's recently appointed Director of Education makes the telling statement that 'during the foundation year a doctor should be given sufficient exposure to surgery to determine their aptitude for the *craft* [my italics]'.[46] Despite the extreme contrasts between surgery in 1505 and 2005, it can still be described legitimately as a craft.

## EXAMINATIONS

### Fellowship

Just as training was shaped by many external as well as internal College influences, it was the logical and inevitable consequence that examinations would have to change also. Largerly unaltered from the 1880s, when it was reintroduced, the FRCSEd Examination was revised, with the introduction of the Primary Examination in Basic Sciences in 1948 'because of the enormous expansion of the scientific basis of surgery' (see Chapter 5).[47] At about the same time, the question of a specialist register was discussed. It was felt strongly that ultimate certification should be made by the College, though more global specialty advisory committees might be set up. This neatly illustrates the growing dichotomy between the increasing fragmentation and specialisation of surgery and the wish of the College to maintain global rights of validation for all surgical areas. This dichotomy would be resolved, but not in the way that the College wished at that point.

It had been agreed that full reciprocity would be welcomed in the interests of maintaining and standardising requirements, and it was also considered that similar reciprocity of examiners would be desirable. By December 1950 a raft of recommendations had been agreed, including reciprocity with the Royal Australasian College, and the necessary alterations which would have to be made to the laws of the College were outlined in February 1951. By April 1955 some agreement had been reached with other British Colleges on the question of reciprocity of the Part I FRCSEd Examination, but the recommendations showed that a measure of independence was desired by the various Colleges in terms of syllabus, examination papers and external examiners.

Most of the changes in the 1960s and 1970s related to marking schemes and the introduction of MCQ papers.[48] The question of MCQs was surprisingly important, for economic as well as pedagogic reasons, and in December 1970 it was agreed to introduce an MCQ into the Primary Fellowship Examination due to the drop in the numbers of candidates, which was perceived to be in part because there was not an MCQ paper. The introduction of this change was advertised widely in the medical press in view of the inevitable delay in implementing the decision. In February 1971 it was noted that only 36 candidates had presented themselves for the College's Part I FRCSEd Examination as compared with 360 in Glasgow where an MCQ examination was already in operation.[49] This brought the dilemma into much clearer focus than any abstract discussion about the merits of this sort of examination.

Apart from the introduction of MCQ papers (and of interviews for failed candidates), no real change was made to the FRCSEd until the mid-1970s, when the point had been reached at which the emerging specialties could be ignored no longer. It was proposed that candidates for the Part II FRCSEd should profess one of the following specialties: general; otolaryngology; or obstetrics and gynaecology (oral and maxillo-facial surgery would be added in 1985 – see the section on the Dental Faculty below). Clinical and written examinations would be undertaken in the professed specialty, though the principles and practice of surgery in general would still be included in the Part II for all specialties. The Examinations Committee was asked to prepare plans for a new Part I FRCSEd Examination embodying the Principles of Surgery in General as well as the Applied Basic Sciences, and an adviser in each of the recognised surgical specialties was appointed, to prepare plans for a new Part II FRCSEd.[50]

In 1980 the College held a meeting of fellows to discuss the future of the Fellowship and its associated training programmes (against the parallel context of repeated government enquiries and proposals for revision of surgical training). The major issues relative to reform centred around the thorny question of whether the

FRCSEd diploma should be regarded as an indication of full competence to practise surgery independently, or as confirmation of the completion of basic training.
By that point the FRCSEd diploma was a necessary prerequisite to the acquisition
of a Senior Registrar post, though this did not guarantee the practical experience
required for independent consultant status and practice. It was considered that
in the longer term there would be three main areas of development and change:
firstly, the training and promotion pyramid in the NHS would need to be reshaped;
secondly, greater emphasis would need to be placed on continuous and periodic
assessment during training; and lastly, reform of the examinations and clarifica-
tion of their relationship both to completion of surgical training and certification
through the JCHST would have to come about.[51]

In terms of results, there seems to have been a downward trend in the rate of
pass for the Part II FRCSEd Examination between 1960 and 1990. In 1965, 40.7
per cent of candidates were successful, in 1975 the figure was as high as 58.6 per
cent, but by 1995 had fallen to 28.3 per cent. This may be explained in part by the
increase in numbers of candidates (813 in 1965, 724 in 1975, but 1,660 in 1995) and
in part by the effects of specialisation, or unfamiliarity with MCQ examinations.[52]
It seems also to confirm that the FRCSEd Examination was no longer adequate as
a measure of full, independent surgical competence.

In the last ten years, more radical change has been implemented. The AFRCSEd,
or Associate Fellowship, was a short-lived, transitional qualification, offered only
between 1998 and 2000, but what has become fully established is the principle
that validation of surgical competence must come in two stages, the first of which
will henceforth be a Membership (MRCSEd) examination, achieved at the end of
basic training. This will be followed by a Specialty Fellowship at the end of higher
surgical training.

A key feature for most of the period covered by this chapter is the requirement
that candidates for Fellowship examinations must demonstrate that they have
undertaken their training in posts recognised by the College as appropriate. This
started in a small way in 1946 with the requirement that one year of the three-year
training period should be spent in an approved post, and the first recorded request
for recognition of such a post came from Warrington General Hospital in 1949. For
reasons not altogether clear, it was not until 1969 that the first application for
recognition came from a Scottish hospital, perhaps surprisingly not a large city
hospital, but Belford Hospital, Fort William. An extensive programme of visitation and validation of posts is now in operation, in which the College is closely
involved.

### Intercollegiate MRCS – the last barrier?

One issue which has exercised the minds of the College Council for many years
has been the question of the merits and/or possibility of introducing an intercollegiate basic surgical qualification, the MRCS. This would remove the element of
competition among the Colleges on the attraction of candidates, who, of course,

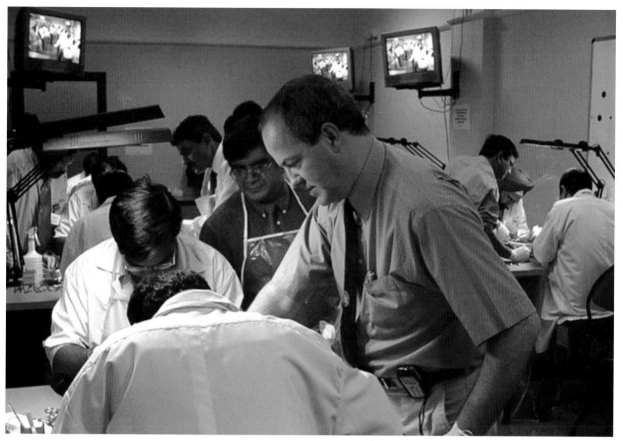

**PLATE 15** *Basic surgical skills course, Delhi, 2003.*

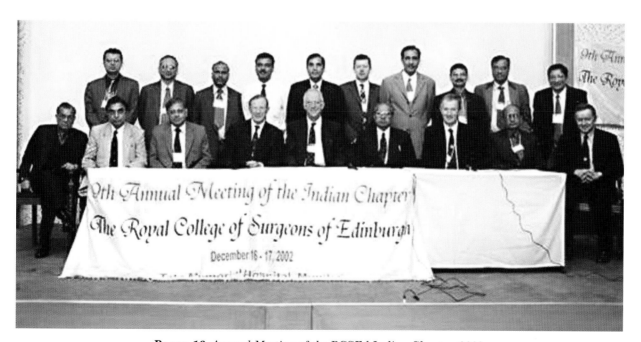

**PLATE 16** *Annual Meeting of the RCSEd Indian Chapter, 2002.*

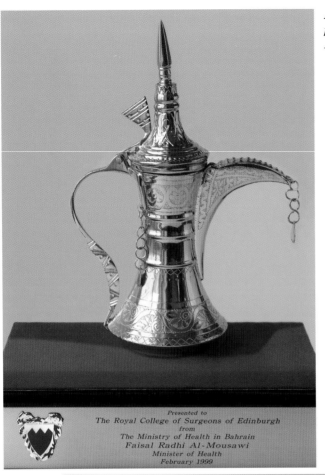

**PLATE 17** *Gift to the College from the Ministry of Health, Bahrain, 1999.*

**PLATE 18** *Gift to the College from the Kuwait Institute for Medical Specializations, 2000.*

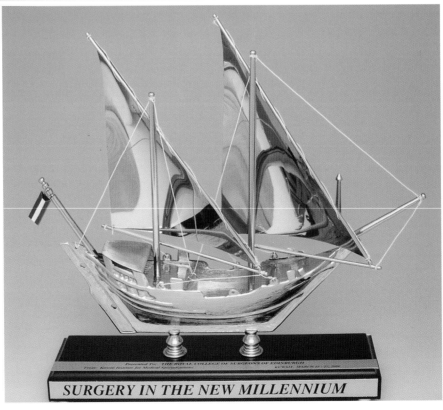

SURGERY IN THE NEW MILLENNIUM

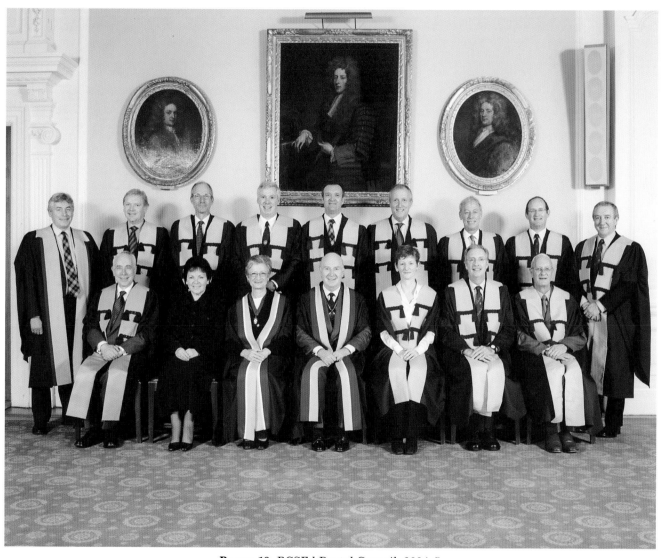

**PLATE 19** *RCSEd Dental Council, 2004–5.*
*Back row: J. F. Montgomery, J. R. Sandy, R. J. Ibbetson, D. J. Birnie, W. P. Saunders, F. J. T. Burke, D. Wray, J. C. Cowpe, J. F. McCord*
*Front row: G. H. Moody (Vice-Dean elect), V. Brown (Administrator), J. R. Goodman (Vice-Dean), J. P. McDonald (Dean),*
*A. C. Shearer, J. W. Frame, R. B. Winstanley*
*Absent: D. H. Felix, M. L. Jones, J. Pirrie, D. R. Thomas*

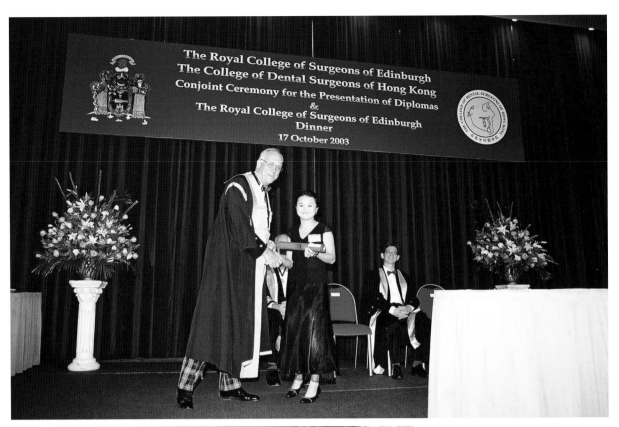

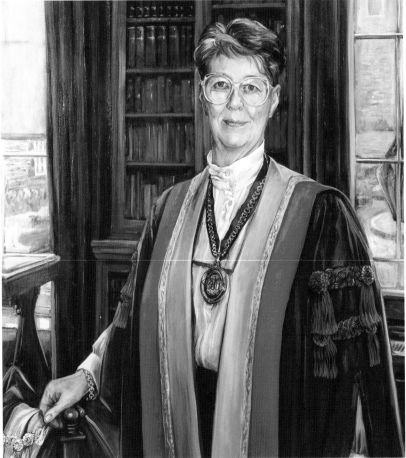

**PLATE 20** *Dental Diploma Ceremony, Hong Kong, 2003.*

**PLATE 21** *Portrait of Professor Dorothy Geddes, first female Dean of the College Dental Faculty and first female dental professor in Britain. (Jane Allison.)*

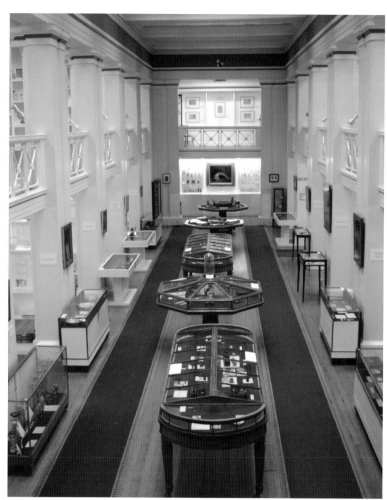

**PLATE 22** *The Pathological Hall of the College Museum.*

**PLATE 23** *The Sir Jules Thorn Museum of the History of Surgery.*

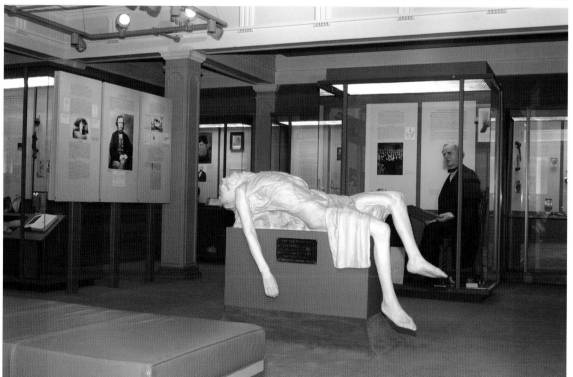

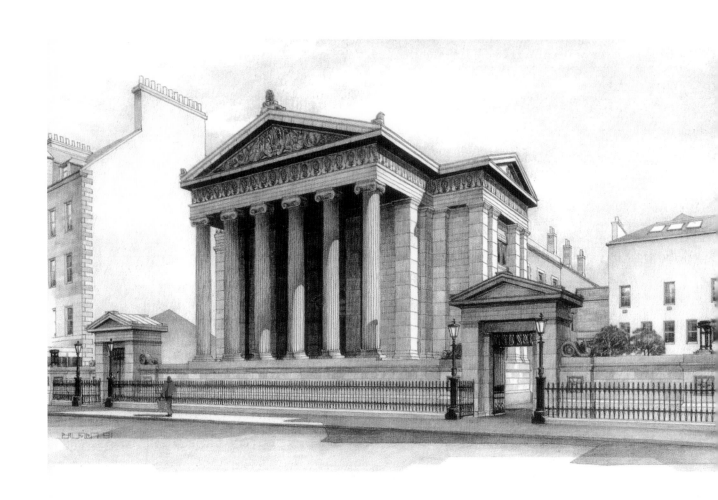

**PLATE 24** *Painting of the Playfair Building by W. J. S. Fulton, 1991.*

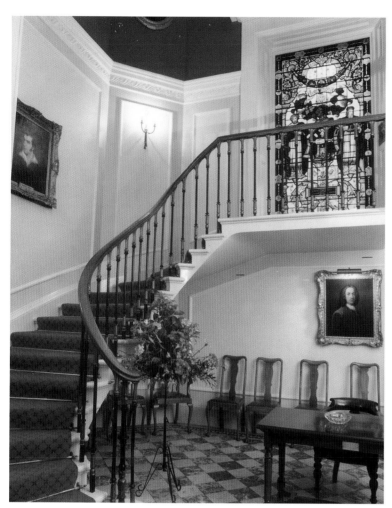

**PLATE 25**
*View of the Playfair Building showing staircase and the stained-glass window installed in 1897.*

**PLATE 26**
*Diploma Ceremony in the Main Hall of the Playfair Building.*

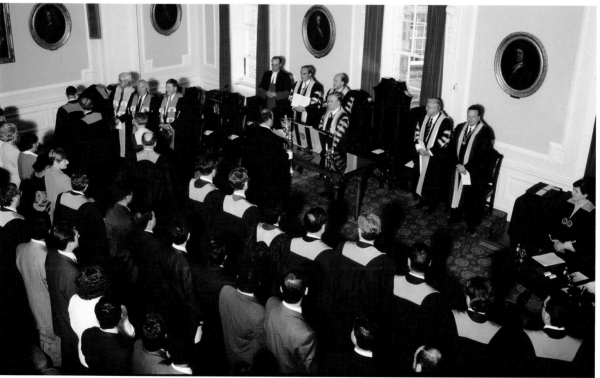

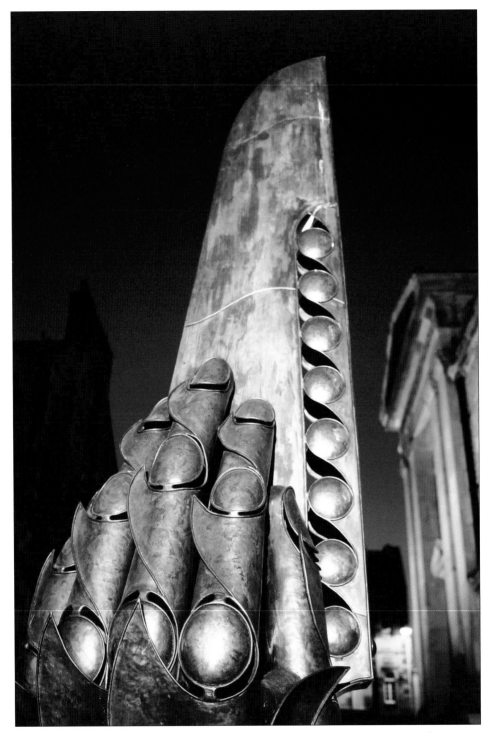

**PLATE 27** *Sculpture,* Hinc Sanitas, *by Denys Mitchell, in the College garden.*

form the life-blood of the financial structure of these bodies. Though Intercollegiate Specialty Fellowships have been available since the late 1980s (see below), with candidates choosing the College of which they wish to become Fellows, there have been considerable difficulties with the establishment of a common basic surgical qualification. As with many of these overtures, the RCSEng has been perceived, rightly or wrongly, as the stumbling block, but agreement has now been reached. In an article in *Surgeonsnews* in 2003, the then President, Sir John Temple, claimed that 'history is in the making', and that after long years of difficult and at times acrimonious relations, 'the four Colleges have agreed in principle the necessary process to establish an intercollegiate basis for the membership examination'.[53] Some of the administrative obstacles have been overcome, and the examinations of all four Colleges will be held on the same date and at the same time, the first examination being held in January 2004. The economic effects on the College remain to be seen.

### Specialty Fellowships and other new examinations

In 1977 the Annual Meeting of the College saw the biggest attendance to date of such meetings, and the main area of debate was the revision of the FRCSEd Examination. It was acknowledged that the College could not go too far alone, without the co-operation of other medical bodies, but it was agreed to introduce longer periods of higher surgical training. The first Specialty Fellowships were introduced shortly thereafter. In a letter to Fellows, the President, Andrew Wilkinson, outlined the proposals, and also indicated regret that the other Colleges had not agreed to proposals to restructure their examinations. It was accepted, perhaps belatedly, that the value of the FRCSEd had diminished in recent times, as in other countries the equivalent qualification was taken at the end of surgical training and labelled its recipient as fully competent to operate as a consultant, whereas the Edinburgh diploma was taken at the beginning of higher surgical training. Proposals had been put forward for a nationwide restructuring of both parts of the FRCS examinations, but complaints were made about the apparent 'loss of unity of purpose' among the Colleges, and the blame for this was laid yet again at the door of the RCSEng. The compromise solution proposed for the College – one that proved far sighted – was to maintain the FRCSEd in its current form, and to introduce a series of Specialty Fellowships, the examinations for which would be taken at the end of higher surgical training. In his strongly worded letter, Wilkinson stated that though there appeared to be some within the profession who would relax the 'stringent standards of practice for which we have successfully striven for nearly 500 years, your Council has no intention of giving way'.[54]

The first of the Specialty Fellowships were in Surgical Neurology (1979) and Orthopaedic Surgery (1980), closely followed by Cardiothoracic Surgery (1982). An FRCSEd in Accident and Emergency Medicine and Surgery was offered in 1982, not as a full Specialty Fellowship but at the same level as those already available in Ophthalmology, Otolaryngology and Gynaecological Surgery.[55] In an article in

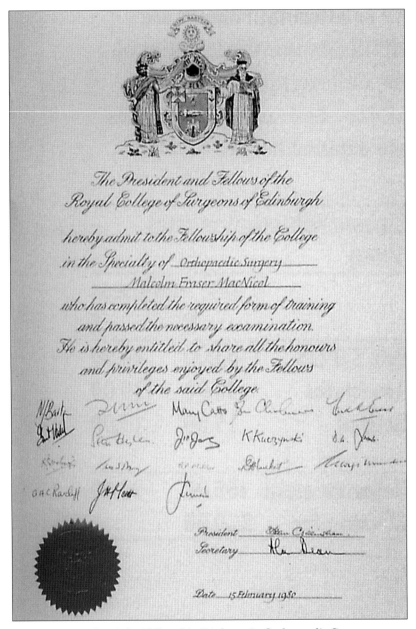

*FIG. 6.2* Specialty Fellowship Diploma in Orthopaedic Surgery,
awarded to Malcolm F. Macnicol in 1980.

the College journal, the Convener of the Examinations Committee, A. C. B. Dean, emphasised that these new examinations would not compete with the work of the JCHST and SACs, but were in line with the aims of these bodies.[56] This move confirmed the FRCSEd Examination as the 'end of the beginning' of surgical training, and Specialty Fellowships would henceforth signal full competence, in conjunction with the necessary acquisition of the CCST under the aegis of the

JCHST. Though the RCPSG had supported the notion of a specialist register to be held by the GMC, it had not yet taken independent steps in this direction, but was quick to participate once the specialty examinations became intercollegiate in nature.[57] It was emphasised, though, that care would be needed with the composition of the intercollegiate boards, so that the Specialty Associations would not have the upper hand.[58]

The geographical origins of the candidates for Specialty Fellowships give some evidence about where specialist training was taking place. A sample of successful candidates in the FRCSEd Orthopaedics Examination between 1979 and 1990 showed that 64 per cent came from the UK and Ireland, 30 per cent from the Antipodes and the remainder from North America. This may not be typical, but it does reflect the key centres of development of specialist training in orthopaedics at the time. Candidates are only accepted for these examinations when they are deemed to have undertaken the full range of required training, and the geographical distribution of the candidates may reflect more advanced training opportunities and facilities in these areas.

Though an intercollegiate path had not been possible at the start, the British Association of Urological Surgeons submitted proposals for a specialist Fellowship and, mistakenly in the view of some, the College agreed to an intercollegiate examination, which was inaugurated in 1987. However, despite any doubts, most of the Specialty Fellowships and Diplomas are now run on an intercollegiate basis under the auspices of the Intercollegiate Specialty Boards.

The College also introduced an innovative Diploma in Sports Medicine in 1991, in the wake of the increasingly professional and scientific nature of many sports; this was awarded jointly by the Scottish Royal Colleges following discussions initiated by the College. This is a good example of scientific progress in one area generating the need for a specialty in another and providing a further opportunity for the College to diversify. This diploma is now administered by the Intercollegiate Academic Board of Sport and Exercise Medicine.

Since its early forays into specialist examinations, the College has introduced a number of new qualifications, including the Diploma in Immediate Medical Care, established in the late 1980s in conjunction with the EPGBM and resulting in a new College Faculty, that of Pre-Hospital Care. The examinations include scenario-type assessments aimed at assessing the core skills required for dealing with medical and surgical trauma, together with coverage of scene management and command and control skills. The majority of candidates are medical practitioners, with small numbers of paramedics and nurses taking the qualification. The Faculty is now about to offer a full Fellowship Examination in Immediate Medical Care.

Rapid advances in communication technology were at the root of the action taken by the College to offer a qualification in Medical Informatics. This is very different from the examinations which test surgical abilities, but would seem to be just as important in the present context. In a relatively short time this has spawned yet another College Faculty, that of Health Informatics, formed in 1998, initially as the Faculty of Medical Informatics, which offers a distance-learning qualification in conjunction with the University of Bath. It is, of course, possible to see this primarily in terms of economics, but innovation would seem to be one of the key requisites for the survival of the College long-term.

Once the specialties were underway, Regional Advisers were appointed in each specialist area, as not all specialties were represented on the College Council at any point. These Advisers also assist surgical trainees working in their geographical areas, as well as informing Council of developments in their specialties which might have an impact on the nature of training requirements and the format of examinations. Though not the first British College to introduce specialty examinations, it may be claimed with reasonable justification that the College was in the vanguard. The key question for historical analysis, though, is whether the College was pioneering in its views on specialty examinations, or whether the consolidation of the specialties themselves forced it into action, in part to try to prevent the proliferation of specialist colleges. In terms of statistics, the pass rates for these examinations have been higher than for the FRCSEd, not surprisingly, given the relatively small numbers involved and the longer and more specialised periods of training undergone by the candidates.[59] Specialty examinations are the way of the future, although 'the model of the traditional British general surgeon has a long and distinguished pedigree'.[60] Perhaps ironically, Surgery in General is a specialty in its own right, though it too may well give birth to system-specific specialties in the future.

### The examinations

When the first candidate recorded in the College minutes took his examination in the early 1580s, all that was required of him was that he answer satisfactorily general questions put to him by the assembled masters at the end of the required period of apprenticeship. A modern examination candidate has to fulfil stringent prior training and supervision requirements, though still has to respond adequately to questions posed face-to-face by examiners. The knowledge required of the aspirant master in the 1580s was restricted and the surgery he could perform was equally limited in scope, but the core aims of the examinations have not changed. In the early eighteenth century, the questions allocated to candidates covered general topics, together with questions on anatomy and prescriptions and, invariably, dressings and bandages. These questions reflected the current state of anatomical knowledge and surgical possibility. Nowadays, though the aims are the same, the questions demonstrate the modern state of knowledge and teaching methods. A few examples will illustrate these points.

When examined in 1712, John Edgar was asked to discuss 'couching of cataract', whereas in the examination held in Chennai in 2001, candidates for the Fellowship in Ophthalmology were asked: 'In cataract surgery, what factors are important in deciding the post-operative refraction to aim for? Discuss the management of unexpected post-operative refractive results.' The aims were the same, but the questions reflected three centuries of change.

In July 1752, entrant master John Balfour gave a discourse on 'modern improvements upon amputated extremities'. Candidates taking the intercollegiate MRCS from 2004 will be faced with MCQ questions such as:

Complications of an above-knee amputation include:
A. Mental depression
B. Sudek's atrophy
C. Myoglobinuria
D. Neuroma formation
E. Amyloid deposition[61]

Amputation is still a major topic, but again the questions are very different. Many similar comparisons may be made, but the point is that the content and scope of the examinations must have a symbiotic relationship with the current state of the 'knowledge' and the requirements of modern surgery. The 'modern improvements' in 1752 were probably concerned with matters of surgical approach and problems of wound healing. In 2004 the coverage is both more scientific and holistic, with consideration of the patient's post-operative psychological state being included at least as a possibility, whether or not it is one of the correct responses.

### Overseas examinations: altruistic outreach or economic necessity?

From the middle of the eighteenth century, the College wielded considerable international influence through its diploma and Licentiateship examinations. During the latter half of the twentieth century this influence took a new direction. Once again, as had been the case throughout most of its long history, the institution depended at least in part on the support, actions and 'patronage' of individuals. In this case, Honorary Fellow P. H. Teng was instrumental in the establishment of the College's first overseas examination centre in Hong Kong. The first diet of the Part I FRCSEd examination took place there 1966, when fourteen of the twenty-nine candidates passed. It was stressed that College 'should not avoid the expense of undertaking examinations in overseas centres',[62] and over the years centres have been established worldwide in many locations, including Bangladesh, Pakistan, Malaysia, Egypt, Saudia Arabia, Sri Lanka and Myanmar, most of which were set up in response to requests from the foreign locations themselves. Among the many College Fellows involved in establishing overseas centres was A. J. Duff, who was largely responsible for the establishment of the centre in Saudi Arabia, where the first Primary Examination was held in Riyadh in 1982.[63] For practical purposes it was also felt that holding the initial examinations overseas would act additionally as a screening mechanism to identify suitable candidates to come to Edinburgh for training, under the Overseas Doctors Training Scheme (ODTS). The Wade Professorship of Surgical Studies was set up by the College to oversee the workings of this Scheme, which relied on individual sponsorship arrangements and a guaranteed

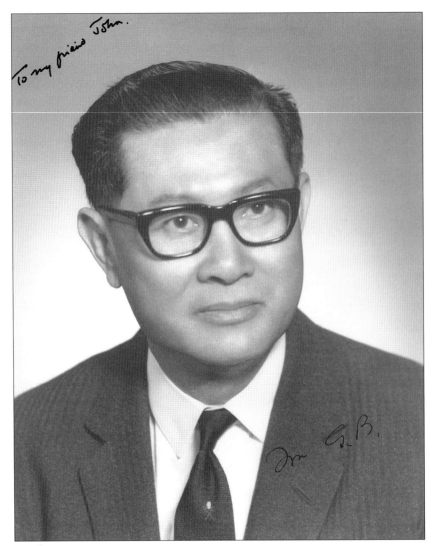

**FIG. 6.3** *Photograph of G. B. Ong, presented to Sir John Bruce. Ong was a key figure in establishing and maintaining contacts between the College and Hong Kong.*

training place for each participant. From 1994 the GMC did not recognise individual consultant sponsorship and henceforth endorsement from one of the Colleges has been necessary in order for applications to be legitimised, while the early 1990s brought in perhaps unforeseen difficulties with the ODTS, as general restructuring of surgical training meant a reduction in the number of available registrar posts. This situation may worsen with the implementation of the EWTD.

Most of the initial overseas examinations were for the Primary or Part I FRCSEd, but in 1970 a Part II FRCSEd examination was held in Hong Kong. This brought immediate opposition from the other British Colleges, and it was agreed that while a special case might be made for Hong Kong, there would be difficulty in mounting final examinations in other overseas centres. In due course, though, a Joint FRCSEd and Joint Fellowship with Hong Kong in Orthopaedic Surgery were introduced, followed by similar qualifications in otolaryngology, paediatrics and urology. On 28 October 1996 a Memorandum of Understanding was signed with the College of Surgeons of Hong Kong, in order to facilitate mutual examination programmes and qualifications. The connections between the College and Hong Kong were strengthened greatly by the influence of the late G. B. Ong, College Fellow and world-renowned general surgeon. A conjoint FRCSEd Part II and M. Med has also been set up with the National University Hospital, Singapore.

Overseas outreach has also produced local initiatives. An Association of Edinburgh Surgeons in Malaysia was formed in 1972, and of the eighty surgeons working in various disciplines in Malaysia at that point, no less than sixty-seven were Fellows of the College.[64] In 1975 College Fellows took part by invitation in a

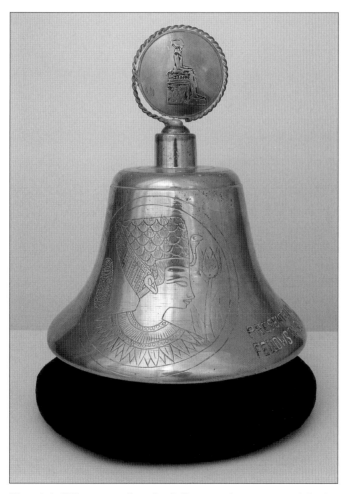

*FIG. 6.4* *Gift presented to the College on the occasion of the first overseas meeting, held in Cairo and Alexandria in 1976.*

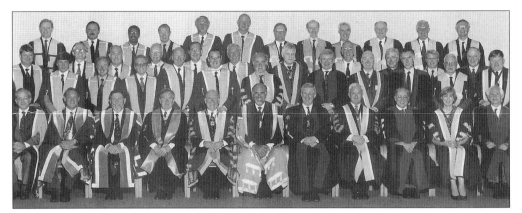

***FIG. 6.5*** *Joint meeting of the Royal College of Physicians and Surgeons of Edinburgh with the College of Medicine of South Africa, 1999.*

basic sciences course in Baghdad, and since then similar activities have taken place in most of the foreign locations at which examinations are held. An Indian Chapter of the College was established in 1976, helped by the influence of Sir James Fraser and subsequent College Presidents and office-bearers. The Indian Chapter organised the first Part B and C FRCSEd examination in India in December 1999 (from 1990 the FRCSEd was divided into Part A and Parts B and C), and it currently hosts a variety of College examinations in various cities, as well as mounting basic skills and other courses.[65]

As well as holding examinations and running courses overseas, the College has travelled abroad for a number of clinical and scientific meetings. The first of these took place in Cairo and Alexandria in 1976 and is regarded as a milestone in the process of raising and maintaining the international profile of the College. Subsequent meetings have been held in various global locations. The exchange of gifts is a feature of international contacts, and the College has received many distinctive gifts over the years.

Most of the other British corporations now hold examinations and training courses overseas, and, increasingly, foreign locations are providing their own surgical training, and setting up their own surgical organisations. That is not to say that the future of the College's overseas programme is in jeopardy. Courses and examinations will continue to be held in these areas, though the nature of these may change in the light of electronic and technological advance.

## WHAT DID THE SURGEONS DO?

### The twentieth-century general surgeon

Until after the end of the Second World War at least, the general surgeons, the main 'product' of the College in terms of the practical working lives of its Fellows, were the typical surgeons of the day. They were truly general surgeons, in that

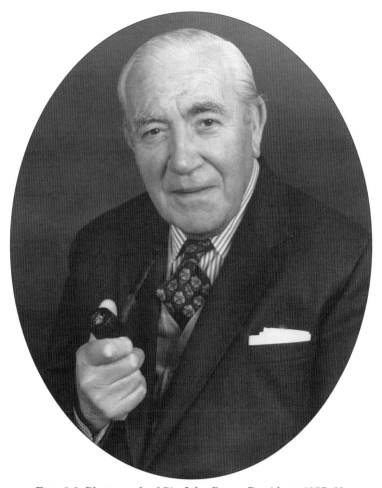

*FIG. 6.6* *Photograph of Sir John Bruce, President, 1957–62.*

they performed the full range of surgical procedures, turning a ready hand to any-thing from an ingrowing toenail to complicated abdominal surgery.

This situation could not last indefinitely. In the post-war years, and with surgery now bathed in the comfort of antibiotics, surgeons were able to develop more advanced and complex surgical techniques, helped by technology, laboratory sciences and the proliferation of the paramedical professions. It would take several decades before computers would play much of a role, and also before minimal-access surgery began to revolutionise certain areas of surgery, but the time was rapidly approaching when one surgeon quite simply could no longer be an expert in the full range of surgical techniques.

One example to represent the many thousands of truly general surgeons produced by the College is Sir John Bruce, who rose to become a knight of the realm and royal surgeon as well as President of the College, Regius Professor of Clinical Surgery and one of the foremost British surgeons, in addition to a distinguished war record. Bruce operated in Edinburgh for many years and evidence of his eclectic surgical interests

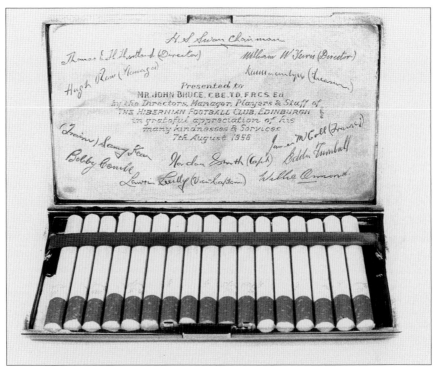

**FIG. 6.7** *Signed cigarette case presented to Sir John Bruce by the Hibernian Football Club, of which he was President.*

comes from the papers he wrote and collected. Bruce wrote papers on breast cancer, stomach surgery, abnormalities of the foot and congenital dislocation of the hip, as well as a number of more philosophically orientated articles on the rationale of surgery and the best methods of surgical training. He collected papers published by others on a similarly wide range of subjects, as well as being involved, during his term of office as President of the College (1957–62), in matters of surgical training, particularly in the late 1960s and early 1970s, when serious concerns were being aired about the relevance and adequacy of surgical training in the modern era. Bruce was surgeon to Hibernian Football Club, and also served as its Chairman, and a sign of the times is seen in the gift made to Bruce by the Club of a silver cigarette case. It bore the engraved signatures of members of the team and club officials, but betrays continuing ignorance of the dangers of its contents. Indeed, many Fellows were photographed on formal occasions with a cigarette as a 'normal' part of the presentation.

Though the College minutes rarely make direct reference to matters of practical surgery, it was noted on 29 July 1958 that 'the President should consult the Lord president of the Court of Session about the legal aspects of obtaining human tissue for grafting and the methods of influencing public opinion'. It was also remarked that Sir Michael Woodruff and Andrew Wilkinson would submit comments on the report by the British Paediatric Association on renal transplants in children. In his

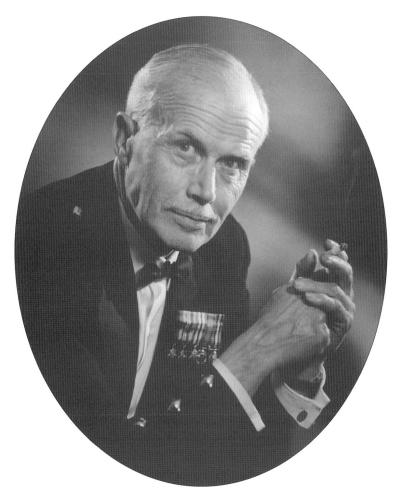

***FIG. 6.8*** *Photograph of J. R. J. Cameron, demonstrating the acceptance of cigarettes in formal portraits at the time.*

autobiography, Woodruff described the first renal transplant operation in Britain, which took place at the RIE, and stated that 'for a newcomer to have any chance of getting renal transplantation off the ground in conservative Edinburgh it was important that our first case should be a resounding success'.[66] Woodruff's pioneering work on transplantation cannot be overestimated.

On 14 July 1961 it was reported that a questionnaire on the current techniques and use of surgical diathermy had been undertaken and that discussions were ongoing about the use of such equipment. The College was also involved in discussions with the Scottish Home and Health Department on the building of operating theatres. Perhaps surprisingly, though, and this was the case right through its history, there is little material in the records relating to a corporate view on particular surgical techniques or advances. The slant taken is usually to discuss the consequences for the College in terms of its training or examinations rather than the techniques for their own sake. The Developments Committee did, though, express 'considerable concern regarding the development of so-called medical gastroenterology and the transfer of endoscopic procedures to physicians'. There was the great danger of the 'surgeon being regarded merely as the final technician or the doctor responsible for the management of emergency conditions'.[67] Demarcation disputes did not end in the seventeenth century.

### The surgical specialties in the later twentieth century

As discussed, signs of surgical specialisation came early in the twentieth century. During the last fifty years much more rapid change has taken place, and in order to set the College and its Fellows in context, it is necessary to look briefly at some of the major specialist areas. *What follows is a representative selection only*, with the primary purpose of illustrating the role of the College in these areas rather than that of the surgeons or their technical innovations. Other areas of surgical specialisation are included by implication in the general conclusions. The process here was influenced by continuing and new features, the latter including much greater technological opportunity, the establishment of specialist wards in hospitals and the consequent and parallel changes to surgical training requirements. There is an obvious problem with naming individuals within the memory span of current Fellows, as accusations of omission or wrongful inclusion are unavoidable. Consequently, very few individual Fellows are named here – the purpose is to highlight general College influences – and it is hoped that the few Fellows who are named will be seen as representing these influences and not singled out primarily as individuals, though, of course, there were many pioneering College Fellows in all parts of the world and in all surgical specialties by this time. The College has always been wary of any of its Fellows being singled out as *primus inter pares*.

Many Fellows were pioneers in the development of urological surgery. Sir Henry Wade, though a typical general surgeon, had been recognised as an expert in urology, producing a seminal paper on prostatic obstruction in 1913, and this was followed by many other publications on urological topics. Successive Fellows have continued the link between the College and the developing specialty. Fellows were also to the fore in the British Association of Urological Surgeons (1945), founded in 1945. David Band and Geoffrey Chisholm were awarded the St Peter's Medal of the Society; Band was President of the Association from 1959 to 1961, and Chisholm from 1986 to 1988, while Sir Henry Wade was one of its first honorary members.[68] Specialty Associations were an important focal point for contact with and potential influence of the main medical corporations.

In orthopaedic surgery, major stimuli were war, epidemic disease and congenital malformations. As mentioned, Harold Stiles was involved in orthopaedics in the EMS Hospital at Bangour in West Lothian,[69] and many Fellows had included orthopaedic procedures in their range of operations as general surgeons. Though Walter Mercer was one of the early specialists, he was still the epitome of the early-twentieth-century general surgeon. In an oration in the *Journal of Bone and Joint Surgery* in 1956 it was said that he could 'nail a fractured neck of the femur more quickly than others; but he can also divide a stenosed mitral valve, resect a lung, or remove a brain tumour' – though it was stated also that he had not 'dibbled and dabbled' in these fields of surgery all at once but had progressed through abdominal surgery, then chest surgery, then neurosurgery and, lastly, orthopaedics.[70] This confirms the transitional nature of the specialists emerging out of the background of general surgery.

William Cochrane, one of the first full-time orthopaedic surgeons in Scotland, was succeeded by Mercer. This, combined with the fact that a Chair of Orthopaedic Surgery had been established at the University of Edinburgh in 1948, stimulated development of the specialty and the specialist training of surgeons. The combination of academic and hospital orthopaedics[71] in most major centres was important in allowing close links between university research and its application. Over the years sub-specialties have evolved in spinal deformity, knee surgery, hand surgery, rheumatology and paediatric orthopaedics. Orthopaedic procedures had invariably appeared as College examination topics and, while amputation was the main procedure examined in early times, this was just as much of a specialist procedure in its day as, say, carbon fibre replacement for ruptured cruciate ligaments is nowadays.[72] The eradication of crippling diseases and the early detection of congenital deformities has changed the face of orthopaedics (and, consequently, orthopaedic examinations). Outside Edinburgh, the major contributions of Fellows such as Sir Robert Jones enabled the influence of the College through its Fellows to widen well beyond the borders of the country as well as the city.

Plastic surgery is another area where the effects of war were considerable. In the post-1945 era, the former EMS hospital at Bangour served as the focus of the specialty until the Unit was moved to St John's Hospital at Livingston in 1990.[73] (This pattern of developing EMS burns units for a post-war role as regional centres was typical of the country as a whole at this time.) As with other specialties, the emphasis was increasingly on training in combination with new science (in areas such as the treatment of the potentially fatal shock associated with severe burns).[74] By 1967, plastic surgery had been incorporated by the JCHST as one of the nine specialties, and significant contributions were made by Fellows at home and abroad.[75] The first diet of the intercollegiate Specialty Fellowship was held in 1986. As with orthopaedics, sub-specialties, particularly hand surgery, have emerged, and there is nowadays considerable public demand for cosmetic surgery, perhaps a rather more controversial aspect of the specialty. All of these will continue to modify the relationship between the College and the specialty in terms of the range and scope of training and examinations.

Similar forces were in operation in cardiothoracic surgery, though complex procedures took a little longer to become safe, given the problems of opening the chest and exposing the lungs to atmospheric pressure.[76] Cardiac surgery required considerable technological advances before it could become 'routine' in any form. The first successful pneumonectomy for lung cancer was performed in 1933, and since then techniques have advanced to the stage where it is now possible to remove a whole lung using 'keyhole' surgery.[77] The nature of thoracic surgery has changed considerably since the eradication of tuberculosis, and cardiac surgery has evolved in line with the technology of heart-lung machines, and cardiac transplantation is now almost a routine procedure.[78] This was one of the first specialties to have a Specialty Fellowship Examination, and once again College Fellows have been involved in developing pioneering techniques in this area in most parts of the world.[79]

In neurosurgery the early specialisation discussed in the previous chapter continued, and the legacy of Dott was the flourishing of neurosurgery in Edinburgh and elsewhere. The computer age has been of considerable significance here, in areas such as diagnostic investigations, stereotactic surgery, the precise location of brain tumours, and treatments for conditions such as Parkinson's disease, in addition to, of course, brain and spinal injuries. The establishment of a Department of Clinical Neurosciences in Edinburgh strengthened the essential link, seen in most specialties, between hospital and academic aspects.[80]

Similar influences can be seen in all of the other specialty areas, including ENT and gynaecological surgery, and a clear pattern emerges, so that the role of the College in relation to the surgical specialties generally took the form of a progression through: recognising that the scope of particular surgical areas was expanding to the extent whereby the general surgeon could no longer operate in all surgical areas; offering specialist options within the FRCSEd qualification; offering a full Specialty Fellowship, supported by appropriate training and examinations; providing support for research and publication; and gaining representation on specialist bodies. These patterns were shaped by a complex combination of influences in terms of both initiative and reaction. Whereas the major influence on the surgical activities of the College in the nineteenth and early-twentieth centuries was the medicalisation of hospitals and the opportunities offered by anaesthetics and antiseptics, and the growing role of national government, key stimuli in the very recent past have been technological advance and the efforts to streamline and recast higher surgical training, in addition to the more practical and scientific features of modern surgery, not to mention the effects of European legislation. What was also important is that many of the emerging specialist surgeons held university chairs in all parts of the UK and abroad, and several also served as College President, enabling a close network of reciprocal influences to be strengthened.

## THE DENTAL COUNCIL AND FACULTY

Though dentistry had long been part of the work of individual College Fellows, and indeed may be cited as the first College specialty, it was not until the 1950s that a separate Dental Council was established within the College. There were dental representatives on the College Council, but in July 1952 discussions opened on the question of whether there should be a Dental Council within the College, or a Dental Faculty, the view being expressed that the dentists wished to have a fuller role in the life of the College. There was, at that time, a well-established tradition for individuals to become qualified in both surgery and dental surgery, and there was provision for FRCSEd candidates to be examined in dental surgery as an option in the second part of the examination. There was therefore a distinctively surgical flavour to the higher levels of the dental profession, and this would prove to be of some significance in the area of oral and maxillo-facial surgery. A major factor had been the necessities of the Second World War – as with many aspects of medicine and surgery – and by the end of hostilities most of the dental pioneers held the HDD RCSEd diploma, including individuals such as Norman Rowe and H. C. Killey, whose *Fractures of the Facial Skeleton* is regarded as the seminal text on this area.[81]

As with most major changes to the structure and functions of the College, it was deemed necessary to consult legal opinion, and the view of counsel was that it would not be possible to set up a Dental Faculty without altering the laws of the College. It was decided in the first instance to establish a Dental Council, and discussions were entered into on the detail, such as library privileges to be granted to members, and the design for an academic gown – visual symbolism had clearly not lost its importance.

The first meeting of the Dental Council took place on 26 February 1954, chaired by the College President, Sir Walter Mercer. Mr F. G. Gibbs was elected as first Convener, and Mr W. Russell Logan appointed Secretary to the Dental Fellows. Within a fairly brief space of time the Convener of the Dental Council became an *ex officio* member of the College Council,[82] and representatives were nominated to serve on a variety of boards on behalf of the Dental Council.[83] Ever mindful of history, a lecture and dinner were arranged to mark the bicentenary of James Rae, in 1963.

As with the College itself, the Dental Council was involved fairly early in its life in government-appointed enquiries into dental staffing and training. In August 1963, for example, a memorandum was submitted to the Shiach Committee on Dental Staffing in Scotland.[84] Similar contacts would be made in the future as the dental wing of the College became inextricably entwined in the mesh of government enquiry, legislation and restructuring in the same way as the surgical side.

Relations with the College Council were not always cordial. There were problems concerning matters such as the voting rights of dental Fellows at College meetings; there was a lukewarm response to the request for the inclusion of a dental section in the College journal; and considerable disquiet was voiced when in 1974 the College expressed the view that oral surgery should be the province of higher surgical training, and not higher dental training.[85] Relations with Glasgow were rather more cordial. The RCPSG set up a Dental Council in 1967[86] and joint meetings between the Edinburgh and Glasgow Dental wings began in 1968.

Throughout the 1970s the Dental Council concerned itself with the difficulties involved in setting up and arranging examinations, training and supervision, with continued friction with the College about who should have oversight of training for oral surgery. The major areas of concern demonstrated by a survey of the minutes of the Dental Council from its inception mirrored very closely those of the College in general, and related to matters of examinations, relations with other Colleges, the element of competition for candidates, and the beginnings of the overseas examination centres. In April 1970, for example, there was detailed discussion on the implications for dentistry in the recommendations of the Royal Commission on Medical Education, and a sub-committee was set up to deal with questions from the GDC on this area.[87]

Relations with the College Council did improve to the extent that by 1982 the recommendation was made that the Dental Council should be renamed the Faculty of Dental Surgery and the term Dean should be used instead of Convener of the Dental Council. It was resolved that 'that the College shall have a Faculty of Dental Surgery which shall consist of Fellows and Associate Members in Dental Surgery; the Convener of the Dental Council shall be Dean of the Faculty of Dental Surgery ex officio'. This was approved by College Council on 2 December 1982, and thus came into being the Dental Faculty, which has since then been organised on very similar lines to the College itself.

It is also, perhaps, a measure of the perceived importance of the dental arm of the College by 1998 that the then President, Arnold Maran, chose to address the Dental Council on matters concerning the College as a whole, not just its dental wing. The thrust of his message was that it would be crucial henceforth for the College to develop 'niche marketing', particularly in three areas, which were Dental Surgery, Pre-Hospital Care and Informatics – all of which now have their own Faculties within the College.

Just as the Dental Faculty was finally established, though, serious implications for the future of dental surgery in Edinburgh arose, with the threat of possible closure of the Dental School at the University of Edinburgh. This, combined with the new legal requirements of the EEC, meant a period of considerable uncertainty for the dental side of the College. There were plans for a new dental hospital and postgraduate institute, but the Dental School closed in June 1994 before these arrangements could be implemented. The Edinburgh Dental Institute eventually opened in late 1998, with responsibilities for postgraduate dental education and training, in which the College has a part to play.

## Dental teaching and examining

In line with the general educational aims of the College and its focus on offering comprehensive postgraduate training, the Dental Council resolved in April 1954 to organise a preparatory course for second part of the FDS RCSEd Examination, despite some objections. There were significant problems in attracting sufficient numbers of students for these courses, but the need for such training seems to be confirmed by the fact that in May 1955, it was noted that all candidates had failed the anatomy part of the Part II FDS examination.[88] The numbers taking the courses gradually built up over time, and, as with the surgical side, these courses are now an integral part of the work of the Dental Faculty. Concern was expressed that progress in the dental specialties was not as fast as that in the surgical specialties, and consideration was given to measures which could be taken to remedy this situation. The closure of the Edinburgh Dental School made practical training opportunities and examination arrangements difficult, and in line with general trends towards distance learning, the Dental Faculty introduced learning packages for the MFDS/MFD RCSEd examinations, the current acronym for which is PASS (Prepare and Study Successfully). These proved to be a popular innovation and economically beneficial to the College.

Most of the concerns of the Dental Council in the early years related to examination regulations and organisation, and by 1956 it had been agreed that individuals who had obtained the HDD RCSEd before 1936 should be admitted FDS RCSEd without examination, and a fair number took advantage of this over the years. There were problems with the College, which initially rejected the Dental Council's list of potential recipients of the FDS RCSEd without examination, claiming that these awards should be given in the same way as Honorary Fellowships, to individuals already fully qualified and in senior posts. There was no minuted response to this, but matters seem to have been settled as there are regular mentions of recipients of the award thereafter.

The first FDS RCSEd examination had taken place in 1949, and was originally divided into two parts covering all aspects of dental surgery. Shortly afterwards, the question of reciprocity of examinations arose along with a proposal for reciprocity of the primary examination.[89] This was eventually achieved among the British and Irish Colleges in 1969.[90] The FDS RCSEd continued in very much the same form until 2002 (the last diet was held in Bahrain in December 2002), when it was replaced by a more flexible and specialised examination structure, based on an initial Membership Diploma, followed by a Specialty Fellowship. From 1997, candidates for the FDS RCSEd qualification had taken an intercollegiate first examination, followed by an examination for entrance to the College to which they wished to belong.

The intermediate Membership qualification for dental surgery and dentistry (MFDS/MFD RCSEd) has become partly intercollegiate, the first diet taking place in 1999. The third part of the three-part examination is still collegiate, giving individual college affiliation at that stage. At the end of higher dental training, candidates take a Specialty Fellowship by assessment as a mark of competence. In this way, as with the surgical side of the College, the initial examination signifies completion of basic training and the Specialty Fellowship the culmination of higher training and full competence to practise in the candidate's chosen specialty area. All of this, of course, has to comply with government rules and European requirements.

### The dental specialties

Several factors combined to induce the Dental Council, and later Dental Faculty, to pursue the issue of specialty examinations. These included the growing requirements of oral surgery (most oral surgeons tended to qualify in both surgery and dentistry, and from the early 1990s this was a requirement), the technological advances in areas such as restorative dentistry, orthodontics and paediatric dentistry and, of course, the more general background factors such as the effects of fluoride and the increasing market for cosmetic dental procedures, as well as the scientific context. The technology of dentistry was just as significant as the technology of surgery in acting as stimulus towards new methods of training and new kinds of examinations.

The growing significance of oral and maxillo-facial surgery (OMS) – coupled with the setting-up of a specialist unit in the RIE and the need for general surgical as well as dental expertise – prompted the Dental Council to approach the College with a proposal that a Part II FRCSEd examination in OMS be established. A Specialty Advisory Board was created and the first examination took place in January 1985, eighteen of the twenty-two candidates being successful. This high pass rate is not surprising, given that the specialty examinations are taken at the end of higher training, and thus the level of competence and experience is commensurately high and the field of candidates already filtered by the earlier, intermediate examinations.

All the way through, both College Council and Dental Council minutes reveal suspicion as to the real motives of the RCSEng. In the mid-1980s there was particular concern when the RCSEng converted its FDS examination to a specialty examination.[91] This spawned much discussion and debate about the future of the Edinburgh dental examinations. The reduction in time after graduation before eligibility and, more importantly, the intention of the RCSEng to become more involved overseas in areas which had 'traditionally been within the sphere of the Edinburgh College' were also worrying moves. It was perhaps not surprising, then, that a few years after the introduction of the new OMS examination, the RCSEng brought in its own examination directed at OMS trainees, the requirements for which were 'considerably less stringent' than those of the College. The College weathered this particular storm, and eventually OMS was fully incorporated into the ambit of the JCHST and JCHTD. It may be that at times the perceived threat from London has been exaggerated, but it has been a concern since the eighteenth century, and will be slow to change.

Over the last three decades the College has offered a proliferation of specialty dental examinations, including:

- Diploma in Restorative Dentistry (1978), superseded by MDS RCSEd in Restorative Dentistry (1993)
- Diploma in Orthodontics (1987), superseded by MDS RCSEd in Orthodontics (1989)
- MDS RCSEd in General Dental Surgery (1990)
- Conjoint MDS RCSEd in Restorative Dentistry with Hong Kong (1996)
- MDS RCSEd in Paediatric Dentistry (1998)
- MDS RCSEd in Surgical Dentistry (1999)
- MDS RCSEd in Oral Surgery (2000)
- MDS RCSEd in Oral Medicine (2000)
- Diploma in Dental Hygiene (2001)[92]

Most of these new qualifications have been introduced in the very recent past, reflecting rapid advances in the science and technology of these areas. There are also Specialist Advisory Committees for Dental Public Health, Oral and Maxillo-facial Surgery, Orthodontic and Paediatric Dentistry and Restorative Dentistry, on which the Dental Faculty is represented.

By the turn of the twenty-first century, as with surgery, the Dental Faculty is in the process of restructuring its examinations to meet the needs of modern dentistry, training and specialisation. The FDS RCSEd examination has been phased out, to be replaced by Membership and Specialty Fellowship diplomas. The College Specialty Fellowships will, therefore, be available to any individual who has completed specialist training and is in possession of a Membership Diploma in that specialty. Arrangements are also being made for those trained overseas to have the opportunity to enter for Specialist Membership Diplomas. These new examinations are designed to provide the best proof of competence in a world of much advanced and increasingly technological dental surgery. The general context is, of course, important here, not least the balance of time required to be spent by the practitioner between treatment of dental caries and the provision of orthodontic and cosmetic treatments, particularly in the light of improvements following fluoridation, however controversial that might have been. Better general dental heath has the natural consequence of reshaping the work of dental practitioners[93] and by extension the scope of College training and examinations.

Just as the main College examinations have reached many parts of the globe, with the foundation of overseas examination centres, so the Dental Faculty is now offering candidates in Amsterdam, Bahrain, Hong Kong, Chicago, India, Singapore and Egypt the chance to take examinations in these centres. The first European examination centre was established in Amsterdam, in 1993. Of these locations, the Chicago centre is perhaps the most interesting, given that the United States has its own complex training structures. The Faculty has recently appointed forty-two new Regional Advisers, of whom thirteen are based overseas, in order to assist the proactive approach of the Faculty in this area.

Nowadays the Dental Faculty is an integral part of the College structure, though operating independently in terms of its Council, examinations and training programmes. Despite the unfortunate loss of dental training for undergraduates at the University of Edinburgh, this aspect of the College's life seems to be flourishing both nationally and internationally. History has not been forgotten, and in anticipation of the quincentenary, the Dental Faculty recommended the establishment of the King James IV Professorships in 1995 – royal approval being required before the title could be used. These professorships are offered in open competition to both surgical and dental Fellows and up to five may be awarded each year, the successful candidates giving a prestigious lecture. Among the topics covered so far have been: 'intracellular signalling pathways in osteoblasts', 'dentistry and the medically compromised patient' and 'the evolution of extra-cranial carotid artery surgery'.

## WOMEN AND SURGICAL TRAINING

The progress of women in surgery has not been easy or straightforward. As discussed in Chapter 5, the College did not admit its first female Fellow until 1920. By the second half of the twentieth century the situation had improved, but still only around 4 per cent of surgeons nationwide were female. Part of the problem lay in the dichotomy between raising children and undergoing full-time surgical training. There has long been the view that part-time training is somehow less valid than full-time training, not just in the field of medicine. The College's view was that part-time work 'did not amount to proper surgical training', but if this were to be accepted by the authorities, then it must not be fragmented and must be continuous for 'whatever time might be deemed necessary by the Royal Surgical Colleges'.[94]

A milestone for the College Council came in 1984, when Miss Caroline Doig, a paediatric surgeon, was elected as its first female member. The College *Newsletter*

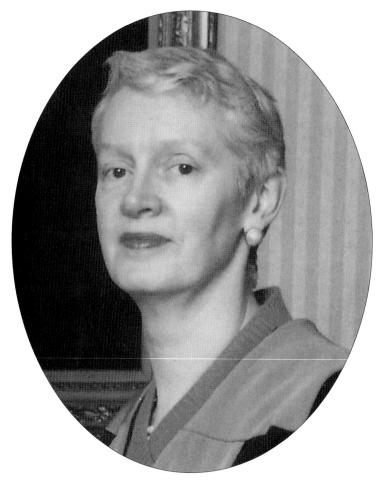

*FIG. 6.9* *Photograph of Miss Caroline Doig, first female member of the College Council, elected in 1984.*

opined somewhat unctuously that 'the College is not as chauvinistic as may have been reported'[95] – though it had taken some sixty-four years since the election of the first female Fellow for this to come about. For most of the period since then there has been female representation on the Council – the current Council including Miss Christine Evans, the first female urological surgeon in Britain, who was the focus of a recent series of television programmes about her work[96] (in 1999 the Council of the RCSEng included four women in a total membership of forty). The first female holder of the College Dental Fellowship, and first female member of the Dental Council, was the late Professor Dorothy Geddes, who in 1992 became the Dean of the College Dental Faculty and the first woman Dental Professor in Britain.

More recently a number of initiatives have been taken by the surgical colleges to try to attract more women to the surgical profession. Miss Janet Wilson was appointed by the College as its adviser to women in surgical training in 1992, and in January 1994 an information day was held for female medical students and junior doctors with the aim of inducing them to consider surgery as a profession. In addition to talks given by a number of practising female surgeons and information about training requirements, some surviving early female College Fellows were either present or sent in biographical accounts of their surgical careers. One of these, Betty Slesser, who gained her FRCSEd in 1946, related that when she applied for a post as a consultant thoracic surgeon, one of the interviewers asked her 'where did you get that bloody awful hat?' Despite her apparent sartorial deficiencies, it had taken her only six years after gaining the FRCSEd to reach consultant status. There was at that time no higher surgical training programme and no specialty examination to be undertaken. Another female Fellow, Lydia Duff, had been employed as a consultant during the Second World War, but 'in 1945 the men came home and I was replaced by a London Consultant, a brilliant and colourful personality, who worked in Salisbury for two years and then cut his wrists'.[97] This latter point neatly illustrates a major problem for female medical practitioners of all sorts in the early post-1945 period, when men returning from war service gained most of the new consultant posts in the early years of the NHS. There was also the important factor of decolonisation and the return of many Scottish and British practitioners from service in India and elsewhere. It must also be remembered that social attitudes towards appropriate gender roles were slow to change, and the College cannot be singled out for particular opprobrium on this account.

More recently the path to consultant status has become much longer and steeper, for men as well as women, and in future, the matter of part-time and flexible training will be determined by European legislation, though concomitant change in attitudes will be necessary. In the general trend of setting up organisations to cater for interest groups, Women in Surgical Training (WIST) was established under the aegis of the RCSEng and the Department of Health in 1991, and aims to assist women wishing to take up a surgical career. WIST has a Scottish representative and offers an information service on surgical careers for women, aiming to double the number of female consultants by 2011, which would mean that 20 per cent of all British consultants would be female by that stage. The American Association of Women Surgeons pursues similar aims to foster surgery as a career for women.[98] There are many problems to be overcome, not least in gaining recognition for flexible or part-time training. There is, or has been, a view that part-time training in many careers is not as 'good' as full-time training. If this is the case, then perhaps it is the organisation of the training rather than its interrupted nature that needs to be addressed. It may be that in these days of global technology and widely available internet facilities, flexible training, at least in the theoretical parts, may be made easier. Some female surgeons have gained a high public profile in television documentaries, and, indeed, situation comedies, but this problem is one which, it would seem, will require to be dealt with on a wider front than that of individual colleges. There may, though, be further difficulties if moves to shorten the period of surgical training are implemented.

## MUSEUM AND LIBRARY

### Museum

The College Museum continues to be a central feature of the Playfair Building and, given the overspilling of many of the College's administrative departments to alternative accommodation in the Hill Square 'campus', this is even more the case, and will continue to be so in view of the Heritage policy being adopted by the College (see below). As discussed in previous chapters, the Museum owes its modern form to the acquisition of a number of key collections during the nineteenth century. The holdings of the Museum are eclectic and modern technology is used in the dissemination of information, while important historical functions are retained. Successive Conservators have maintained and developed the various collections of dental as well as general surgical material, and in the last few decades a number of significant new initiatives have been undertaken. Following the end of hostilities in 1945, the Museum was gradually restored – the specimens had been rescued from their basement storage in 1943 – and under the Conservatorship of J. N. J. Hartley, a concentrated effort was made to improve the standards of conservancy of the specimens. A small demonstration room for use in postgraduate courses was made available and a photographic service for Fellows was instituted. Ultimately postgraduate teaching was relocated in the accommodation occupied formerly by the School of Medicine of the Royal Colleges and an agreement made between the College, the RCPEd and the University, which strengthened the work of the EPGBM. The changes to medical education in general and surgical training in particular meant that by the 1980s the Museum was apparently in relative stagnation in terms of teaching activity as opposed to holdings, though efforts continued to be made to 'modernise' the approach. Professor D. E. C. Mekie succeeded to the Conservatorship in 1955, and during his term of office, which lasted until 1974, the General Catalogue was revised and the display collections refined, the Barclay Room being the location of selected specimens reflecting the contribution of

Edinburgh surgeons. Preparation of a multi-volume *Colour Atlas of Demonstrations in Surgical Pathology* was undertaken, though only the first two volumes were published,[99] and histopathology and radiology (Bruce Dick) collections were added. Over the years the physical space occupied by the Museum and its associated laboratories and workshops has been modified as necessary.

In terms of historical work, the Museum received considerable financial support from the Sir Jules Thorn Charitable Trust, to enable the establishment of a museum dedicated to the history of Edinburgh surgery, which would be open to the general public, though at that point the future of the Museum itself was in some doubt – not for the first time, as the original library and museum collections were lost to the University in 1763 when the College was going through a period of particular economic stress. During the last decade of the twentieth century, though, during the Conservatorship of Professor D. L. Gardner (who followed Dr A. A. Shivas and Dr I. S. Kirkland) the College made a considerable sum available to the Museum, which allowed for the basement store to be upgraded, for the Barclay Hall to be rebuilt and to upgrade teaching and cataloguing facilities.[100] The Museum area now has accommodation for meetings as well as for displays and general Museum functions.

After several years of difficulties and delays,[101] and under the general supervision of I. S. Kirkland, I. F. MacLaren and J. A. Ross, the Sir Jules Thorn Exhibition of the History of Surgery opened its doors to the public in January 1992, though it had been officially opened by Mrs A. J. Rylands, daughter of Sir Jules Thorn, in April 1989, and this has proved to be a particularly successful exercise in attracting the interest of the general public in the history of surgery and of the College itself.

For the dental side of the College, the Menzies Campbell collection was another significant donation, in the tradition going back to John Barclay. Despite considerable difficulties in satisfying the minute organisational and display requirements of Dr Menzies Campbell, particularly concerning what was deemed to be the correct means to label and display the collection, it was handed over to the College on 30 June 1965. The collection was finally set up and displayed to optimum advantage in part of the refurbished Barclay Room in May 1994. The dental collections of the College were enhanced by the extended loan of historical material from the Edinburgh Dental School, which closed in September 1994, and by this time Dr P. R. Geissler had been appointed as Dental Conservator. All of this has ensured that the dental parts of the College Museum are organised to best advantage.[102]

In recent years the Museum has constructed an electronic database catalogue and has been closely involved in mounting exhibitions, particularly during the Edinburgh International Festival. These have attracted wide public interest, and have covered such diverse areas as the paintings of Sir Roy Calne, fifty years of surgery and Lister's contributions to antisepsis.[103] One novel appointment was that of an artist in residence, Mr Michael Esson, in 1994, and ten of his etchings were given to the Museum that year. Similar ventures in the future would be interesting. In tandem with this, though, and keeping the strong thread of continuity

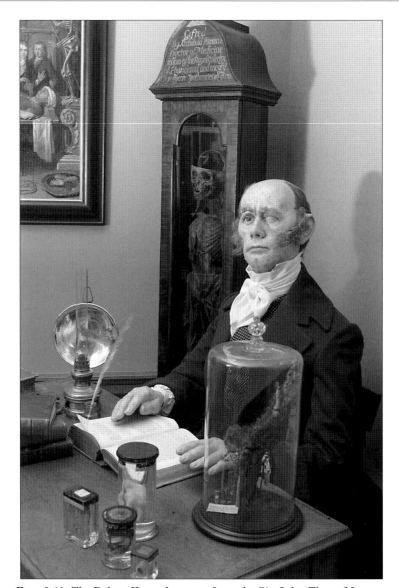

**FIG. 6.10** *The Robert Knox showcase from the Sir Jules Thorn Museum of the History of Surgery.*

going, *pace* postmodernism, the flow of donated items remains as eclectic as ever. The gifts for 1993–4, for example, included a portable field surgeon's pharmacy kit, a stereotactic frame, a 'modern surgical gown, mask, and other equipment to protect against HIV', and a nineteenth-century dental surgery cabinet, while the haul for 1996 boasted a 'fitted case of instruments from Hitler's yacht' and a box of seven aneurysm needles.

In terms of the relationship of the Museum to the College, in the recent past this appears to have been somewhat tense, with the demise of the Museum Committee in 1997 and the transfer of some recently appointed staff to other

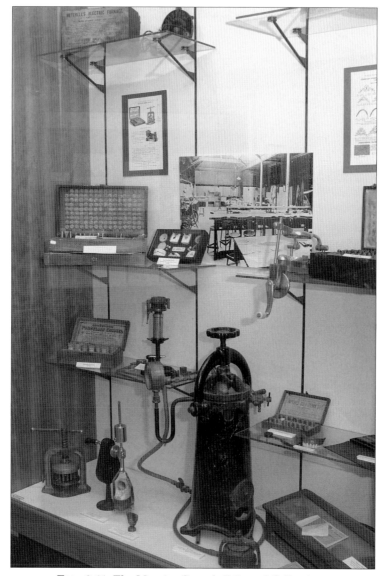

*FIG. 6.11* *The Menzies Campbell Dental Collection.*

departments of the College. This was probably due in part to the wider context of the much-changed role of historic institutional museums in surgical education (which is, of course, the prime concern of the College). It is likely, though, that the recent decision to extend the College's Heritage activities will give the Museum renewed stimulus, albeit in different directions.

## Library

The major activities undertaken by the College Library in this period have been concerned with adding to the 'live' stock of contemporary surgical texts and journals available to visiting Fellows and examination candidates, together with embracing the electronic age and at the same time conserving older books, manuscripts and ephemera held by the College.

In 1969, though at that point the survival of the Library was not in question, some disquiet was expressed about the position of the College regarding the proposal to set up a medical library at the University. It had been suggested that the College was opposed to the move, but as noted in the minutes, 'These rumours were disturbing, since it was obvious that such an appeal would be practicable only if it was signed by and had the wholehearted support of the major Edinburgh Medical institutions.' It was stressed that the College was not going back on its word and the President did not wish it to be thought that the College withheld its support for the project, 'but its position in regard to its own library was unlike that of the other main signatories and this would have to be adequately explained either in the Report or in a covering letter distributed with the appeal'.[104] There were evidently still some suspicions as to the motives of the University, though the disputes of the nineteenth century were long in the past.

In the more recent past the College Library has both pioneered developments in electronic technology and responded to new developments elsewhere, particularly in the areas of electronic communication, electronic journals and electronic literature searching. From relatively small-scale beginnings with a single electronic link with Edinburgh University Library in the early 1980s, the Library now boasts an award-winning internet café and provides a range of electronic teaching and learning aids, including CD and video, as well as offering electronic searching and the full range of library facilities. Before the establishment of the Faculty of Health Informatics, the College Librarian organised IT courses for surgeons. The establishment of the College website was also initiated from the Library and this has developed into a key aspect of the College's communication network with its Fellows, Licentiates, Members and other institutions. In 1999 the College Library was a finalist in the Bangemann Challenge in Stockholm, which recognised practical and functional information technology projects which benefited people and communities. The Librarians of the British medical and surgical colleges have also established a Royal College Librarians' Group, with the aim of exchanging ideas and developing library policies.

Parallel to this, though, the Library staff has continued the work of conserving the historic books and reorganising the College archive of manuscript and other material. Dr A. H. B. Masson was appointed Honorary Archivist in the early 1980s and oversaw the renovation of storage facilities, consequent on the receipt of advice from the staff of the NLS. More recently the Library has inaugurated an 'adopt-a-book' scheme, to allow individual subscribers to meet the cost of conserving single books. In these ways both the ancient and modern aspects of the Library will be maintained. The archive contains donated papers of many famous and flourishing surgeons, including Lister, Bell, Bruce and others.

Academic and institutional libraries tend to have similar atmospheres, although having different functions. The RCSI library, for example, caters for

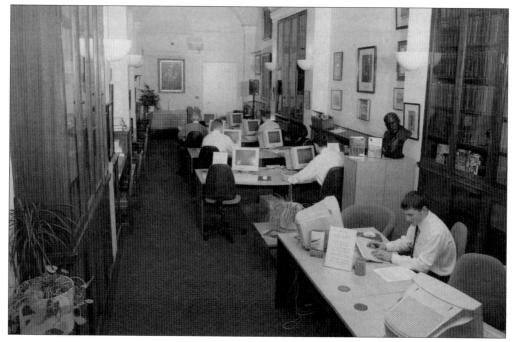

**FIG. 6.12** *The College internet café.*

undergraduates as well as postgraduates, and the library of the RCPSG has developed a more central role in postgraduate education than that of the College. This was particularly the case from the late 1940s, when the RCPSG had to carve out a new niche for itself in order to ensure its survival, and its library facilities were expanded to cater for this.[105] The College has a key role in postgraduate training, but rather more indirectly, as much of this teaching is organised by the Lister Institute and EPGBM, although the College runs many courses and skills workshops.

Over the last half-century the College Library has both embraced the technological age and conserved its historic roots – mirroring the general aims and functions of the College itself. Its future will be shaped by the same influences as those which will shape the future – long or short-term – of the College. Virtual libraries and electronic journals are proliferating, surgical training is changing and becoming shorter, and the Library will henceforth be part of the College's Heritage network. There would, though, still seem to be a place, and a need, for a physical space in which real as opposed to virtual texts can be consulted, and where the manuscript heritage of the College is preserved. There is something of a dichotomy here, between the requirements of a modern library providing a modern service and the very different concerns relating to preservation of historic collections.

## HERITAGE

As part of the drive to preserve the past for the future, the College has taken the decision to establish a Heritage Trust (Surgeons Lodge Ltd), in order to maximise

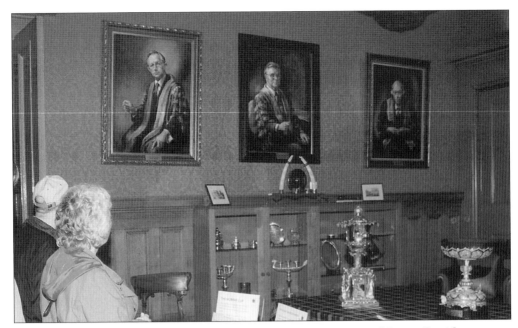

**FIG. 6.13** *Visitors to the College on Doors Open day. Portraits of former Presidents T. J. McNair, Professor Sir Robert Shields and Sir James Fraser hang on the wall, and the cabinets house many of the gifts received by the College from other countries.*

the potential of the College's physical assets in terms of conservation and more open public access, and to enable the Playfair Building to be an educational asset in its own right.[106] A conservation plan is in preparation, and this will inform the next stage of planning – which will, of course, require major funding. The acquisition of Heritage Lottery funding and Trust status will also place some restrictions on the uses to which the Playfair Building may be put, and it would seem that in order to develop the Heritage aspect fully, it is equally important that the plans for expansion of teaching facilities in the recently acquired Forbes Laboratory come to fruition. There is perhaps something of a trade-off here. The original building was very much a working building, the hub of the College and its activities. A complex combination of influences has forced it to expand into the surrounding areas of the campus, quite naturally. A basement chemical laboratory was adequate at the end of the seventeenth century, but is no longer so. In order for the College to ensure that each of its future Fellows 'knawes everything that he werkes', it must provide very different facilities, very different examinations and very different training. All of this means that of course the Playfair Building is no longer adequate. And this is nothing new. Each of the homes which has been occupied by the College since its early days has been acquired because of growing pressures on its previous location. The fact that it is now possible to retain a building but develop around it is rather different, and should allow the history to remain as well as allow the College to survive and prosper. There is also a more public face to this aspect of the College, and in recent years the buildings have been opened to the public on the annual Doors Open days.

## CONCLUSION

In the relatively short period covered by this chapter the College has undergone significant change. The context is one of global communication and rapid technological advance, combined with increasingly prescriptive regulations for surgical training. Many aspects of the College's activities in training and examination are carried out in conjunction with other bodies, and the recent advent of the intercollegiate MRCS means that all of its major examinations are intercollegiate. This has added to the number of interacting spheres of contextual influence which continue to shape its role and actions. The College has to relate to, and interact with, other medical corporations, government departments, government enquiries, European legislation, the universities, the specialist bodies and the hospitals. Centuries ago the main struggle was to gain acknowledged possession of surgical knowledge and practice in Edinburgh. Nowadays the priority is to be innovative in its use of this knowledge rather than merely having it. All of the surgical colleges require similar curricula, they operate intercollegiate examinations and work to the same standards, and there is no longer a tug-of-war with the universities about initial training. The College has to deal with a variety of outside agencies at the same time as trying to maintain a distinctive identity. It has made a number of initiatives in training in the light of new requirements, and also in the development of its heritage side, with the aim of maintaining its distinctiveness and, therefore, ensuring survival. The social, political and medical construction of the College in 2005 is complex and the future is not entirely in its own hands.

## NOTES

1. College Fellow, 1997.
2. There is a concise account of modern Scottish politics in Hutchison, I. G. C., *Scottish Politics in the Twentieth Century* (Basingstoke, 2001).
3. *Health in Scotland* (Scottish Executive, 2002) outlines the main strategies.
4. Ross, J., 'Memoirs of an Edinburgh Surgeon', (unpublished, Royal College of Surgeons of Edinburgh, 1988), p. 154.
5. By 1970 the College was represented on over twenty boards and committees, as well as being involved in the JCHST and the EPGBM.
6. *Our Changing Democracy: Devolution of Scotland and Wales* (Cmnd. 6348) (HMSO, 1975).
7. College Minutes, 26 March 1976.
8. College Minutes, 23 April 1976.
9. College Minutes, 17 October 1977.
10. College Minutes, 15 July 1954.
11. College Minutes, 17 November 1979.
12. College Minutes, 19 July 1950.
13. Hull and Geyer-Kordesch, *The Shaping of the Medical Profession*, p. 27.
14. The last diet under the old regulations took place in 1999. After that it came under the

auspices of the United Examination Board. Any candidates wishing to take the examination in Scotland would still be awarded the TQ.

15. *The Report of the Inter-Departmental Committee on Medical Schools* (Ministry of Health. Department of Health for Scotland, London, 1944) [The Goodenough Report].

16. Hull and Geyer-Kordesch, *Shaping of the Medical Profession*, p. 50.

17. College Minutes, 16 July 1976.

18. The Director of Standards speaks for the College on all medical, medico-legal and public liaison matters; the Director of Training provides representation on Intercollegiate Boards and PMETB; the Director of Education oversees the educational activities of the College; the Director of Communication will seek to improve communication with the College's 16,000 Fellows worldwide.

19. Masson, *Portraits, Paintings and Busts*; Masson, *A College Miscellany*; Kaufman, *Musket Ball and Sabre Injuries*; Chalmers, J., *Audubon in Edinburgh and his Scottish Associates* (National Museums of Scotland, 2003); Macintyre and MacLaren, *Surgeons' Lives* (forthcoming); Geissler, *Royal Odonto-Chirurgical Society*.

20. Letter to Fellows from Professor G. Chisholm, in his capacity as Chairman of the JCHST, November 1993, relating to proposals for restructuring of surgical training and the various registrar grades.

21. College Minutes, 19 October 1966.

22. RCSEd, *Annual Report 1971–2*, p. 2.

23. RCSEd, *Annual Report 1972–3*, p. 2.

24. Sir James Fraser was appointed in 1969 to the Inaugural Chair of Clinical Science in Surgery; in 1980 to the post of Postgraduate Dean and Director of Edinburgh Postgraduate Board for Medicine; and in 1990 to the office of College Regent. During his presidency he was able to rehabilitate Surgeons' Square, including the restoration of St Michael's Church to become the Symposium Hall, opened in 1982.

25. College Minutes, 15 October 1969.

26. College Minutes, 12 June 1970.

27. Cuschieri, A., 'The laparoscopic revolution', *J. Roy. Coll. Surg. Edinb.*, 34 (1990), p. 295.

28. Watson, F., 'The role of virtual reality in surgical training in the UK' (unpublished M.Sc. thesis, University of Sheffield, 2000).

29. Ibid., p. 19.

30. Chaudhry, A., Sutton, C., Wood, J., Stone, R. and McCloy, R., 'Learning rate for laparoscopic surgical skills on MIST VR, a virtual reality simulator: quality of human-computer interface', *Annals of the Royal College of Surgeons of England*, 81 (1999), pp. 281–6.

31. El-Khalili, N. H., 'Surgical training on the World Wide Web' (unpublished Ph.D. thesis, University of Leeds, 1999).

32. Hughes, F. E., 'Proficiency training for space flight', in Royal College of Surgeons of England, *Surgical Competence: Challenges of Assessment in Training and Practice* (RCSEng, 1999), pp. 73–81.

33. Jackson, B., 'Why do we need to assess competence?', in ibid., pp. 6–16.

34. Levy, L. F., 'Personal View', *BMJ*, 285 (1982), p. 1271.

35. Driscoll, P., 'Challenges in Surgical training', *Surgeonsnews*, 3 (2) (2004), pp. 56–7. See also Roscoe, T. and Bacon, N., 'Why should surgeons use the internet?', *Surgeonsnews*, 3 (2) (2004), pp. 54–5.

36. College Minutes, 8 February 1974.

37. *Royal Commission on Medical Education* (HMSO, London, 1968) (Cmnd. 3569) [The Todd Report], p. 23.

38. *Royal Commission on the National Health Service* (HMSO, London, 1979) [The Merrison Report], p. 368.

39. *Staffing the Service. The Next Decade. Report to the Scottish Joint Consultative Committee and the Scottish Home and Health Department Following Review of Hospital Medical Staffing Estimates in Scotland* (Edinburgh, 1987) [The Shaw Report], p. 115. It was

emphasised that each specialty would require different training arrangements, and several College Fellows were involved in the various sectional committees which produced the report.

40. *Postgraduate Medical and Dental Education in Scotland. Report of Advisory Group Chaired by Dr Kenneth C. Calman* (Scottish Office, 1991), p. 41.

41. Department of Health, Press Release 95/260, 26 May 1995.

42. Department of Health, *Hospital Doctors. Training for the Future* (London, 1993), under the chairmanship of Sir Kenneth Calman.

43. *The Appointment of the Chair and Scottish Members of the Postgraduate Medical Education and Training Board* (Scottish Executive, 2003).

44. Ibid.

45. Chikwe, J., de Souza, A., Pepper, J. R., 'No time to train the surgeons', *BMJ*, 328 (2004), p. 418.

46. Rowley, D., 'A vision for surgery – the future of UK surgical training', *Surgeonsnews*, 3 (1) (2004), p. 42. This appointment means that all postgraduate education, continuing education and professional development will be collegiate based.

47. Maran, A. G. D., 'Revised Edinburgh Fellowship Examination', *J. Roy. Coll. Surg. Edinb.*, 35 (1990), p. 137.

48. College Minutes, 8 May 1964. It was agreed that a new close marking system should be introduced in Part II of the Fellowship examination. Under this scheme the marks ranged from 3 to 8, with 6 being the pass (with relevant provision for compensation).

49. College Minutes, 5 February 1971.

50. College Minutes, 26 November 1976.

51. Cook, J., 'The changing pattern of surgical education 1955–1980', *J. Roy. Coll. Surg. Edinb.*, 25 (1980), pp. 293–8.

52. Figures drawn from College Examination Statistical returns to the GMC.

53. *Surgeonsnews*, 2 (1) (2003), p. 74.

54. RCSEd, *Annual Report 1997–8*, p. 26.

55. As early as 1965, the College Minutes note concern at the trend for consultants to be appointed in Accident and Emergency departments who did not have a higher surgical qualification. College Minutes.

56. Dean, A. C. B., 'Specialty Fellowship Examinations', *J. Roy. Coll. Surg. Edinb.*, 30 (2) (1985), pp. 141–2.

57. Hull and Geyer-Kordesch, *Shaping of the Medical Profession*, pp. 224–7.

58. College Minutes, 16 January 1987. The RCPSC introduced a Specialty Fellowship in Plastic Surgery.

59. In 1985–6, for example, nineteen out of twenty-five candidates were successful in the Orthopaedic Fellowship (76 per cent, though the average was more often between 30 and 40 per cent), and in the same year four of the eight candidates were successful in the Surgical Neurology examination.

60. Blandy and Lumley, *Royal College of Surgeons of England*, p. 132.

61. RCSEd website, specimen MRCS questions.

62. College Minutes, 7 February 1969.

63. Important contributions came from, among others, H. Sin-Yan Fang, James Gibson, Arthur Hodgson and Alexander McFadyen.

64. College Minutes, 17 March 1972.

65. 'The Indian Chapter', in *Royal College of Surgeons Annual Report 2002–3*, pp. 38–40.

66. Woodruff, M., *Nothing Venture, Nothing Win* (Edinburgh, 1996), p. 139. For details of this operation, see pp. 139–40. See also Woodruff, M., 'Transplantation: a personal recollection', in P. Terasaki (ed.), *History of Transplantation in Thirty-Five Recollections* (Los Angeles, 1991), pp. 184–98. It is of interest that the College's Honorary Archivist, Dr A. H. B. Masson, was one of the anaesthetists at this operation.

67. RCSEd, *Report of Developments Committee 1987/88*, pp. 7–8.

68. For a full account of the Association, see Blandy, J. and Williams, J. P., *The History of the British Association of Urological Surgeons* (London, 1995).

69. For a fuller account of the work of the EMS, see Dingwall, *History of Scottish Medicine*, pp. 200–7. Stiles and his colleagues at Bangour carried out many orthopaedic procedures, including tendon transplantation and reconstruction of limbs. Hendrie, W. F. and Macleod, D. A. D., *The Bangour Story. A History of Bangour Village and General Hospitals* (Aberdeen, 1991), p. 32.

70. Watson-Jones, R., 'Homage to Sir Walter Mercer', *Journal of Bone and Joint Surgery*, 38B (1) (1956), p. 435.

71. In addition to individual interest and the need to cope with war trauma there were, of course, the problems of congenital deformity and crippling conditions caused by poverty or epidemic disease. Following a public appeal, the Princess Margaret Rose Hospital was opened in 1933 and this helped to raise the profile of Edinburgh as a major orthopaedic centre.

72. Macnicol, M. F, Penny, I. D. and Shephard, L., 'Early results of the Leeds-Keio anterior cruciate ligament replacement', *Journal of Bone and Joint Surgery*, 73 (3) (1991), pp. 377–80.

73. Hendrie and Macleod, *Bangour Story*, pp. 109–26.

74. Details are in Miss A. B. Sutherland's notes, available in the College Archive.

75. These included Alexander Buchan, Thomas Gibson, Anne Sutherland, John Tough and Alexander Wallace.

76. I am grateful to Mr P. Walbaum for information on developments in cardiothoracic surgery. See also Barry, J. P. S., Adams, A. P. and Fleming, P. R., *The History of Cardiothoracic Surgery from Early Times* (London, 1996).

77. For example, Craig, S. R., Hamzah, M. and Walker, W. S., 'Video-assisted thoracoscopic pneumonectomy for bronchial carcinoid tumor in a 14-year-old girl', *Journal of Pediatric Surgery*, 32 (7) (1997), pp. 1724–6.

78. I am personally indebted to Mr E. W. J. Cameron FRCSEd for his expertise in cardiothoracic surgery.

79. Including Iain Aird, Bruce Dick and Philip Walbaum.

80. See a fuller account in Miller, J. D. and Steers, A. J. W., 'Surgical neurology and clinical neurosciences in Edinburgh, Scotland', *Neurosurgery*, 39 (1) (1996), pp. 151–9. I am grateful to Mr J. F. Shaw for information on the development of neurosurgery.

81. Rowe, N. L. and Killey, H. C., *Fractures of the Facial Skeleton* (Edinburgh, 1968).

82. College Minutes, 19 December 1962.

83. These included the Dental Consultants and Specialists Committee, the General Dental Council, the Central Committee on Higher Training in Dentistry, the Dental Manpower Committee and the Dental Consultants and Specialists Committee.

84. College Minutes, 5 August 1963. *Report to the Secretary of State for Scotland by Review Committee on Dental Staffing Structure* (1964) [The Schiach Report].

85. College Minutes, 1 February 1974.

86. Hull and Geyer-Kordesch, *Shaping of the Medical Profession*, p. 207. It acquired Faculty status in 1990.

87. Dental Council Minutes, 24 April 1970.

88. College Minutes, 22 September 1955.

89. Dental Council Minutes, 19 April 1956.

90. Dental Council Minutes, 14 March 1969.

91. Dental Council Minutes, 23 September 1985.

92. I am grateful to Mrs Violet Brown, Dental Faculty administrator, for this information.

93. Craig, G. C., 'Fluorides and the prevention of dental decay: a statement from the Representative Board of the British Dental Association', *British Dental Journal*, 188 (12) (2000), p. 654.

94. College Minutes, 21 May 1976.

95. RCSEd, *Newsletter*, July 1984.

96. Foster, J., 'Christine Evans – the Barbara Woodhouse of Urology', *Surgeonsnews*, January 2004, pp. 94–5 (title of article by the editor, David Tolley). 'Under the knife with Miss Evans' was a documentary series first transmitted by Channel 4 in July 2002.

97. RCSEd, Women in Surgery Symposium, 21 January 1994.

98. McCarthy, M. C., 'The Association of Women Surgeons', *Archives of Surgery*, 128 (6) (1993), pp. 633–6.

99. Mekie, D. E. C. and Fraser, J. (eds), *Colour Atlas of Demonstrations in Surgical Pathology* (London, 1983, 1986).

100. Design assistance was received from the Edinburgh College of Art and a number of new staff appointed, including a graphics artist and computer expert (though these posts were later absorbed into the general College structure). I am grateful to Professor D. L. Gardner for discussion on these points. Following Professor Mekie, Dr I. Kirkland and Dr A. Shivas served as Conservators.

101. This is evident from the large volume of correspondence held in the College archive.

102. Full details of developments in the main College *Annual Reports* and the series of reports produced by Professor D. Gardner, Honorary Conservator, during the 1990s.

103. Gardner, D. L., *Surgery Comes Clean. The Life and Work of Joseph Lister 1827–1912* (Edinburgh, 2002).

104. College Minutes, 27 June 1969.

105. Hull and Geyer-Kordesch, *Shaping of the Medical Profession*, pp. 117–19.

106. I am grateful to Ms Dawn Kemp, Director of Heritage, for information on heritage developments.

# 7

# The College buildings – symbols of a Famous and Flourishing Society

It was a matter of congratulation that they now possessed a meeting place worthy of their status as members of a literal and scientific body.[1]

During its lifetime the College has occupied a number of rented and purpose-built premises. It was important to have a specific location for meetings, not least for the visual symbolism which this would convey, both to members of the College itself and to the community in general. This sort of symbolism is important nowadays, but in earlier times was even more so. This chapter will assess the various buildings inhabited by the College over the years, their symbolism and adaptation to changing circumstances.

## Humble beginnings – Dickson's Close and Kirkheugh

The early-modern period was visual, in all aspects. Symbolism was not confined to the portrayal of kings in Roman uniforms, or the extension of royal palaces in the classical style; it was there in all aspects of life, in an age when communication was difficult and the written word was available only to a minority of the population. Buildings were the outward symbols of their inhabitants and their status within society, but there were other pressures. Incorporations gathered corporate possessions; they needed storage space and a convenient meeting house, for practical as well as symbolic purposes. The surgeons and barbers were no different. They met initially in the house of the current deacon, or occasionally in the 'ile' of St Giles, perhaps the same 'ile' that housed the Incorporation's altar dedicated to St Mungo.

This peripatetic life continued until 1647 when, during the turbulent period of the Civil War, 'three rowmes of ane tenement' in Dickson's Close were rented by the Incorporation at a cost of £40 per annum. Expenses for this move included £36 for 'half a dozen of chares' and 6s 'for carrying the skeleton to the Convening House'.[2] The first meeting was held there in August 1647. Early in 1650 the Incorporation moved to new accommodation in a tenement belonging to Robert Hardie at the 'foot

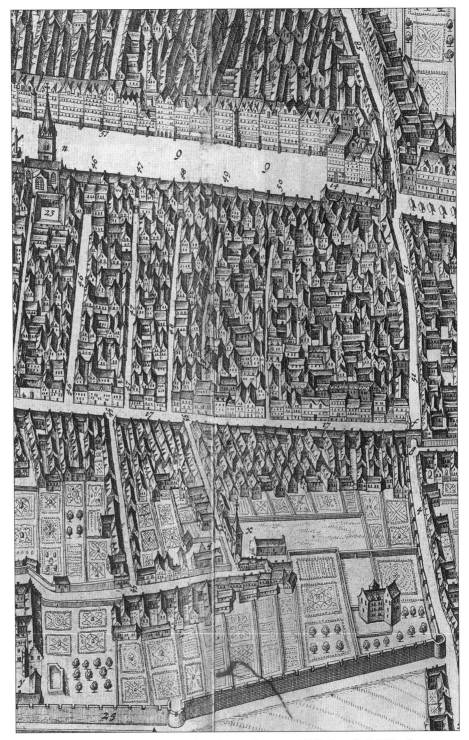

**FIG. 7.1** *Extract from Gordon of Rothiemay's map of Edinburgh (1647), showing Curryhill House (bottom right) and Dickson's Close (no. 47). (National Library of Scotland.)*

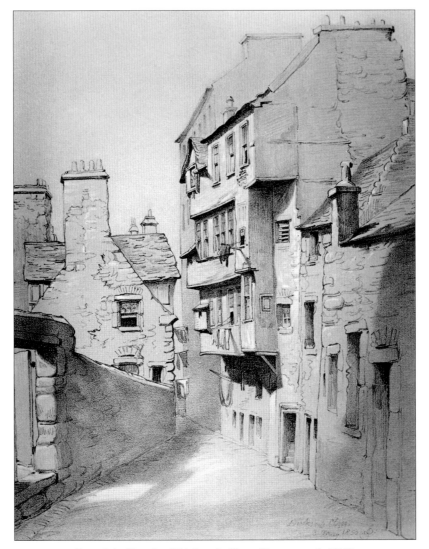

**FIG. 7.2** *Sketch of Dickson's Close (Drummond, 1879).*

of the Kirkheugh'. This proved not to be a wise move. The rooms were apparently unsuitable and the surgeons tried to give up the lease after a few months, but the landlord refused to allow the Incorporation to remove its goods from the building. There were also problems with looting by occupying Cromwellian troops, and on 4 March 1651 a representative of the Incorporation was sent to the Kirkheugh to 'see what of the Calling's goods being in the Convening House . . . were extant, to the fore, unplundered or away taken by the English soldiers'. The situation seems eventually to have been resolved, and the Incorporation paid only £20 of the £41 due for rent, but for the next few years it was forced to use cramped accommodation comprising 'two front rooms in John Scott's house' and a 'chamber' owned by Thomas Kincaid, both masters of the Incorporation. Thus for the first 150 years of its existence, the Incorporation lacked a stable physical environment. It would seem to be the case that for any institution to develop strong internal structures and functions, a permanent location is important, not just as a public statement, but also as a means of allowing its corporate functions to develop. Uncertainty of location was, for the Incorporation, a growing burden by the middle of the seventeenth century.

### First signs of permanence – Curryhill House

Always mindful of its quest for academic status, which in itself would require something more visually significant than the front room of one of its members, the Incorporation was quick to grasp the opportunity which came in 1656 to acquire 'a suitable site in a desirable neighbourhood'. This was Curryhill House, which cost the Incorporation 3,000 merks.[3] Situated at the south-east corner of the Flodden Wall, Curryhill House 'lay between the yard of umquhile Andrew Henrysoun upon the west, the town wall of the burgh . . . upon the east and south, the auld dyke and fosse of the said yard and Kirkyard of the brethren of the Blackfriars of the burgh of Edinburgh . . . with full entry through the High School yards as the same was possessed by Mr Samuel Jonstoun'.[4] It comprised a 'large half-quadrangular four-storeyed house with dormer windows, a circular turnpike stair with a conical roof on its north front and surrounded by a spacious garden'. This was much more appropriate to the needs of a 'famous and flourishing society'.[5] This land had in the past belonged to the Black Friars, and subsequently became the home of two brothers, both Court of Session judges, who each adopted the judicial title Lord Curriehill. This was not a purpose-built home, but was much better than the cramped, temporary accommodation to which the surgeons had become accustomed, and considerable outlays on renovations were necessary. In the short term, new walls were built, a garden laid out at a cost of £200 Scots, and in 1664 a gardener was employed to 'furnish the yaird with all kind of medicinall herbes and flowers that can be had anyqr'.[6]

At that time the Incorporation did not have many – or any – of the trappings of the learned society; all that would come with the next building. Curryhill House was a more impressive edifice, though, reflecting something of the status to which the Incorporation had risen within the hierarchy of the burgh trades. Various alterations were made to the structure but by the late 1660s it was considered inadequate and dangerous, and the boxmaster was instructed to 'take down the house qr it is faultie and lyke to fall and to take off the sclaits for preservation'. In 1669 plans were drawn up for a new building, to which most of the masters pledged donations.[7] Though apparently reasonably solvent financially at this point, as witnessed by records of moneylending transactions, the costs of renovating Curryhill House and the expensive disputes with the physicians and others meant that these plans had to be shelved. It seems also that there were two buildings on the site – Curryhill House itself and a house which had been built by the Town Council, originally meant for the use of the Professor of Divinity. The records note

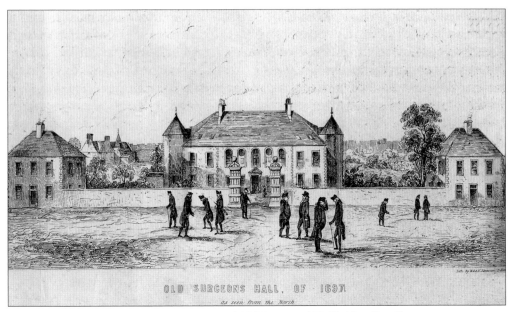

**FIG. 7.3** *Line drawing of Old Surgeons' Hall. After Sandby.*

that the 'Convening House' had been lent to the Presbyterian congregations of the Tron and College Kirk parishes, while the Incorporation continued to meet in the 'ordinary house'. This latter was renovated in 1704 to accommodate the Incorporation's Officer, following the construction of the new hall. In any event, the building was clearly becoming increasingly unsound and inappropriate for its purposes.

### 'Old' Surgeons' Hall

The next major move – as would be the one following that – was forced on the Incorporation by external influences as well as the desire to acquire more suitable premises. As discussed in Chapter 3, in the early 1690s a member of the Incorporation, Alexander Monteith, had petitioned the Town Council to grant him bodies for dissection. Whether for altruistic intentions or merely to prevent one of their number from branching out on his own, the Incorporation swifly petitioned the Town Council on its own account with a similar request, which was granted on condition that a new hall was built, containing an anatomical theatre, by Michaelmas 1697. This was early notice but the Incorporation took little action for two years and indeed ordered a new roof for its current house in 1694. By 1696, though, it was clear that some action would have to be taken, and on 2 June the masters 'unanimously agreed for the building of the house'. A committee was appointed to consider the available options, and eventually the decision was made to construct a hall *de novo* on the site of Curryhill House. It was designed by architect James Smith, who submitted an estimate for building and finishing, apart from glass-work, of £500 sterling. The foundation stone was laid in August 1696, and a guinea placed under it by the Deacon – 'conform to the ordinary custom used in such cases'. Despite minor problems with the need to insert extra windows and a note that the 'chimely in the laboratorie was too little',[8] by the following year it was at least partly ready for use, as Monteith was able to rent part of the basement as a chemical laboratory at £10 per annum, the laboratory also to be available for the use of entrant apothecaries undergoing trials.

The Hall has been described as 'originally a two-storey and nine-bay piend-roofed block with semi-octagonal towers at the ends'.[9] It was noted by Maitland in his history of Edinburgh to be 'a beautiful building, wherein is a collection of natural Rarities, and a Bagnio'.[10] As well as the best decoration that could be afforded, with quantities of Dutch marble and French glass, a chimney piece and door surrounds were carved by 'a stranger (possibly a French Huguenot) now upon the place who was very skillfull and could work very well in carving of timber'.[11] The interior of the Hall was embellished with a series of portraits of the masters of the Incorporation, executed by Sir John Medina and his apprentice William Aikman. These lozenge-shaped paintings, some forty in number, provide a unique visual catalogue of the masters around the turn of the eighteenth century.[12] Very much in line with the aesthetic aspirations of learned societies, the importance of these images is confirmed by a minute of 1720 which states that five recalcitrant surgeons who had not yet had produced a portrait must do so immediately, on pain of losing the right to book apprentices. The College archives also contain the bill from Andro Sim of Calton for hanging the paintings, the cost being £1 18s 6d, deemed by Sim to be 'a guid bargain at six pence per piece'.[13] By December 1697 the finishing touches were being made to the Hall. It was reported that the building committee would 'commune with Tradesmen for lyning and perfecting the great hall', and that the boxmaster was ordered to pay the relevant tradesmen for 'work not contained in the contract and all other things as he shall think requisit'.[14] A Turkish bath, or bagnio, was built on the site and was intended to bring in money as well as follow trends in medical treatment (see Chapter 3). The bagnio was not a commercial success, though, and by 1740 the enterprise was discontinued. In this and in many other aspects of the College activities, the masters pursued what they perceived to be appropriate goals within the social, political, economic and cultural context of the time. They appeared, or claimed, to be self-motivated and of course they were, but these motivations were also shaped and influenced by the discourse and attitudes of the time.

The Hall was a considerable drain on the Incorporation's finances, and large sums were again borrowed from La Perle. Ongoing financial difficulties meant that the Incorporation was forced to consider selling or renting out various parts of the building at intervals. The problems had increased substantially with the separation from the barbers in 1722. The barbers had enjoyed little or no influence in the affairs of the Incorporation, but their quarterly dues and entrance fees had been a welcome source of income. In February 1728 the minutes record that:

It was moved by the Treasurer that since the Callings affairs were in such a situation as required the most frugal economy it would be considered how far it might tend to their interest to sett [rent out] the wester pavilion and accommodate the officer within the under roumes of the Hall. Which motion having been accordingly considered by the Calling, they approved thereof and ordered to make such Reparations as might sufficiently accommodate the Officer in the under roumes of the Hall.[15]

Various parts of the building were rented out and the surgeons had to make do without the full use of their purpose-built accommodation. The following year, matters had not improved, as it was now decided to try to sell the bath house and other buildings in order to cope with mounting debts. The minutes record in the evocative language of the day that:

> The Calling for certain weighty reasons agreed that their large house yeards and two pavilions should be exposed to sale the second week of July next ... And remitted to the Deacon and his Councill to draw ane advertisement and cause insert the same in the Edinburgh newspapers for that purpose. And impowered the same Committee together with the Committee appointed for falling upon ways and means to extinguish the Callings Debts to condescend upon the place Day and hour of Sale.[16]

No suitable purchaser was found, however, and a similar attempt to sell the entire building in 1733 was equally unsuccessful. On that occasion the building was advertised as 'the large beautifull and well aird house commonly called the Surgeons Hall with the Bagnio two pavilions and Gardens all well enclosed with home dykes and hedges having a water pype led with several other conveniences'.[17] It was reported that officials of the Incorporation had attended the sale, but that unfortunately no offers had been received for any part of the buildings.

It was decided eventually that the main hall should be retained in the possession and occupation of the surgeons and that other parts of the building should be rented out as residential accommodation. It was perhaps fortunate that no buyer came forward to purchase the whole building, as this would have robbed the Incorporation of one of the most important outward manifestations of the learned society. In the event, sections of the building were inhabited variously by the Rector of the High School, who rented the east pavilion for five years at £100 Scots per annum; by Mr William McDougall, merchant, who occupied the east gable at £18 sterling; and in 1740 the west gable was leased by Lord Elchies, Senator of the College of Justice, for twelve years at £27 sterling yearly rental.[18] Lord Elchies was not the most careful of tenants, though, as it was noted in 1745 that 'the servants of the Honorable Lord Elchies had broken and spoilt most of their Chaires, and used them even in the kitchen ... upon the bottoms whereof the impression of pots and pans was visible'.[19]

The next remedial attempt came in the early 1760s, when it was considered to be of potential benefit if at least parts of the properties were sold outright and the areas of unbuilt ground feued off. This would have the advantage of bringing in an annual income in the form of feu duty, which would not be liable to depletion on account of expenditure for building repairs. Figures from a summary of finances relating to properties between 1722 and 1760 had shown that out of a total income from rental of £2,043, some £897 had been spent on repairs, leaving a net income of £1,146.

The areas of ground to the east and west of the Hall were set to roup 'during the running of an half-hour glass' on 9 May 1764, when the north-east area was feued to an architect, William Mylne, who proceeded to construct two houses on the vacant ground. Efforts to dispose of land in this way continued, and by 1786, when most of the area surrounding the Hall had indeed been disposed of, the houses built on the land came to be known as Surgeons' Square, 'the cradle of modern surgery in Edinburgh'.[20] The properties were certainly occupied by a number of high-profile surgical individuals, including John Thomson, John Bell and Robert Knox, and it seems a little ironic that the Incorporation's severe financial difficulties helped to achieve this concentration of surgeons and their houses in the immediate area of the Hall, thus reinforcing the importance of surgeons and surgery in the town.

Though it has been considered that no anatomical teaching took place in the Old Hall after Monro *primus* moved to the sanctuary of the University in 1726, it appears that at least one lecturer, John Aitken, did carry out teaching there, as did John Bell.[21] Following the removal of the College to its new premises in 1832, the Hall was pressed into service as a temporary cholera hospital during the outbreak that year. Following this, the old anatomy theatre was used for teaching by Robert Knox, and in June 1833 the building was sold to the managers of the RIE.

## The Playfair Building

By the 1820s the College Fellows had begun to reconsider their physical surroundings yet again. Various parts of the Hall had been let out at different stages in order to try to revive the College's flagging finances, though by 1745 there had apparently been enough spare cash to expend on fire insurance, the policy to be issued by the Edinburgh Friendly Insurance.[22] By the early nineteenth century, though, the building was becoming increasingly uninhabitable. There were also considerations of prestige and the growing desire of the College, however poverty-stricken it might be, to acquire a building suitable for its status as an eminent scientific society and in tune with the buildings and intellectual intent of classical Edinburgh and the ambience of New Town elegance, in contrast to the unsavoury state of the Old Town.[23] In February 1822 the College set up a fourteen-man committee to investigate the possibilities of rebuilding on the present site, adapting an existing building elsewhere or commissioning an entirely new, purpose-built hall.[24] Only two weeks later the committee reported that it had consulted William Playfair about the possibility of acquiring and renovating Minto House.[25] Playfair had advised against developing the College's existing building in High School Yards, but had indicated that the ground would be suitable on which to build *de*

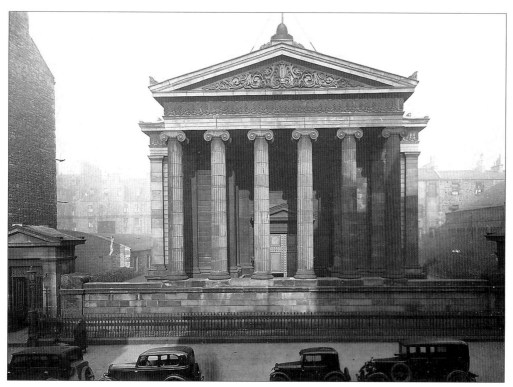

**FIG. 7.4** *Photograph of the Playfair Building, c. 1920s.*

*novo.* By April that year the Fellows resolved to commission Playfair to furnish designs for a new building on the current site, with or without an integral classroom, and also to look at possible alternative sites on Calton Hill and in the New Town. Playfair was one of the foremost architects of his time, and prior to his engagement by the College he had designed Dollar Academy (1819), the Edinburgh City Observatory on Calton Hill (1819), several of the streets and crescents of the New Town, and the Royal Scottish Academy (1822) (following the successful completion of the College, Playfair went on to design Donaldson's Hospital for the Deaf (1842), the National Gallery of Scotland (1850) and even his own funeral monument). The College had therefore chosen an architect with considerable pedigree, whose elegant buildings were in exactly the sort of style and configuration which would enhance the status of the College when it was housed in a similar building.

As well as the visual symbolism of possessing such an impressive building, the College had been forced to consider its accommodation as part of the terms of its acquisition of the Barclay museum collection (see Chapter 5), a condition of which was the construction or provision of suitable accommodation. The College acquired a house in Surgeons' Square in 1818 for this purpose, but there were delays in fitting it up appropriately. Overtures were made to politicians and government to try to gain financial support (the RCSI had been successful in this area). David Hay wrote to Lord Melville in 1825 to solicit his patronage for a petition to the Treasury, 'the object we humbly contend to be one of great national importance', the not too subtle point being made that 'the late Viscount Melville, who was Honorary Fellow of the College, attended his patronage to us on various important occasions'. The petition to the Treasury claimed that 'without the aid of His Majesty's government they will be unable to place their Museum in a situation where it can be accessible or of much utility'.[26] The petition was not successful.

Discussions continued and various proposals were considered, including extension of the existing building, purchase of the Old High School building, and Minto House (now the Royal Museum of Scotland), until in 1828 the option of developing the site of the Royal Academy for Teaching Exercise (a riding school) arose. Playfair reported on this site, and in February 1829 the College received his rough plans, followed in April of that year by more detailed designs at an initial costing of £11,500.[27] The project went ahead, and the minutes reveal that the Fellows were concerned by now with detail and matters of decoration, and, of course, cost. The main contract, with Messrs Young and Trench, was signed on 23 November 1829.

The foundation stone was laid on 3 March 1830 by the President, William Wood, and *The Scotsman* reported the occasion in detail:

> On Saturday the foundation stone of the new building for the Royal College of Surgeons, was laid by the President in presence of many of the members of that body, in the ground lately occupied by the Royal Menage, Nicolson Street. The bottles deposited in the stone, contained copies of the Royal Charter of Foundation, the Deed of Gift of the Barclayan Museum and a copy of each of the newspapers published in Edinburgh, etc. These documents were prepared for preservation by Mr Dunn, philosophical instrument maker. The building is to be executed from a plan by Mr Playfair; and, when completed, we have no doubt, it will add to that Architect's well earned and deservedly high reputation. The elevation to the street will present a portico, upwards of forty feet in breadth and fifty feet in height, composed of six Grecian Ionic columns. The length of the building, from west to east, will be 190 feet. As far as can be judged from the plans, this building will combine elegance of design with ample accommodation for the Royal College, and prove another classic decoration to our northern metropolis. The estimated expense of the edifice is about £10,000, and has been contracted for by Messrs Young and Trench, who built St Stephen's Church.

A container was placed under the foundation stone with:

- Copy of charters, royal grants and Acts
- Present Laws of the College
- Printed regulations for examination candidates
- Copy of Trust Deed of the Barclay Museum
- Copy of Settlement by Barclay Trustees
- Copy extract matriculation of College Arms

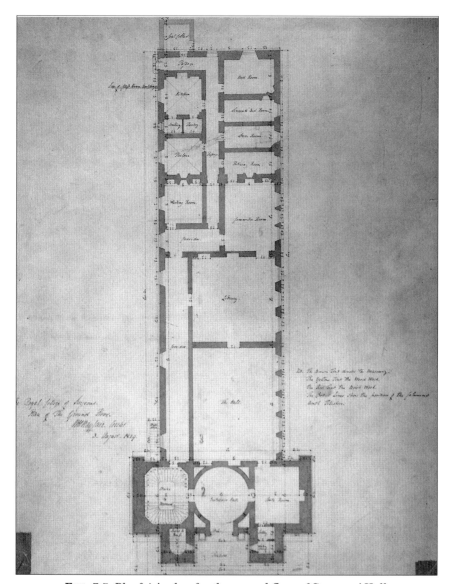

***FIG. 7.5*** *Playfair's plan for the ground floor of Surgeons' Hall.*

- Copies of Licentiate and Fellow's Diplomas
- Impressions in wax of the College seals
- Museum admission tickets
- Edinburgh Almanack
- Latest printed statement of funds
- Copies of all Edinburgh newspapers

In October 1830 there was anxious debate about whether fir should be used instead of oak for the museum floors. Playfair had preferred oak for this purpose but he had been asked to cut costs wherever possible. (It was agreed, though, to spend an extra £200 on ornamentation of the ionic portico to make it appear more Corinthian. The outward face of the College and its impact were still thought worthy of the best.) By this time also, though, costs were mounting, and a further £3,000 had to be found. It was agreed to borrow this sum from the Widows' Fund and Auxiliary Widows' Fund. During the period of building, the Incorporation met in the premises of the Royal Medical Society (which had in its early days rented accommodation from the College).

The building has been described as a 'pure Greek revivalist temple to medicine'[28] and as a 'T-plan Ionic temple', containing a 'round two-storey coffer-domed vestibule'.[29] The College held its first meeting in the new Hall on 16 May 1832, at which it was stated that 'it was highly creditable to them to have applied so large a portion of their funds to the establishment of a museum, by which the acquisition of professional knowledge would be greatly facilitated'. The total cost of the project thus far was noted as £12,043 6s, but shortly thereafter had risen to £13,257 18s 7d.

The Hall was opened formally on 7 July 1832, in the presence of dignitaries including representatives of the RCPEd and the Medical Departments of the Army, Navy and East India Company. The occasion was reported in *The Scotsman* a few days later, it being noted that 'all who have seen this edifice pronounce it to be one of the greatest ornaments of our city, and a most successful effort of the skill of its accomplished architect'.[30] In a display of comradeship from its sister College, the Vice-President of the Royal College of Physicians, Dr Davison, 'proposed the prosperity' of the College 'in a speech of the most eloquent and classical description, which called for the repeated plaudits of his auditors.'

It was not just the external appearance of the building which was planned in great detail. Playfair also designed the interior as well as the furniture and fittings for the College, in order that the scheme should be coherent as a whole and not just provide an outer shell. He designed furniture for all the ground floor rooms, including the Hall of Meeting, Library and students' room. Particularly elegant chairs were designed for the use of the office-bearers of the College.[31]

The Fellows' wish to have a building which reflected their status was very much in line with the public face of exclusivity which they had been developing since 1505, though they may not have been able – or thought it necessary – to articulate the concept. The late eighteenth century had seen the increasingly public facets of science and other knowledge, and, perhaps paradoxically, the freedoms brought about by the Enlightenment generated their own constraints, controls and the need to offer some public visual evidence of the growing intellect, professionalism and knowledge of the College and its Fellows.

In a highly detailed study of the architectural transformation of Edinburgh in the nineteenth century, focusing mainly on the financial aspects, Richard Rodger states that 'a critical mass of professional expertise was concentrated in Edinburgh as a direct result of the guarantees enshrined in the Act of Union'.[32] The College may not have been involved in the legal or religious professions, but nevertheless it was part of this 'critical mass' and this must be seen as a factor in its desire to acquire a building with the right kind of visual symbolism. Gone were any hints at the Scottish baronial style as in the 1697 building – this was full-blown Greek revival and purposely so.[33]

This was not the end of the matter by any means. Regular modifications and repairs had to be made to the building and innovations adopted, including electric light and telephones. In 1863 it was decided to install gas lighting in the Museum, and on 7 February 1895 the Secretary wrote to the Town Council seeking permission to install electric lighting in the College.

By the turn of the twentieth century the Playfair Building was proving yet again to be increasingly inadequate and too inflexible to cater for the needs of a burgeoning organisation, particularly the Museum. The 400th anniversary celebrations had demonstrated the inadequacy of the building, not least its lack of adequate toilet facilities. Proposals for alterations were discussed at a College meeting on 16 July 1907 and a committee formed to consider the matter and draw up plans with the architect, Balfour Paul. Despite some opposition – including the suggestion that the Barclay collection should be disposed of (not the last time the Museum would be under threat) – agreement was eventually reached, and substantial internal rearrangements were completed by 1909. These included the reconstruction of the upper floors of two houses in 9 Hill Square adjacent to the new museum hall, which had been constructed from the upper floors of 7 Hill Square. The *BMJ* reported that:

> The Council room, which occupied the greater part of the ground storey, has been vacated as such, divided into two, one part being added to the library, and the other part forming a reception room. The western portion of the old museum devoted to the Barclay collection, has been converted into the new Council Room. To provide for the Barclay collection certain tenement houses have been converted into additional museum spaces. The design of the original museum has been followed in the arrangement of the galleries, but glass shelves have been introduced so as to give good light. The flooring of the galleries has been formed of glass with the same object.[34]

To maintain the historical lineage of the buildings, the lintel which had been preserved from the door of Old Surgeons' Hall was incorporated into the door of the then Journal Office in 1957, having been returned to the College by Sir William Turner, College President, in 1883 and stored in the College since that time.

## MORE RECENT BUILDING PROJECTS

Throughout most of the more recent period the College has pursued a policy of acquiring, where possible, most of the property in and around Hill Square, in order to provide accommodation for an increasing range of College activities and their administration. Council was frequently concerned with the juggling of various bits of accommodation in order to make more efficient use of the space and to cope with

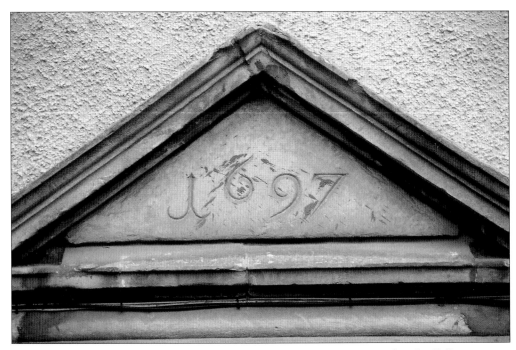

**FIG. 7.6** *Door lintel from Old Surgeons' Hall, which was returned to the College in 1883 and incorporated into the present building in 1957.*

new demands, such as a photographic office. In 1961 the glass front doors and new Council Room were completed, and at the meeting of the College Council on 17 October 1962, alterations to the Library and kitchens, dampness in a house in Hill Square owned by the College, heating, ventilation and minor adjustments to the Museum were discussed, together with the proposed redecoration of the Hall, the appearance of the Museum staircase and 'essential' repairs to properties in Hill Square.

It was decided in the late 1970s, during the presidency of John Gillingham, to go ahead with work to convert the adjacent St Michael's church into a symposium hall, given the relatively healthy financial position of the College at that time as a result of good investments and fruitful appeals. This church had been built by Thomas Hamilton in 1847 as Roxburgh Free Church and from 1887 it became St Michael's Episcopal church. The internal space was not ideal for its purpose, but by judicious planning and careful conservation the church was indeed converted.[35] The financing of this project was assisted by a donation of £10,000 from Marks and Spencer, in the light of the name of the church, and, rather more substantially, by the gift of £350,000 from the Saudi Arabian royal house, specifically for this aspect of the College's redevelopment programme. The King Khalid Bin Abdul Aziz Symposium Hall, designed by James Parr and Partners, was handed over to the College formally on 5 October 1982. On 28 June 1983 the Patron visited the College and unveiled a plaque commemorating the successful completion of the Symposium Hall and the Postgraduate Residence.

The conversion of the church was only part of an ambitious scheme, which

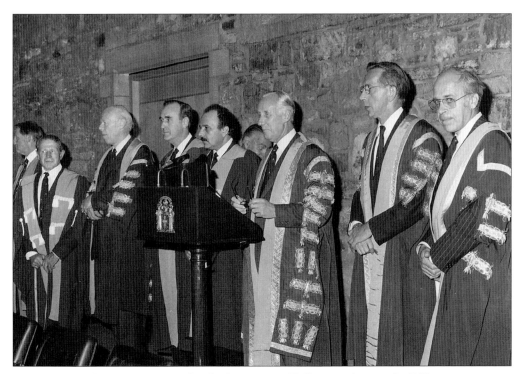

**FIG. 7.7** *Opening ceremony for the Symposium Hall, 1982. Among the Fellows present are A. I. S. Macpherson, Sir James Fraser, A. J. Duff, F. J. Gillingham and T. J. McNair.*

included the construction of residencies for postgraduate students. The initial plan had been to convert St Michael's church for this purpose, but this proved not to be feasible and attention was turned to properties in Hill Street. A public appeal raised some £925,000 and tenement houses were donated by the town council, but this was not without controversy as Robin Cook, then an Edinburgh MP, opposed the plans, claiming that the housing should have been refurbished by the council and let out to tenants.[36] Six months later, though, *The Scotsman* felt able to state that: 'students at the Royal College of Surgeons of Edinburgh will be able to live in a row of Georgian houses, attend lectures in a tiered symposium hall modelled on the great hall of Padua, and stroll to classes across an elegant new Surgeons' Square'.[37] In 1987 the redundant Salvation Army Hall was purchased, and eventually demolished to allow landscaping of the College grounds.

In addition to the work on the Symposium Hall, conversion work took place in Hill Square, funded by a generous donation from the Sir Jules Thorn Charitable Trust, to set up a museum of the history of surgery and of the College (see Chapter 6), and a continuous process of adaptation and acquisition of premises around the Square has been undertaken, in order develop and maximise the efficient use of the campus. By 1992 the Playfair Building had undergone a full restoration, with the original type of gas lamps and iron railings refitted. Ever interested, the local press took the view that 'a grand old lady has emerged as a stunning beauty after

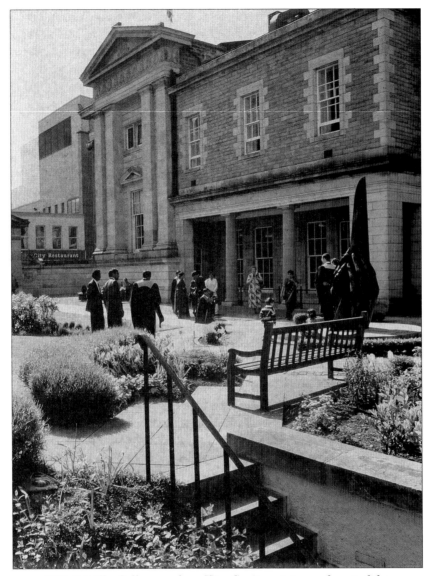

*FIG. 7.8* *The College gardens,* Hinc Sanitas *statue and part of the Playfair Building.*

a lengthy facelift'.[38] The ceremony to mark the close of the restoration programme took place on 24 September 1992. In 1994 the distinctive statue by Dennis Mitchell, entitled *Hinc Sanitas*, was placed in the College gardens.

## BUILDING FOR THE FUTURE – DREAMS AND REALITIES

In the lead-up to the celebrations of the College quincentenary, Council has been considering how best to improve the practical facilities in the College and to develop more and better means of delivering the surgical training courses which have become one of its pivotal activities. A new Careers Centre has recently been established in the Adamson Building – enabled by a generous bequest from Mrs Patricia Adamson, in memory of her late husband, Bill Adamson, a Fellow of the College – in nearby premises acquired from the BMA, and ambitious plans were drawn up to construct 'New Surgeons' Hall'. The intention was to provide a 'versatile, multipurpose facility', containing a large surgical skills training laboratory with the relevant preparation and storerooms, together with classrooms and study areas for students. The major problem with this, as with all other such ambitious plans nowadays, is, of course, finance. It had been estimated that the total cost of building and furnishing New Surgeons' Hall would be some £15,000,000 and an appeal was launched for this purpose with the hope of receiving substantial donations from 'individual, Trust and corporate philanthropists'.

The plans for New Surgeons' Hall were drawn up for a number of reasons, some of which are absolutely the same as they have always been, but others having more to do with surgical life and organisation in a very different atmosphere. There are three main aspects to this. Firstly, the elegant Playfair Building is just that – elegant but no longer suitable for the work of a modern organisation. Secondly, the College has perceived its major function in the future to lie in the area of education, and the present facilities for training are increasingly inadequate. Thirdly, and not the least important, if the ambitious new building could be built, it would be doubly symbolic – of the long and mostly distinguished history of the Incorporation and College, and of the anticipated direction of its future life and activities. The building was designed to be modern, functional and adaptable, but also to sit harmoniously with the adjacent Playfair Building, which is set to become the focus of the heritage aspects of the College. It is important, not just from the point of view of present and future historians, that the old be retained, cherished and preserved, but also from the much longer-term perspective of the College, however long its future existence as an independent surgical body may be.

Unfortunately, though, the most altruistic and far-sighted plans depend on money. In the nineteenth century, the College had to borrow from the Widows' Fund to make up the shortfall in the cost of the Playfair Building, but it has proved to be impossible to acquire the funding to build New Surgeons' Hall at present. All is not lost, though, as the College has been able to acquire the adjacent Forbes Laboratory. Though externally perhaps a little utilitarian in aspect, this is a building with a history and with connections to the College. It was owned by the College until it was sold off in the 1980s. It had been renovated in 1904 to accommodate the Incorporation's Officer, and prior to that it had, among other things, acted as a base for the first Scottish Antarctica Expedition led by William Speirs Bruce in 1902, and also housed the Scottish Oceanographical Laboratory. The building is deceptively large and internally flexible enough to be adapted to meet at least some of the needs of a modern surgical training laboratory. There are also plans to continue campus development with the redevelopment of the postgraduate residence to form 10 Hill Place which, in combination with the enlarged and greatly modified Symposium Hall, will offer a commercial hotel opportunity as well as providing facilities for College events and needs.[39]

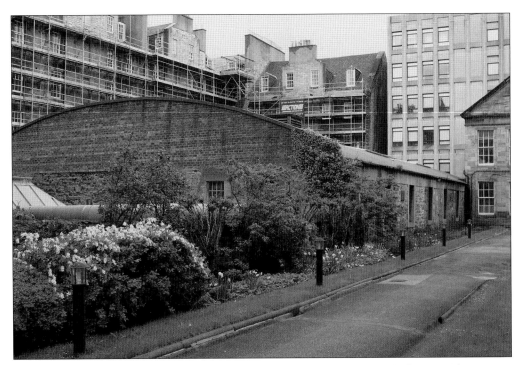

**FIG. 7.9** *The Forbes Laboratory, which is to be extensively modified to provide new training facilities.*

Medical coporations elsewhere led similar peripatetic lives in the early periods of their existence. The FPSG, founded in 1599, met in a variety of locations including the Deacon's house, the church, the Regality Hall or Crafts' Hospital.[40] Coincidentally, it was in 1697 that the FPSG took the first steps towards acquiring purpose-built accommodation. It moved through premises in Trongate and St Enoch Square, to the present building in St Vincent Street, acquired in 1862.[41] The RCSEng and RCSI are housed in similarly impressive buildings. The Irish College managed to attract a grant of £6,000 from the government towards the building of a new hall in 1805 and, like most such buildings, was modified over the years according to circumstance.[42] After sojourns in Fountain Close and George Street, the RCPEd moved to its new hall in George Street, still in the fashionable New Town, in 1846. Designed by Thomas Hamilton in the classical style, it has been described as 'spectacular' in effect, 'although it is perhaps not unfair to say that it is more Victorian than Roman'.[43] The home of the RCSEng, constructed with government support to a design by George Dance from 1805, and rebuilt by Charles Barry (who also built the Houses of Parliament) in the 1830s, suffered severe damage during the Second World War, although the classical portico from Dance's 1813 building was preserved.[44]

The importance of buildings to institutions of this sort has not, perhaps, been a major consideration for historians, but the combination of symbolic wish and practical necessity has ensured that many institutions have been housed in very

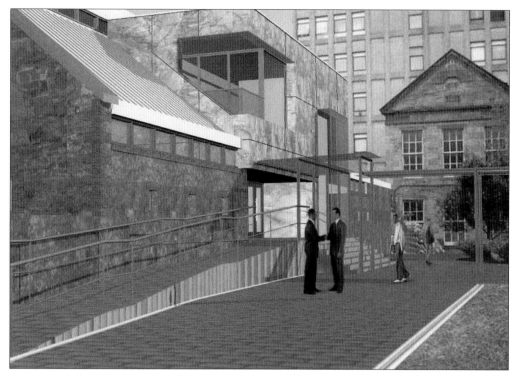

***FIG. 7.10*** *Architectural drawing of proposed alterations to the Forbes Laboratory.*

visible and architecturally significant buildings. Most of the medical corporations are currently housed in elegant buildings, though economic pressures and the needs of modern medical education may mean that this situation cannot continue indefinitely. Historic buildings certainly lend gravitas to institutions, but they are generally inflexible and difficult to adapt to changing circumstances.

The Incorporation made use of a series of buildings, increasing in opulence with each one, but each one appropriate to the particular circumstances of the time. The minutes do not contain any directly articulated awareness of the wider symbolism of their homes, but this is implicit in their actions throughout and in all of their buildings. Just as the coat of arms, matriculated in 1672, was important, and equally so the ornate badge worn by the Officer from 1697 and later the academic gowns worn by the Fellows, so the importance of physical place, or *genius loci*, was clearly acknowledged.

## NOTES

1. John Gairdner, President, 16 May 1832.
2. Creswell, *Royal College of Surgeons*, p. 46.
3. Ibid., pp. 48–50.
4. Ibid., p. 48. It seems that part of the site was acquired as a result of a bequest to the Town Council of 26,000 merks by Mr Bartholomew Somervell, of which 6,000 merks were to be used for building a house bearing his name and arms. This house was to be for the

use of the Professor of Divinity, but appears to have been acquired by the Incorporation along with the original Curryhill house.

5.  See Dingwall, *Physicians, Surgeons and Apothecaries*, pp. 58–9; Grant, J., *Cassell's Old and New Edinburgh* (London 1884), i, p. 382; ii, p. 241.

6.  College Minutes, 5 August 1664.

7.  Ibid., 18 May 1669. Each master present agreed to donate or lend £100 towards the costs of this enterprise.

8.  Ibid., 2 October 1696.

9.  Gifford, J., McWilliam, C. and Walker, D. (eds), *The Buildings of Scotland: Edinburgh* (London, 1984), p. 186.

10. Maitland, *The History of Edinburgh*, p. 182.

11. College Minutes, 16 April 1697.

12. Details of the individual Medina portraits in Masson, *Portraits*.

13. Creswell, *Royal College of Surgeons*, p. 94.

14. College Minutes, 17 December 1697. A recent Edinburgh University undergraduate essay has covered the building of the Old Hall in considerable detail. Williams, M., 'A Report on the History of Old Surgeons' Hall, Edinburgh' (unpublished MA essay, 2004).

15. College Minutes, 22 February 1728.

16. Ibid., 27 March 1729.

17. Ibid., 15 November 1733.

18. See the detailed account in Creswell, *Royal College of Surgeons*, pp. 55–62.

19. College Minutes, 27 July 1745.

20. Creswell, *Royal College of Surgeons*, p. 59.

21. Kaufman, *Medical Teaching in Edinburgh*, pp. 19–20. This book includes several chapters covering the occupants of Surgeons' Square.

22. College Minutes, 15 May 1745. This was a period when the concept of insurance against misfortune was becoming more common, a particular misfortune being fire.

23. For a full account of the development of the New Town, see Youngson, A., *The Making of Classical Edinburgh* (Edinburgh, 1967).

24. College Minutes, 2 February 1822.

25. Kaufman, *Medical Teaching in Edinburgh*, pp. 3, 125.

26. NAS, GD51/5/708/1, Letter from David Hay to Lord Melville, 31 January 1825; GD51/5/708/2, Petition to Treasury.

27. College Minutes, 2 February and 7 April 1829. Further discussions are noted in October, and within a few months discussion took place as to the items to be placed in a box under the foundation stone of the new hall.

28. McKean, C., *Edinburgh. An Illustrated Architectural Guide* (Edinburgh, 1992), p. 74. The Museum is described as containing 'awesome exhibits'.

29. Gifford et al., *Edinburgh*, p. 244. This also describes the Balfour Paul reconstruction which took place in 1908–9.

30. *The Scotsman*, 14 July 1832.

31. See Masson, *A College Miscellany*, for illustrations of these and other Playfair artefacts.

32. Rodger, R., *The Transformation of Edinburgh. Land, Property and Trust in the Nineteenth Century* (Cambridge, 2001), p. 13. See also Allen, N. (ed.), *Scottish Pioneers of the Greek Revival* (Edinburgh, 1984).

33. For a discussion of Greek revival, see Mordaunt Crook, J., *The Greek Revival. Neo-Classical Attitudes in British Architecture 1760–1870* (London, 1995).

34. *BMJ*, 9 October 1909, p. 1094. On 20 December 1909 the same source reported on the occasion when Lord Rosebery, descendant of Gilbert Primrose, gave a speech at a College dinner.

35. Maloco, A. and Dear, D., 'Symposium Hall for the Royal College of Surgeons of Edinburgh', *Edinburgh Architectural Association Review*, 12 (1984), pp. 105–15 discusses the conversion from the architectural point of view. The architects were James Parr and Partners.

36. *Edinburgh Evening News*, 5 April 1979.
37. *The Scotsman*, 7 December 1979.
38. *Edinburgh Evening News*, 28 August 1992.
39. Foster, J., 'The Forbes Laboratory', *Annual Report 2002–2003* (Royal College of Surgeons of Edinburgh, 2003), p. 37.
40. Geyer-Kordesch and Macdonald, *Physicians and Surgeons in Glasgow*, p. 88.
41. Hull and Geyer-Kordesch, *The Shaping of the Medical Profession*, pp. xxi–xxx, describes the various domiciles of the RCPSG.
42. Widdess, *The Royal College of Surgeons in Ireland*, p. 60.
43. Youngson, *Making of Classical Edinburgh*, p. 280.
44. Blandy and Lumley, *The Royal College of Surgeons of England*, pp. 19, 25, 71–2. The College made a donation towards the post-1945 restoration project.

# 8

# Conclusion: the College –
# past, present and future

We have made the transition from a Club to a major organisation, not without some difficulties, but successfully and more importantly without changing our essential character.[1]

The College has been shaped by many forces and influences over its first 500 years. Their manifestation, though, has changed significantly in the light of changing contextual influences. Surgeons and surgery at the start of the next half-millennium are very different, at least on the surface, from what they were in 1505, as are the City of Edinburgh, the Scottish nation, Great Britain and the world. It is possible, though, to trace common elements throughout this lengthy and often turbulent period. This is not to take a Whiggish approach to the explanation of the historical process. Nor is it to abandon causality completely in favour of the undiluted postmodernist approach, in which causality is anathema. Nor is it, though, to dismiss the postmodernist view out of hand. To the early masters of the Incorporation, 'diligently and avisitly examinit and provit' meant the same as it does nowadays, but in a very different and more limited context. At first sight, the simple surgical procedures and restricted anatomical knowledge which formed the basis of surgical tests in 1505 bear little relation to the specialty Fellowship examinations taken by potential new-millennium Fellows. The key point is, though, that each was and is entirely appropriate to its age, and must be interpreted in the light of the contemporary context. The end result may appear to have been a seamless path from 1505 to 2005 in terms of the development of surgical examinations, but influences varied according to the changing context. Similarly, the interaction of medical and public spheres, the relationship between surgeon and patient, and the social construction of the medical world in which the College operated have been subject to different influences over time.

The same is true of other factors, particularly the general background context. In earlier times the small number of surgeons and barbers in Edinburgh had to deal mainly with the Town Council and the pursuit of unauthorised practice by individuals who had not taken the freedom of the Incorporation. As time went on, concerns were widened to encompass the actions of the physicians, the patronage of royalty and politicians, and more recently the increasingly detailed and prescriptive requirements of government.

In other areas too, the fate of the College has depended greatly on what was happening elsewhere. For 400 years it has operated in the context of Great Britain, not Scotland, and for a more limited period, against the wider backcloth of Empire. Its global context has now become as wide as it can get. The combination of instant communication and almost unbelievable technological advance means that consideration must be given to the extent to which Scotland or Scottish factors have anything at all to do with the shaping of the modern College or the careers of its Fellows, who come from, and work in, many cultural contexts worldwide. This brings matters back to the question of identity and distinctiveness.

The original identity of the College was that of a typical urban craft. Its modern identity is more difficult to define. It can still be viewed in some ways as a craft which provides training and validation for entrant members. There are, though, much more complex and difficult contextual considerations. Surgeons, as other medical practitioners, are subject to national registration, national standards, national politics and a national health service. They have far greater opportunities to cure patients than they had half a millennium ago; they have access to all sorts of technology, diagnostic and paramedical support services; they operate in purpose-built buildings; they still demonstrate the caring ethos; and they share, in modern terms, the original aims of the Incorporation. There is perhaps much less nowadays that is identifiably Scottish in all of this, particularly in the light of the distribution of adherents to the College. Currently, of the circa 17,000 Members and Fellows worldwide, 1,560 are in Scotland, but over 7,000 in England and a similar number in the rest of the world.[2]

Is there a place for institutions such as this at the beginning of the twenty-first century? In some ways they sit uneasily in the modern context of management, global communication and thrusting business enterprises. They are led by surgeons, not by business professionals. The President and other office-bearers serve for limited periods of time, and a presidency of only three years may not be long enough to see ambitious plans brought to fruition, plans which may not necessarily be shared by the next President, who, quite naturally, wishes to make his (and it is to be hoped at some point, her) stamp on the College and leave an attributable legacy. This has the inevitable, if unintentioned, effect of producing uncertainty at times. The situation has been alleviated to a great extent, though, by the much more extensive, permanent management and administrative structures which have developed in the last decade or so.

In the wider context, what does a historic institution such as this mean? Its original purpose was to maintain the exclusive rights of its members. Nowadays the regulation, registration, and scope of surgical training are determined at national level. There is no longer the need for the College to prosecute unqualified individuals; there is no longer the need to supervise barbers; there is no longer the need to fight for custody of surgical knowledge. A key function of the original masters was to train apprentices, so that they would be able to practise the best surgery that could be offered, within the not inconsiderable constraints of limited anatomical knowledge, superstition and the lack of anaesthetics or the means to effectively control infection. The regulation of surgical training may now be out of the College's control; the training which it offers through its education department is, as yet, not, and this remains a key function.

On most counts, the case for the future of the College articulates itself with ease. But there are potential problems for any institution which wishes to retain its history, its national and international status and, importantly, the finance to do these things. Three major problems would appear to be facing this and the other Colleges at present. The first is the question of whether there should be a single British College of Surgeons, which would, probably, be based in London (though an alternative may be a multi-campus 'virtual' British College).[3] Problems of history, civic rivalry and politics are deeply embedded in any question of amalgamation of the two Scottish Colleges, let alone the creation of a single British College.

The second problem is that most surgical corporations provide a similar range of educational offerings. The College must, therefore, be seen to be providing something that cannot be obtained from other sources. Linked to this is the third problem, that of continuing to attract examination candidates, both to Edinburgh and to the overseas examination centres run by, or in conjunction with, the College. As these centres increasingly organise their own training and examinations and set up their own institutions, further opportunities here may be limited. In addition to the growth of local expertise, the almost immeasurable possibilities of global internet communication mean that surgical training, at least in its theoretical aspects, can be delivered at a great distance and without the necessity for a physical location.

The College does, though, have strengths and attributes which should enable it to survive. It has the great legacy of an impressive history. However much it may be denied, many individuals continue to be impressed by the gravitas of a long history. Institutions with long histories continue to attract candidates and members. To be a Fellow of the Royal College of Surgeons of Edinburgh is still regarded in many quarters and distant parts of the globe as a distinction to be sought after. To be Fellow of an institution whose earlier members included Syme, Lister and many other famous names still has meaning. Tradition is not everything, and no institution should sit back on the laurels of its long history, but it is still a considerable advantage. Adherents to institutions nowadays, though, expect rather more in return for their loyalty, and prestige alone is not sufficient to guarantee allegiance and support.

As the College, the city, the nation and the medical world enter the second millennium, the College enters the second half of its first millennium with aims and characteristics which are at the same time very similar to, and very different from, those of the original Incorporation. The two major phases of its history span almost equal periods – the Incorporation from 1505 to 1778 and the College from 1778 to 2005. The Enlightenment period, during which the Incorporation achieved royal status, was something of a general as well as intellectual watershed for

Edinburgh, Scotland and Europe. It can of course be argued that the College started life as an enlightened incorporation, given the stated aims of its masters right from the start. The 'Famous and Flourishing Society' was seen as just that from the start. The insistence on literacy in 1505 was far-sighted, and helped to set the Incorporation apart from the other groups which sat around the Deacon convener's table in the Magdalen Chapel to thrash out matters which affected the trades as a whole. The Incorporation was something of a hybrid institution – at once a typical manual trade and a learned society; at once on the 'wrong' side of the merchant/craft divide and the educated equal of the professions. This hybrid beginning resulted in the masters adopting a rather ambivalent stance at times. Though they relied on Town Council and craft support, their very clear aim was to leave the ranks of the manual trades and join those of the learned professions, and they used an extensive network of patronage and contacts with the elite and royal in society to foster these aims. It was perhaps inevitable as well as convenient that the transition to Royal College took place within the particular ambience that was Enlightenment Edinburgh. The academic trappings which had been built up by the Incorporation already helped to mark it out as a body which embraced learning as well as manual skills. That the surgical procedures which it was possible to undertake in the middle of the eighteenth century were limited was certainly true, but was not really the major issue at that point. The Royal Charter did not come because complex surgery was now possible; what was probably more important was the status built up by the Incorporation over the years as surgeons to successive monarchs and their armies, political patronage, and relationships with high-status individuals from all of the important walks of Scottish elite life, not least the increasingly powerful legal profession.

The second, or College, phase has been much more complex – at least on the surface – and apparently much less in the direct control of the College itself. The College had to adapt and function within a very different and often much more difficult background, involving the fate and fortunes not only of Edinburgh and Scotland, but also of Britain, the temporary British Empire and ultimately the entire compass of the known world. Allied to this have been the much more rapid advances in the sciences and surgical technology and the greatly increased role of government in the regulation of the profession. By the end of the twentieth century the modern College Fellow operates very differently, in a very different context and in all corners of the globe. However, many of his or her aims are the same as those articulated by those who petitioned the Town Council for a charter five centuries ago.

Visual symbolism has been important throughout the history of the College and in some ways is just as important in the twenty-first century. It has a coat of arms, its Fellows wear distinctive gowns,[4] and the College mace precedes the Fellows on formal occasions. Buildings were also important in this way. Homeless at first, by the mid-seventeenth century Curryhill House had been acquired, followed by a new Hall opened in 1697, and the present, classical building opened in 1832. These developments have been discussed in greater detail in the foregoing chapters, but it is important in any summing-up of the College to revisit and highlight the visual symbolism of this and any other learned organisation. In earlier centuries, symbolism helped the illiterate to learn about the world, the church, society and politics; it gave the Incorporation a physical location and corporate focus. By the turn of the nineteenth century the symbolism had rather different purposes. Status had been achieved, and physical grandeur, as practised and aspired to by big government and local government in civic buildings, was the background to the specific design of the new College building. Symbolism is just as important in 2005.

In all of these ways it can be seen that throughout the history of this and other professional organisations, the outward, visual factors have been just as important as what was going on inside these buildings. It is all part of the rather hybrid nature of these organisations that history and ancient tradition go hand-in-hand with modern management structures. This dichotomy is not unproblematic, but it does seem that both aspects still have their place.

The future of surgical education is, it seems, a future ordered by acronyms – national organisations with national remits, which have responsibility for the modernisation, validation and supervision of postgraduate medical training. While the medical corporations will be represented on these bodies, they will not be in the majority.

So what must the College do to maintain its identity and, importantly, influence on the future of surgical training? Whatever the nature of the encroaching acronyms, the College has the advantage of long history and of a physical presence (as a base for Fellows, both resident and non-resident), rather than being simply a paper or electronic organisation. Some observers may consider that these factors no longer have relevance in the modern, global age. This may be the case, but as long as there is demand for a symbolic, physical, focus point, surgeons will be attracted to membership. However, as has been the case for most of its long history, it will not be enough for the College to rest on the laurels of its lengthy pedigree and historical presence. A number of initiatives have been taken, or will be taken, mainly in the rapidly developing area of surgical training in the laboratory. Surgical skills have been taught by, and in conjunction with, the College for many years; nowadays the requirements are more complex and demand expansion of laboratory facilities in order to provide training on simulators and other non-patient devices. To this end, new training facilities are under development, and innovations will also be necessary in assessment procedures, knowledge-based testing and workplace assessments, and progress is already being made in these areas.[5]

What the College is seeking to do for the future is to provide first-class, life-long surgical education, first-class educational facilities, and examinations which are appropriate to the nature, scope and potential of modern surgery as well as complying with the requirements set out by the supervisory bodies. The College is a registered charity and is developing its Heritage side with the aim of widening public awareness of its activities. Departments are now much more co-ordinated and clear plans for the future are in place. The original aims and objectives of the College have not changed. Though management, planning, finance and other economic matters are crucial to the survival of the College, its prime function still remains that of ensuring that surgeons are trained and qualified to the highest and most rigorous standards possible. The seeing hand depicted in the College's coat of arms now sees by complex technological means, but it still must see as clearly as possible.

The future is somewhat uncertain. This is not new. At several points during the last 500 years the survival of the College was equally uncertain. This was mainly because of financial difficulties or lack of numbers, but more recently the main threat seems to be the increasing dominance of national organisations and the difficulties of maintaining three surgical colleges in the UK. However, providing that the College continues to adapt to the changing context and altered pattern of external influences, there is no reason why it should not continue to flourish famously, either independently or within a different, British context.

## NOTES

1. Arnold G. D. Maran, RCSEd *Annual Report 2000*.
2. Figures from RCSEd Membership Department.
3. Conversation with John Smith, President, 23 December 2003.
4. Prior to 1911 only the President, Vice-President and Treasurer wore robes, faced with red. It was decided to acquire new robes, in 'College Blue', and one of the first occasions on which these were paraded was the coronation of George V in 1911.
5. Conversation with Professor Sir John Temple, then President, 23 June 2003.

# Appendix I

# Text of Seal of Cause, 1505

Text from an entry in the Town Council Records, entitled 'The Copye of Ye Barboris Seall of Cause as Followis.[1]

To all and sindrie to quhais knauledge thir present letteris sall cum, the prouest baillies and counsale of the burgh of Edinburgh, greiting in God euirlesting: Witt your vniuersities that the day of the dait of thir presentis comperit befoir me, sittand in jugement in the Tolbuith of the said burgh, the kirkmaister and brether of the Sueregianis and Barbouris within the samyn, and presentit till me their bill and supplicatioun desiring ws for the louing of God, honour of oure Souerane Lord and all his lieges, and for worschip and policy of this burgh, and for the gude reull and ordour to be had and maid amangis the saidis craftis in tymes to cum, that we wald grant and consent to thame the previlegis reullis and statutes contenit in their said bill and supplicatioun quhilk efter follows:

To you my loirdis provest baillies and worthy counsall of this gude tovne, right humblie meins and schawis your daylie servitouris the kirkmaister and brether of Chirurgeonis and Barbouris within this burgh, that quhair we beleve itt is weill knawen till all your wisdomis quhow that we vphald ane altar situat within your College Kirk of Sanct Geill in the honour of God and Sanct Mongow our patrone, and hes na importance to vphald the samyn but oure sober oulklie penny and vpsettis, quhilk ar small in effect till sustene and vphald oure said altar in all necessary thingis convenient theirto, and because we ar and ever was of gude mynde till do this gude tovne all the staid pleasour and seruice than we can or may, baith in walking and wairding stenting and bering of all vther portabill charges within this burgh at all tymes, as vther nichtbouris and craftis dois within the samyn, we desire at your lordship and wisdoms till geve and grant to ws and oure successouris thir reulis statutes and previlegis vndir written, quhilkis are consonant to resoun, honour till oure Souerane Lord and all his lieges, proffeitt and lowabill to this gude tovne: In the first, that we micht have yeirlie chosin amangis ws ane kirkmaister and ourisman to quhome the haill brether of the craftis foirsaid sall obey for that yeir: Item, that na maner of persoun occupie nor vse ony poyntis of our saidis craftis of Surregenie or Barbour craft within this burgh bott gif he be first frieman and burges of the saymn, and that he be worthy and expert in all the poyntis belangand the saidis craftis diligentlie and avysitlie examinit and admittit be the maisters of

295

the said craft for the honorabill seruying of oure Souerane Lord his lieges and nychtbouris of this burgh, and als that euerie man that is to be maid freman and maister amangis ws be examinit and previt in thir poyntis following, that is to say, that he knaw anatomell, nature and complexion of euery member humanis bodie, and inlykewayes he knaw all the vaynis of the samyn, that he may mak flewboth-omell in dew tyme, for euery man aucht to knaw the nature and substance of euery thing that he werkis, or ellis he is negligent; and that we may have anis in the yeir any condampnit man efter he be deid to mak antomell off, quhairthraw we may haif experience, ilk ane to instrict vtheris, and we sall do suffrage for the soule; and that na barbour, maister nor seruand, within this burgh hantt vse nor exerce the craft of Surregenrie without he be expert and knaw perfytelie the thingis abouewritten: and quhat person sal happin to be admittit frieman or maisteris to the saidis craftis, or occupies ony poynt of the samyn, sall pay at his entry for his vpsett five pundis vsuall money of this realme of Scotland to the reparatioun and vphalding of oure said altar of Sanct Mongow for deuyne seruice to be done thairatt, with ane dennar to the maisteris of the saidis craftis at his admissioun and entres amangis ws; exceptand that euery frieman maister of the saidis craftis ane of his lawful gottin sonnes to be frie of ony money payment, except the dennar to be maid to the maisteris of the said craft efter he be exeminit and admitted by them as said is: Item, that na maisteris of the said craft sall tak ane prenteis or feit man in tyme cuming to vse the Surregeane craft without he can baithe wryte and reid, and the said maister of ony of the saidis craftis that takis ane prenteis sall pay at his entres to the reparatioun of the said alter tuenty schillingis; and that na maister of the said craft resset nor resave any vther maisteris prenteis or seruand quhill the ische of his termes be run, and quha that dois in the contrair thairof, as oft as he failyies, sall pay xx s. to the reparatioun of the said alter but favouris. Item, euery maister that is resauit frieman to the said craft sall pay his oulklie penny with the priestis meit as he sall happen to cum about, and euery seruand that is feitt man to the maisteris of the said craft sall pay ilk oulk any half-peny to the said alter and reparatioun theirof; and that we haif powar to cheis ane chaiplane till do devyne seruice daylie at our said alter at all tymes quhen the samyn sall vaik, and till cheis ane officiar till pas with ws for the ingathering of oure quarter payment and oulklie pennies, and to pass befoir ws on Corpus Christy day and the octauis theirof, and all vther generall processionis and gatherinis, siclike as vtheris craftis hes within this burgh; and that ane of the maisteris of the foirsaid craftis, with the chaiplane and officiar of the samyn, pas at all tymes neidfull lift collect and rais the saidis quarter payments fra euery persoun that aw the samyn, and gif ony dissobeyis that we may poynd and distrenye thairfoir all tymes haifand ane officiar of the tovne with us: Item, that na man nor freman of the said craft purches ony lordschip incontrair the statutes and rewlis aboue written, in hindering or skaithing of the craftis foirsaidis or commoun weill thairof, vnder the payne of tynsall of their friedomes. Item, that all the maisteris friemen and brether of the said craft reddelie obey and cum to their kirkmaister at all tymes quhen thay sal be requyritt thairto be the said officiar for to heir quarter comptis, or till avyse for ony thing concerning the commoun weill of the saidis craftis, and quha that disobeyis sall pay xx s. to the reparatioun of the said altar; and that na persoun man nor women within this burgh mak nor sell ony aquavite within the samyn except the saidis maisters brether and friemen of the saidis craftis vnder the pane of escheit of the samyn but fauouris. Beseking heirfoir your lordschippis and wisdoms at the reuerence of God that ye will avise with thir oure sempill desyris statutes rewlis and privileges abouewritten, and grant ws the samyn ratefeit and apprevit be you vnder your seill of cause, and with the grace of God we sall do sic seruice and plesour to the Kingis grace and gude tovne that ye salbe contentit thairof, and your delyuerance heirintill humblie I beseik.

The quhilk bill of supplicatioun with the reullis statutis and privileges contenit thairentill being red befoir ws in jugement, and we thairwith beand ryplie and distinctlie avysit, thinkis the samyn consonant to resoun and na hurt to our Souerane Lordis Hienes, ws, nor nane vtheris his lieges thairintill, and theirfoir we consent and grantis the samyn to the foirsaidis craftis of Surregenry and Barbouris and to thair successouris, and in sa far as we may or hes powar, confirmis ratefeis and apprevis the saidis statutes reullis and privilegis in all poyntis and articles contenit in the supplcatioun abouewritten; and to all and syndrie quhome it efferis or may effere we mak it knawin be thir our letters; and for the mair verificatioun and strenth of the samyn we haif to hungin our commoun seill of cause, at Edinburgh, the first day of the moneth of July the yeir of God ane thousand five hundreth and five yeiris.

## NOTE

1.   Comrie, *History*, i, pp. 162–4, from the Records of the Burgh of Edinburgh.

# Appendix II

# Text of Ratification of Seal of Cause by James IV, 1506

---

By King James the Fourth, in Favours of the Surgeons and Barbers of Edinburgh. October 13 1506.

James, by the Grace of God, King of Scots, To the provost and bailies of our burgh of Edinburgh, that now are or shall happen to be for the time, and to all other and sundry our officers, leidges, and subjects, whom it effeirs, to whose knowledge these our letters shall come; greeting. Forasmuch as the craftsmen of Surgery and Barber craft, within our said burgh of Edinburgh, have made certain statutes and rules to be had and kept among them, for the honourable serving our lieges, in their crafts and reparation of their altar in the College-kirk of St Geill within our said burgh, and upholding divine service at the same in time coming, as is contained at length in the letters of ratification and confirmation, made by the provost, bailies, and council of our said burgh, under their common seal of cause, made to the said craftsmen thereupon, shown and produced before us, and a part of the lords of our council. We therefore understanding, that the said statutes are made for keeping of good rule among the said craftsmen, and upholding of divine service, and are not prejudicial nor hurting or us nor our lieges, ratifies, approves, and for us and our successors, by these our letters, authorises, and confirms the said statutes and rules, to be observed, used, and firmly kept among the kirkmaster and craftsman of Chirurgery and Barber crafts foresaid, that now are or shall happen to be within or said burgh in time coming, in all points and articles contained in the said letters under the common seal of the said burgh, given to them thereupon, and after the tenor, form and effect of the same. Wherefore, we charge strictly, and command you, all and sundry, our provost, bailies, and others, our officers, leidges, and subjects foresaid, that none of you take upon hand to do or attempt any thing in contrair, or breaking of the said statutes and rules, or of this our confirmation given thereupon in anywise in time coming, under all highest pain and charge that after may follow. Attour, if any of the said craftsmen disobeys, or acts in contrair the said statutes in any ways, that ye, the said provost and bailies, present and to come, in our name and authority, compel them to obey and fullfill the said statutes as effeirs, in all things after the form of your said letters, as ye will answer to us thereupon, and under the pains foresaid.

Given under our Privy Seal, at Edinburgh, the 13th day of October 1506 years, and of Our reign the 17th year.

*Registrum Secreti Sigilli Regem Scotorum* (ed. M. Livingston et al., Edinburgh, 1908), no. 344, notes: 'A letter maid to the Craftsmen of Syurgery and Barbor Craft, within the burgh of Edinburgh, ratifieand and approvand the statutes and rewlis maid amangis thaim anentis the serying of the Kingis Liegis and uphaldin of their altar in Sang Geilis Kirk. Subscripta per regem.'

# Appendix III

# Deacons/Presidents

There is no reliable information on Deacons prior to 1535. Elections took place at various times during the year and the first date given for each individual is the year during which he was first elected. Prior to 1600, in Scotland the year began on 1 March. The spelling of names was particularly flexible in the early centuries.

| | | | |
|---|---|---|---|
| 1535–6 | Lancelot Barbour | 1589–91 | James Henryson[1] |
| 1536–7 | Anthony Brussat | 1591–2 | James Craig |
| 1537–8 | no record | 1592–4 | Henry Lumsden |
| 1539–40 | George Leithe | 1594–5 | James Rig |
| 1540–2 | no record | 1595–6 | John Naismith |
| 1543–55 | William Quhite | 1596–8 | Henry Lumsden |
| 1555–7 | Alexander Bruce | 1598–1600 | Andro Scott |
| 1557–8 | Nowie [Noyer] Brussat | 1600–1 | James Henryson |
| 1558–9 | Alexander Bruce | 1601–2 | Henry Aikman |
| 1559–60 | Patrick Lindsay | 1602–3 | Gilbert Primrose |
| 1560–2 | Robert Henryson | 1603–5 | James Skaithmure |
| 1562–5 | James Lindesay | 1605–6 | Henry Lumsden/James Kinloch[2] |
| 1565–6 | John Chalmer | | |
| 1566–7 | Nowie Brussat | 1606–8 | Andrew Scott |
| 1567–8 | Alexander Bruce | 1608–10 | James Kinloch |
| 1568–9 | Nowie Brussat | 1610–12 | Henry Aikman |
| 1569–70 | Alexander Bruce | 1612–14 | David Pringle |
| 1571–2 | no record | 1614–16 | James Henryson |
| 1572–3 | Robert Henryson | 1616–18 | Andrew Scott |
| 1573–4 | Nowie Brussat | 1618–19 | James Henryson |
| 1574–8 | Gilbert Primrose | 1619–20 | James Kinloch |
| 1578–80 | Robert Henryson | 1620–1 | James Brown/Andro Scott[3] |
| 1580–3 | Gilbert Primrose | 1621–2 | Andro Scott |
| 1583–4 | Robert Henryson | 1622–4 | David Pringle |
| 1584–6 | Henrie Blyth | 1624–6 | Henry Aikman |
| 1586–7 | James Craig | 1626–7 | John Pringle |
| 1587–8 | James Henryson | 1627–9 | Andrew Scott |
| 1588–9 | James Lindsay | 1629–31 | Lawrence Cockburne |

| | | | |
|---|---|---|---|
| 1631–2 | John Ker | 1706–8 | John Mirrie |
| 1632–3 | John Spang | 1708–10 | Alexander Nisbet |
| 1633–5 | James Rig | 1710–12 | Henry Hamilton |
| 1635–7 | John Pringle | 1712–14 | John Monro |
| 1637–9 | David Douglas | 1714–16 | John Lauder |
| 1639–40 | John Pringle | 1716–18 | John McGill |
| 1640–1 | David Douglas | 1718–20 | John Lauder |
| 1641–2 | James Rig | 1720–2 | Robert Hope |
| 1642–4 | John Scott | 1722–4 | John Knox |
| 1644–6 | Alexander Penicuik[4] | 1724–5 | John Kirkwood |
| 1646–8 | David Douglas | 1725–6 | John Kennedy |
| 1648–51 | James Borthwick | 1726–8 | John Kirkwood |
| 1651–2 | David Kennedy[5] | 1728–30 | John Kennedy |
| 1652–5 | William Burnet[6] | 1730–2 | John Lauder |
| 1655–7 | Thomas Kincaid | 1732–4 | John McGill |
| 1657–9 | James Clelland | 1734–6 | John Kennedy |
| 1659–61 | James Borthwick | 1736–7 | John Lauder |
| 1661–3 | William Burnet | 1737–9 | William Mitchell |
| 1663–5 | Walter Trumble [Turnbull] | 1739–40 | George Cunningham |
| 1665–7 | Arthur Temple | 1740–2 | Alexander Nisbet |
| 1667–9 | Thomas Carter | 1742–4 | George Langlands |
| 1669–71 | Arthur Temple | 1744–6 | George Lauder |
| 1671–3 | Samuel Cheislie | 1746–8 | George Cunningham |
| 1673–5 | John Jossie | 1748–50 | Adam Drummond |
| 1675–7 | William Borthwick | 1750–2 | George Cunningham |
| 1677–9 | George Stirling | 1752–4 | James Russell |
| 1679–80 | James Nisbet | 1754–6 | Robert Walker |
| 1681–3 | William Borthwick | 1756–8 | Thomas Young |
| 1683–4 | Walter Turnbull | 1758–60 | William Chalmer |
| 1684–5 | David Pringle | 1760–2 | John Balfour |
| 1685–7 | Thomas Edgar | 1762–4 | Alexander Wood |
| 1687–9 | John Baillie | 1764–6 | James Rae |
| 1689–91 | George Stirling | 1766–8 | James Brodie |
| 1691–2 | John Reynolds | 1768–70 | Robert Smith |
| 1692–3 | James Crawford | 1770–2 | David Wardrobe |
| 1693–5 | Gideon Elliot | 1772–4 | William Inglis |
| 1695–7 | Alexander Monteith | 1774–6 | Andrew Wood |
| 1697–9 | Thomas Dunlop[7] | 1776–8 | Alexander Hamilton |
| 1699–1700 | Alexander Monteith/ | 1778–80 | James Gibson[10] |
| | Gideon Elliot[8] | 1780–2 | William Chalmer |
| 1700–1 | Gideon Elliott | 1782–4 | William Inglis |
| 1701–2 | Alexander Monteith[9] | 1784–6 | Thomas Hay |
| 1702–4 | James Hamilton | 1786–8 | Forrest Dewar |
| 1704–6 | Henry Hamilton | 1788–90 | Andrew Wardrop |

| 1790–2 | William Inglis | 1877–9 | Sir Patrick Heron Watson |
| 1792–4 | Thomas Wood | 1879–82 | Francis Brodie Imlach |
| 1794–6 | Thomas Hay | 1882–3 | Sir William Turner |
| 1796–8 | James Russell | 1883–4 | John Smith |
| 1798–1800 | Andrew Wood | 1885–7 | Douglas Argyll Robertson |
| 1800–2 | James Law | 1887–9 | Joseph Bell |
| 1802–4 | John Bennet | 1889–91 | John Duncan |
| 1804–6 | John Rae | 1891–3 | Robert Cunynghame |
| 1806–8 | William Farquharson | 1893–5 | Peter MacLaren |
| 1808–10 | Andrew Inglis | 1895–7 | Sir John Struthers |
| 1810–12 | Andrew Gillespie | 1897–9 | John Chiene |
| 1812–14 | James Law | 1899–1901 | James Dunsmure |
| 1814–16 | Sir William Newbigging | 1901–3 | Sir John Halliday Croom |
| 1816–18 | James Bryce | 1903–5 | Sir Patrick Heron Watson |
| 1818–20 | Alexander Gillespie | 1905–7 | Charles MacGillivray |
| 1820–2 | John Wishart | 1907–10 | Sir Joseph Cotterill |
| 1822–4 | William Wood | 1910–12 | Sir George Berry |
| 1824–6 | David Hay | 1912–14 | Francis Caird |
| 1826–8 | David MacLagan | 1914–17 | Sir James Hodsdon |
| 1828–30 | William Wood | 1917–19 | Robert Johnston |
| 1830–2 | John Gairdner | 1919–21 | George Mackay |
| 1832–4 | John Campbell[11] | 1921–3 | Sir David Wallace |
| 1834–6 | William Brown | 1923–5 | Sir Harold Stiles |
| 1836–8 | Sir George Ballingall | 1925–7 | Arthur Logan Turner |
| 1838–40 | Adam Hunter | 1927–9 | Alexander Miles |
| 1840–2 | Richard Huie | 1929–31 | James Ferguson |
| 1842–4 | Andrew Fyfe | 1931–3 | John Dowden |
| 1844–6 | James Simson | 1933–5 | Arthur Sinclair |
| 1846–8 | Samuel Pagan | 1935–7 | Sir Henry Wade |
| 1848–9 | John Argyll Robertson | 1937–9 | William Stuart |
| 1849–51 | James Syme | 1939–41 | Harry Traquair |
| 1851–3 | James Combe | 1941–3 | John Struthers |
| 1853–5 | Archibald Inglis | 1943–5 | Robert Johnstone |
| 1855–7 | Andrew Wood | 1945–7 | James Graham |
| 1857–9 | Robert Omond | 1947–9 | Francis Jardine |
| 1859–61 | Sir Andrew MacLagan | 1949–51 | Walter Quarry Wood |
| 1861–3 | Patrick Newbigging | 1951–7 | Sir Walter Mercer |
| 1863–5 | Benjamin Bell | 1957–62 | Sir John Bruce |
| 1865–7 | James Dunsmure | 1962–4 | James Mason Brown |
| 1867–9 | James Spence | 1964–7 | George Scott |
| 1869–72 | James Gillespie | 1967–70 | James Cameron |
| 1872–3 | William Walker | 1970–3 | Sir Donald Douglas |
| 1873–5 | James Simson | 1973–6 | James Ross |
| 1875–7 | Sir Henry Littlejohn | 1976–9 | Andrew Wilkinson |

| 1979–82 | F. John Gillingham | 1994–7 | Sir Robert Shields |
| 1982–5 | Sir James Fraser | 1997–2000 | Arnold Maran |
| 1985–8 | Thomas McNair | 2000–3 | Sir John Temple |
| 1988–91 | Geoffrey Chisholm | 2003– | John Smith |
| 1991–4 | Patrick Boulter | | |

## NOTES

1. Elections from this point took place in September each year.
2. Lumsden died in May 1606.
3. Scott took over from Brown in November 1620.
4. There are no entries in the Minute Books between May 1645 and April 1646, perhaps because of the current outbreak of plague, but when the records recommence, Pennycuik is listed as Deacon.
5. The election took place in December because of political turmoil.
6. No election is noted in the records but Burnet is still cited as Deacon.
7. Gideon Elliot was chosen but refused to accept office.
8. Monteith was removed by order of the Privy Council in November 1699.
9. Robert Clerk was elected but declined to take office.
10. President in the year the Incorporation received its first Royal Charter.
11. President when the Playfair Building opened.

# Appendix IV

# Chronology

The following chronology includes major general events and key dates in the history of the College (*references to the College are given in italics*).

| | |
|---|---|
| 1410 | Foundation of St Andrews University |
| 1451 | Foundation of Glasgow University |
| 1462 | London Barber-Surgeons' Charter |
| 1488 | James IV crowned at Scone on 26 June |
| 1495 | Foundation of King's College, Aberdeen |
| 1503 | James IV married Margaret Tudor on 8 August |
| 1505 | *Seal of Cause granted to Incorporation of Surgeons and Barbers by the Town Council of Edinburgh on 1 July* |
| 1506 | *James IV ratified the Seal of Cause on 9 October* |
| 1513 | James IV killed at Flodden along with many Scots nobles and clergy |
| 1518 | Charter given to London physicians by Henry VIII |
| 1532 | College of Justice founded by James V |
| 1540 | Foundation of Company of Barber-Surgeons of London |
| 1542 | Death of James VI at Solway Moss, birth of Mary, Queen of Scots, on 8 December |
| 1560 | Reformation in Scotland, first meeting of General Assembly |
| 1561 | Mary, Queen of Scots arrived in Scotland |
| 1566 | Birth of the future James VI and I |
| 1567 | *Letter of exemption granted to the Incorporation by Mary, Queen of Scots* Coronation of infant James VI at Stirling Castle on 29 July |
| 1575 | University of Leiden founded |
| 1576 | First Bible printed in Scotland |
| 1581 | *Surviving Incorporation records begin* |
| 1583 | Foundation of the 'Tounis College' (University of Edinburgh) |
| 1587 | Execution of Mary, Queen of Scots on 8 February |
| 1593 | Foundation of Marischal College, Aberdeen |
| 1599 | Faculty of Physicians and Surgeons of Glasgow founded |
| 1600 | Year started on 1 January in Scotland from this point Birth of Charles I on 19 November |
| 1603 | Accession of James VI to English throne, Union of the Crowns of Scotland and England |

*1605*    *Centenary of foundation of Incorporation*
*1613*    *Incorporation's privileges ratified by James VI*
1617    Worshipful Society of Apothecaries founded in London
1625    Accession of Charles I
1633    Coronation of Charles I at Holyrood
1638    National Covenant, prayer book riot and start of Bishops' Wars
1644    Solemn League and Covenant signed
*1645*    *Two apothecaries entered the Incorporation – the first surgeon-apothecaries* Last major outbreak of plague in Scotland
*1647*    *First formal examination regulations set out in Incorporation records*
          *Incorporation rented accommodation in Dickson's close*
1649    Execution of Charles I
1650    Edinburgh Castle surrendered to Cromwell on 24 December
1654–8  Cromwellian protectorate
*1656*    *Incorporation purchased Curryhill House*
          *Incorporation physic garden laid out*
          Incorporation of Surgeons and Barbers founded in Glasgow
*1657*    *Foundation of Fraternity of Apothecaries and Surgeon-Apothecaries*
1660    Restoration of monarchy with Charles II
          Foundation of Royal Society in London
1667    Royal College of Physicians of Ireland founded
1681    Royal College of Physicians of Edinburgh founded
          Advocates' Library founded
          Publication of Stair's *Institutions of the Laws of Scotland*
*1682*    *Decreet of Separation between Surgeons and Apothecaries*
1685    Accession of James VII
1687    Order of the Thistle established by James VII
1688    Death of James Renwick, the last Covenanter to be executed
          Deposition of James VII
1689    Crown of Scotland offered to William and Mary
1690    Presbyterian settlement
1692    Massacre of Glencoe on 13 February
*1694*    *Incorporation received patent from William and Mary confirming privileges*
          *Alexander Monteith petitioned Town Council for bodies for dissection*
1695    Darien Scheme to set up trading colony in Panama
          Foundation of Bank of Scotland
*1697*    *Completion of new Hall and anatomy theatre*
1698    Start of Darien expedition
*1699*    *Incorporation library and museum collections begun*
          First edition of *Edinburgh Pharmacopoeia*
1702    Accession of Queen Anne
*1705*    *Robert Elliot appointed Professor of Anatomy by Town Council*
          *Two-hundredth anniversary of the Incorporation*

1706    Last Scottish parliament held
1707    Union of Parliaments of Scotland and England
*1708    Adam Drummond appointed Professor of Anatomy by Town Council*
1711    Birth of philosopher David Hume
1714    Death of Queen Anne and accession of George I
1715    Jacobite uprising led by Earl of Mar, battle of Sherriffmuir
*1717    John M'Gill appointed Professor of Anatomy conjointly with Drummond*
*1720    Alexander Monro primus appointed Professor of Anatomy*
1721    Robert Walpole appointed first Prime Minister
*1722    Final separation of Edinburgh Surgeons and Barbers*
*1723    Examination syllabus expanded to include Botany and Materia Medica*
1725    Malt Tax riots in Glasgow
        Grave-robbing scandal in Edinburgh
*1726    Foundation of Medical School at Edinburgh University. Appointment of
        Drs Innes, Plummer, Rutherford and Sinclair as Professors of Physic*
1727    Foundation of Royal Bank of Scotland
        Death of George I and accession of George II
        Last execution for witchcraft in Scotland
1729    Opening of the first Infirmary in Robertson's Close
1736    Porteous riots in Edinburgh
        Royal Charter awarded to Infirmary
1737    Foundation of Royal Medical Society by Edinburgh medical students
1741    Opening of new Infirmary
1745    Jacobite uprising
1746    Battle of Culloden
1747    Experiments by James Lind on treatment of scurvy
1752    Adoption of Gregorian calendar
1755    Webster's census of Scottish population
1759    Birth of Robert Burns
1760    Accession of George III
*1763    Incorporation's library and museum collections transferred to
        Edinburgh University*
1766    James Craig won competition for design of Edinburgh New Town
1769    Publication in Edinburgh of first volume of *Encyclopaedia Britannica*
*1771    First College Diploma examination*
1772    Slavery declared illegal in Britain
1776    American Revolution
        Edinburgh Public Dispensary founded
*1778    Incorporation received Royal Charter from George III, henceforth Royal
        College of Surgeons of Edinburgh*
1784    Foundation of Royal College of Surgeons in Ireland
1789    French Revolution
1790    Completion of Forth and Clyde canal
1791    Henry Dundas appointed Home Secretary

1793    Start of war between Britain and France

1794    Foundation of Glasgow Royal Infirmary

1796    Discovery of smallpox vaccine by Jenner

1800    Foundation of Royal College of Surgeons of England (Company of Surgeons from 1745)

1801    First national census

1803    Start of Napoleonic Wars

*1804*    *Appointment of John Thomson as Professor of Surgery of the Royal College of Surgeons*

*1805*    *Three-hundredth anniversary of the College*

1811    Birth of James Young Simpson

1815    End of Napoleonic Wars

        *Consolidation of College Diploma examinations into Licentiateship Diploma*

        Apothecaries Act

1817    Publication of first edition of *The Scotsman*

1820    Accession of George IV

1822    Visit of George IV to Edinburgh

1823    First issue of *Lancet*

1824    Great fire of Edinburgh, 15–17 November

1826    Royal Commission on the Universities of Scotland

1828    Burke and Hare trial

1829    Execution of William Burke

1830    Accession of William IV

1832    Reform Bill to extend franchise

        Foundation of British Medical Association

*1832*    *Opening of College's new Playfair Hall*

        *Anatomy Act*

        Cholera epidemic

1833    Reform of local government with Burgh Reform Act

1837    Accession of Queen Victoria

1842    Publication of Chadwick's *Report on the Sanitary Condition of the Labouring Population of Scotland*

        Outbreaks of typhoid and typhus

1843    Disruption in Church of Scotland, foundation of Free Church

        Royal College of Surgeons of London became Royal College of Surgeons of England

1845    Poor Law (Scotland) Amendment Act

        Potato famine in Europe

*1846*    *Robert Liston performed first operation in a British hospital under ether anaesthesia on 21 December*

*1847*    *First use of chloroform as an anaesthetic by James Young Simpson on 12 November*

*1848*    *Old Surgeons' Hall used as Cholera Hospital*

1850    Birth of Robert Louis Stevenson
        *Reintroduction of separate examination for College Fellowship*
1851    Great Exhibition
        *College received new Royal Charter*
        *Final separation from the Town Council*
1854    Crimean War
        Compulsory registration of births, marriages and deaths in Scotland
1855    Arrival of Florence Nightingale at Crimea
*1858*  *Medical Act and establishment of General Medical Council*
1859    Royal Commission on Scottish Universities
        *Institution of Double Qualification with Royal College of Physicians*
        Publication of Darwin's *Origin of the Species*
1860    Universities (Scotland) Act
1861    American Civil War
1862    General Police and Improvement (Scotland) Act
        *Appointment of Henry Littlejohn as Medical Officer of Health in*
        *Edinburgh*
1863    Factory Act
1865    Report on the sanitary condition of Edinburgh published
1867    Public Health (Scotland) Act; isolation hospitals allowed
1868    Reform Act (Scotland), giving franchise to all male householders
*1872*  *Education (Scotland) Act*
*1878*  *Dentists Act*
*1879*  *Institution of Dental Diploma and foundation of Edinburgh Dental*
        *Hospital and School*
        Compulsory notification of infectious diseases
1881    Foundation of University College, Dundee
*1882*  *Isolation of tubercle bacillus by Koch*
*1884*  *Triple Qualification examination instituted*
        *Re-establishment of Fellowship examination which had been*
        *discontinued in 1850*
*1886*  *Medical Act Amendment Act allowing joint regional boards*
*1888*  *First female pass in the Triple Qualification*
1889    Universities (Scotland) Act
*1895*  *Foundation of the School of Medicine of the Royal Colleges*
        Discovery of X-rays by Roentgen and wireless telegraphy by Marconi
1898    Foundation of Royal Army Medical Corps
1899    Boer War commenced
1890    Infectious Diseases Notification Act
1901    Accession of Edward VII
*1905*  *Beginnings of postgraduate medical teaching*
        *Four-hundredth anniversary of the College*
        Royal Commission on the Poor Law
1908    Old Age Pensions instituted

| | |
|---|---|
| 1910 | Accession of George V |
| 1911 | National Insurance Act |
| 1912 | Death of Joseph Lister |
| 1913 | Mental Deficiency and Lunacy (Scotland) Act |
| | Establishment of Highlands and Islands Medical Service |
| 1914 | Easter rising in Dublin |
| | Outbreak of First World War |
| 1915 | Midwives (Scotland) Act |
| 1917 | Women over 30 enfranchised; Russian Revolution |
| 1918 | Armistice day, 11 November |
| 1919 | Foundation of Ministry of Health and Scottish Board of Health |
| *1920* | *Admission of first female Fellow* |
| 1926 | General strike |
| 1928 | Announcement of discovery of penicillin on 30 September |
| | Voting age for women reduced to 21 |
| 1929 | Royal College of Physicians and Surgeons of Canada founded |
| | Royal College of Obstetricians and Gynaecologists founded |
| 1934 | Foundation of Scottish National party |
| 1936 | Accession of Edward VIII |
| | Cathcart Report on Scottish health services |
| 1937 | Abdication of Edward VIII and accession of George VI |
| 1938 | Empire Exhibition in Glasgow |
| 1939 | Outbreak of Second World War |
| *1941* | *Polish School of Medicine instituted in Edinburgh University* |
| 1942 | Beveridge Report |
| 1943 | Hetherington Committee Report |
| 1945 | Goodenough Report |
| | Victory in Europe day, 7 May |
| | Labour victory in General Election, 12 April |
| 1946 | Appointment of first full-time Director of Postgraduate Studies in Edinburgh |
| 1948 | Establishment of the National Health Service |
| | *Primary Fellowship examination introduced* |
| *1949* | *Closure of School of Medicine of the Royal Colleges* |
| | *FDS RCSEd examination introduced* |
| 1950 | Medical Act to bring in pre-registration year |
| *1951* | *Agreement for intercollegiate reciprocity of Primary Fellowship examinations* |
| 1952 | Accession of Queen Elizabeth II |
| | Inaugural meeting of Joint Committee of Scottish Royal Colleges |
| *1953* | *Foundation of Edinburgh Postgraduate Board for Medicine* |
| *1954* | *HRH Prince Philip, Duke of Edinburgh became Patron to the College* |
| | *College Dental Council founded* |

1955   *First issue of College Journal*

1956   Suez conflict

1960   End of National Service

1962   Royal College of Physicians and Surgeons of Glasgow confirmed by new charter

1965   *Pfizer Building opened*

1966   *First College overseas examination held in Hong Kong*

1967   *Lister Institute opened*

1968   Todd Report

1969   *Joint Committee on Higher Surgical Training*

1970   *Scottish Council for Postgraduate Medical Education formed*

1970   *Foundation of International Federation of Surgical Colleges*

1971   Decimalisation introduced in Britain

1973   Britain entered European Common Market
       *Conference of Royal Colleges and Faculties in Scotland established*

1975   First North Sea oil piped to shore
       *Further Royal Charter granted to College*

1976   *Indian Chapter of College founded*

1976   *First overseas meeting held in Cairo and Alexandria*

1979   Devolution vote in Scotland, failed to gain required majority
       Margaret Thatcher elected first female British Prime Minister

1980   *First College Specialty Fellowship examination*

1982   Falklands War
       *College Dental Faculty established, superseding Dental Council*

1984   *Appointment of first female member of College Council*

1987   Shaw Report on SHO training

1990   Gulf War

1999   *Women in Surgical Training organisation founded*

1992   *Opening of Sir Jules Thorn Exhibition of the History of Surgery*

1993   Calman Report

1996   Stone of Destiny returned to Scotland

1997   *Specialist Medical Order to establish Specialist Training Authority*
       Referendum on devolution, approved Scottish parliament

1999   Scottish parliament met on 12 May
       *First MFDS/MFD RCSEd examination*

2002   *Foundation of Postgraduate Medical Education and Training Board*

2003   Iraq conflict

2004   *Implementation of European Working Time Directive*
       *Intercollegiate MRCS introduced*

2005   *Quincentenary of foundation of College*

# Bibliography

## MANUSCRIPT SOURCES

### Company of Barber Surgeons of London

Court Minute Books.

### Edinburgh City Archive

Burgh Court Acts and Decreets.
Council Records 1750–1860.
Dean of Guild Court Books.
Macleod D104, 25, Burgh Court Process v. Martin Eccles.
Moses Bundle 32/1321 – Petition by Alexander Pennycuik of Newhall.
Moses Bundle 135/5321, Accompt of Medicaments and Drugs furnished to the Poor of
    Edinburgh by Thomas Gibson, from January 1710 to January 1711.

### Edinburgh University Library/Lothian Health Services Archive

Da31.5, Senatus Minutes, 1733–1900.
Dc2.76/24, Operations Performed in the Theatre of the Royal Infirmary 6 November 1836
    to 30 April 1837.
Dc3.93, Cases Observed at the Edinburgh Infirmary in the Year 1754–1755 by J. A. H.
    Reimarius.
History of the Edinburgh Postgraduate Board for Medicine 1905–50.
LHB1, Minutes of the Managers of the Royal Infirmary of Edinburgh.
P46/7/1–7, Descriptions of surgical cases by Robert Liston.

### National Archives of Scotland

CC8/8, Commissariot Court, Register of Testaments.
GD1/699/4, Records relating to the Royal College of Surgeons of Edinburgh, 1927–1936.
GD51/2/697/1, Letter from David Hay to Lord Melville (1828).
GD51/5/649, Letter from James Russell to Henry Dundas (1797).
GD51/5/670, Letters from James Law to Robert Dundas (1808).
GD51/5/708, Letter from David Hay to Lord Melville and Petition to Treasury (1825).
GD158/926, Account of post mortem on Lady Polwarth undertaken by Patrick Telfer,
    Chirurgeon, 12 December 1701.

GD214/60, Papers relating to the dispute between the University and the Royal College of Surgeons regarding the use of the University Library by members of the College and the books deposited in the Library under an agreement in 1763 (1825).

## National Library of Scotland

Adv. Ms. 33.5.20, Memoirs for compiling the history of the Royal Coledge of Physitians at Edinburgh done from the records by Sir Robert Sibbald.
MS 3157, Depositions of the Chirurgeons and Apothecarys upon the Earl of Atholls death 1579.
MS 3774, Medical Casebook, 1733–1735.

## Royal College of Physicians of Edinburgh

Minute Books.

## Royal College of Physicians and Surgeons of Glasgow

Minute Books.

## Royal College of Surgeons of Edinburgh

Charters.
College Business Papers.
College Laws (RCSEd 7/1).
College Letterbooks (RCSEd 3/1–2).
College Minute Books.
Dental Council Minute Books.
Dental Examination records (RCSEd 6/5).
Dental Faculty Minute Books.
Douglas Guthrie papers.
Examination records (Diplomas, Fellowships, Specialty Fellowships, Overseas examinations) (RCSEd 6/8–9).
Gifts and Deposits Collections, including papers of individual Fellows.
Menzies Campbell Collection correspondence.
Records of the Extra-Mural School and School of Medicine of the Royal Colleges.
Records of the Society of Barbers (SB 1–7).
Records of the Widows' Fund.
Sir Jules Thorn Museum papers.
Triple Qualification records (RCSEd 6/1).

## Royal College of Surgeons of England

Council Minute Books.

## Royal College of Surgeons of Ireland

Minute Books.

## PRINTED PRIMARY SOURCES

Aristides, *Letter to Sir Willam Rae of St Catharine's, Baronet, Lord Advocate of Scotland* (Edinburgh, 1829).

Bell, J., *Memorial Concerning the Present State of Military and Naval Surgery. Addressed Several Years Ago to the Right Honourable Earl Spencer; First Lord of the Admiralty; and Now Submitted to the Public* (Edinburgh, 1800).

Bryant, T., *A Manual for the Practice of Surgery* (London, 1879).

Chadwick, E., *Report on the Sanitary Condition of the Labouring Population of Great Britain*, ed. M. W. Flynn (Edinburgh, 1965).

*Committee on the Scottish Health Services Report* (HMSO, 1936) (Comnd. 5204) [The Cathcart Report].

Cullen, W., *Synopsis Nosologiae Methodicae* (Edinburgh, 1772).

Dalrymple, J. (Viscount Stair), *The Institutions of the Laws of Scotland* (Edinburgh, 1681).

Department of Health, Press Release 95/260, 26 May 1995.

Dickson, T. and Paul, J. B. (eds), *Accounts of the Lord High Treasurer of Scotland* (Edinburgh, 1877–1916).

Eccles, W., *An Historical Account of the Rights and Privileges of the Royal College of Physicians, and of the Incorporation of Chirurgions in Edinburgh* (Edinburgh, 1707).

Erlam, H. D., 'Alexander Monro primus', *University of Edinburgh Journal*, 17 (1953–5), pp. 77–105.

Floyer, J., *An Enquiry into the Right Use and Abuses of the Hot, Cold and Temperate Baths in England* (London, 1697).

*Grants and Acts of Parliament in Favours of the College and Corporation of Surgeons of Edinburgh 1505–1696.*

Hamilton, A., *Elements of the Practice of Midwifery* (London, 1775).

Hamilton, A., *Outlines of the Theory and Practice of Midwifery* (Edinburgh, 1784).

Harvey, W., *Exercitatio Anatomica de Motu Cordis et Sanguinis in Animalibus* (Frankfurt, 1628).

*Health in Scotland* (Scottish Executive, 2002).

*Hints submitted to the Court of Contributors to the Royal Infirmary of Edinburgh by a Member of the Court* (Edinburgh, 1821).

*Hospital Doctors. Training for the Future* (Department of Health, London, 1993) [The Calman Report].

Jex-Blake, S., *Medical Women. Two Essays: I. Medicine as a Profession for Women. II. Medical Education of Women* (Edinburgh, 1872).

Jex-Blake, S., *Medical Women. A Thesis and a History. I. Medicine as a Profession for Women. II. The Medical Education of Women. I. The Battle in Edinburgh. II. The Victory Won* (Edinburgh, 1886).

Johnston, W. T., *'The Best of Oure Owne'. Letters of Archibald Pitcairne, 1652–1713* (Edinburgh, 1979).

*Laws and Regulations of the Royal College of Surgeons with Chronological Lists of Members, Presidents, Deacons and Honorary Members* (Edinburgh, 1793).

*Laws of the Royal College of Surgeons of Edinburgh* (Edinburgh, 1885).

*Letter to the Lord Advocate Disclosing the Accomplices, Secrets and Other Facts Relative to the Late Murders; With a Correct Account of the Manner in Which the Anatomical Schools are Supplied with Subjects, by the Echo of Surgeons Square* (Edinburgh, 1829).

Liston, R., *Letter to the Ladies and Gentlemen Contributors of the Royal Infirmary of Edinburgh 15th December 1821* (Edinburgh, 1821).

Livingston, M. et al. (eds), *Registrum Secreti Sigilli Regum Scotorum* (Edinburgh, 1908– ).

Lowe, P., *Discourse of the Whole Art of Chirurgerie* (London, 1597).

Maclagan, D., *Case of Sudden Death from Rupture of the Superficial Fibres of the Heart* (Edinburgh, 1845).

Marwick, J. D., Wood, M. and Armet, H. (eds), *Extracts from the Records of the Burgh of Edinburgh 1428–1716*, 12 vols (Edinburgh 1871–1967).

*Modernising Medical Careers. The Response of the Four UK Health Ministers to the Consultation on Unfinished Business: Proposals for Reform of the Senior House Officer Grade* (Department of Health, London, 2003).

Newbigging, William, *Case of Inguinal and Popliteal Aneurism Cured by Tying the External Iliac Artery* (Edinburgh, 18–?).

*Our Changing Democracy: Devolution of Scotland and Wales* (Comnd. 6348) (HMSO, 1975).

*Postgraduate Medical Education and Training: The Postgraduate Medical, Education and Training Board: Statement on Policy* (Department of Health, London, 2002).

RCSEd, *Annual Reports*.

RCSEd, *Newsletters*.

RCSEd, *Report of Developments Committee, 1987–8*.

*Regulations to be observed by Candidates for the Qualifications in Medicine and Surgery Conferred Conjointly by the Royal College of Phyisicians of Edinburgh, the Royal College of Surgeons of Edinburgh and the Faculty of Physicians and Surgeons of Glasgow* (Edinburgh, 1887 and subsequent editions).

*Remarks on the Expediency and Practicality of a Union of the Royal Colleges of Physicians and Surgeons in Edinburgh* (Edinburgh, 1821).

*Report of the Committee of Inquiry into the Regulation of the Medical Profession* (Comnd. 6018) (HMSO, 1975) [The Merrison Report].

*Report of the Committee on Social Insurance and Allied Services* (Comnd. 6404) (HMSO, 1942) [The Beveridge Report].

*Report of the Inter-Departmental Committee on Medical Schools* (Ministry of Health, London, 1944) [The Goodenough Report].

*Report of the Royal Commission on Medical Education* (HMSO, London, 1968).

*Report of the Royal Public Dispensary for the City and County of Edinburgh* (Edinburgh, 1822).

*Report of the Royal Public Dispensary for the City and County of Edinburgh* (Edinburgh, 1845).

*Report of the Surgeons of Edinburgh Vaccination Institute* (Edinburgh, 1809).

*Report on the State of the Widows' Fund of the Royal College of Surgeons of Edinburgh as at Lammas 1868* (Edinburgh, 1868).

*Report to the Secretary of State for Scotland by Review Committee on Dental Staffing Structure* (Edinburgh, 1964) [The Schiach Report].

*Royal Commission on Medical Education* (Comnd. 3569) (London, 1968) [The Todd Report].

*Rules and Regulations of the Royal Infirmary of Edinburgh with an Appendix Containing the Charter of 1736 and the Edinburgh Royal Infirmary Act 1870* (Edinburgh, 1881).

*Social Insurance and Allied Services. Report by Sir William Beveridge* (HMSO, London, 1942) [The Beveridge Report].

Spence, J., *Lectures on Surgery* (Edinburgh, 1864).

*Staffing the Service. The Next Decade. Report to the Scottish Joint Consultative Committee and the Scottish Home and Health Department Following Review of Hospital Medical Staffing Estimates in Scotland* (Edinburgh, 1987) [The Shaw Report].

*States of the Affairs of the Royal College of Surgeons of Edinburgh and of the Widows' Fund with Lists of Members, Office Bearers, Acts of Parliament, etc. 1824–1890*.

Strachan, J. M., 'The non-resident Fellowships of the Royal College of Surgeons of Edinburgh', *EMJ*, II (1856–7), p. 475.

Stuart, J. et al. (eds), *Exchequer Rolls of Scotland* (Edinburgh, 1878–1908).

*The Appointment of the Chair and Scottish Members of the Postgraduate Medical Education and Training Board* (Scottish Executive, Edinburgh, 2002).

*The National Health Service in Scotland* (Department of Health for Scotland, 1959).

*The Supervision of Higher Professional Training in Medicine and Dentistry: Guidelines for Regional Postgraduate Medical Education Committees and Specialty Advisers* (United Kingdom Councils for Postgraduate Medical Education, 1984).

Thomson, J., *Outline of a Plan for the Regulation of the Surgical Department of the Royal Infirmary Submitted to the Consideration of the Managers of that Institution* (Edinburgh, 1800).

Thomson, J., *Report of Observations Made in the British Military Hospitals in Belgium after the Battle of Waterloo; with Some Remarks upon Amputation* (Edinburgh, 1816).

Vesalius, A., *De Humani Corporis Fabrica Liber Septem* (Basle, 1543).

Wheatley, H. B. (ed.), *Diary of Samuel Pepys* (London, 1893).

# NEWSPAPERS

*Caledonian Mercury.*
*Edinburgh Advertiser.*
*Edinburgh Evening News.*
*Edinburgh Gazette.*
*Sunday Times.*
*The Scotsman.*

# SECONDARY WORKS

## Books

Alexander, E., *First Ladies of Medicine. The Origins, Education and Destination of Early Women Medical Graduates of Glasgow University* (Glasgow, 1987).

Allan, D., *Virtue, Learning and the Scottish Enlightenment* (Edinburgh, 1993).

Allen, N. (ed.), *Scottish Pioneers of the Greek Revival* (Edinburgh, 1984).

Anderson, R. D., Lynch, M. and Phillipson, N., *The University of Edinburgh. An Illustrated History* (Edinburgh, 2003).

Bannerman, J., *The Beatons. A Medical Kindred in the Classical Gaelic Tradition* (Edinburgh, 1986).

Barfoot, M., 'To ask the suffrages of the patrons: Thomas Laycock and the Edinburgh Chair of Medicine, 1855', *Med. Hist.*, supplement no. 15 (1995).

Barrell, A. D. M., *Medieval Scotland* (Cambridge, 2000).

Barry, J. P. S., Adams, A. P. and Fleming, P. R., *The History of Cardiothoracic Surgery from Early Times* (London, 1996).

Beier, L. M., *Sufferers and Healers: The Experience of Illness in Seventeenth-Century England* (London, 1987).

Blair, J. S. G., *History of Medicine in the University of St Andrews* (Edinburgh, 1982).

Blair, J. S. G., *The Royal Army Medical Corps 1898–1998* (RAMC, 1998).

Blandy, J. P. and Lumley, J. S. P. (eds), *The Royal College of Surgeons of England. 200 Years of History at the Millennium* (London, 2000).

Blandy, J. P. and Williams, J. P., *The History of the British Association of Urological Surgeons* (London, 1995).

Bonner, T., *To the Ends of the Earth. Women's Search for Education in Medicine* (Massachusetts, 1992).

Brockliss, L. and Jones, C., *The Medical World of Early Modern France* (Oxford, 1997).

Brown, K. M., *Kingdom or Province? Scotland and the Regal Union, 1603–1707* (London, 1992).

Burrage, M. and Torstendahl, R. (eds), *Professions in Theory and History* (London, 1980).

Bynum, W. F., *Science and the Practice of Medicine in the Nineteenth Century* (Cambridge, 1995).

Bynum, W. F. and Porter, R., *Medical Fringe and Medical Orthodoxy 1750–1850* (London, 1987).

Cameron, C. A., *History of the Royal College of Surgeons of Ireland and of the Irish Schools of Medicine Including Numerous Biographical Sketches: Also a Medical Bibliography* (Dublin, 1886).

Campbell, R. A. and Skinner, A. S. (eds), *The Origins and Nature of the Scottish Enlightenment* (Edinburgh, 1982).

Catford, E. F., *The Royal Infirmary of Edinburgh 1929–1979* (Edinburgh, 1984).

*Centenary Brochure of the Edinburgh Dental School and Royal College of Surgeons Licence in Dental Surgery* (Edinburgh, 1979).

de Certeau, M., *The Writing of History*, trans. T. Corley (New York, 1988).

Chitnis, A. C., *The Scottish Enlightenment: A Social History* (London, 1976).

Clark, G., *A History of the Royal College of Physicians of London Vol. II* (Oxford, 1966).

Colley, L., *Britons. Forging the Nation, 1707–1837* (Yale, 1992).

Colston, J., *The Incorporated Trades of Edinburgh* (Edinburgh, 1891).

Comrie, J. D., *History of Scottish Medicine*, 2 vols (Oxford, 1932).

Conrad, L. L. et al., *The Western Medical Tradition 800BC–1800AD* (Cambridge, 1995).

Cope, Z., *The Royal College of Surgeons of England. A History* (London, 1959).

Corfield, P., *Power and the Professions in Britain 1700–1850* (London, 1995).

Craig, W. S., *History of the Royal College of Physicians of Edinburgh* (Oxford, 1976).

Creswell, C. H., *The Royal College of Surgeons of Edinburgh. Historical Notes from 1505 to 1905* (Edinburgh, 1926).

Croft Dickinson, W., *Scotland from Earliest Times to 1603* (London, 1961).

Crofton, E., *The Women of Royaumont. A Scottish Women's Hospital on the Western Front* (East Linton, 1997).

Cunningham, A. and French, R. (eds), *The Medical Enlightenment of the Eighteenth Century* (Cambridge, 1990).

Dalyell, J., *Fragments of Scottish History* (Edinburgh, 1798).

Denison, E. P., Ditchburn, D. and Lynch, M. (eds), *Aberdeen Before 1800. A New History* (East Linton, 2002).

Devine, T. M., *The Scottish Nation, 1700–2000* (Edinburgh, 1999).

Dingwall, H. M., *Late Seventeenth Century Edinburgh. A Demographic Study* (Aldershot, 1994).

Dingwall, H. M., *Physicians, Surgeons and Apothecaries. Medical Practice in Seventeenth Century Edinburgh* (East Linton, 1995).

Dingwall, H. M., *A History of Scottish Medicine* (Edinburgh, 2003).

Dobson, J. and Milnes Walker, R., *Barbers and Barber-Surgeons of London* (London, 1979).

Dow, D. (ed.), *The Influence of Scottish Medicine* (London, 1986).

Dow, F. D., *Cromwellian Scotland, 1651–1660* (Edinburgh, 1976).

Duncan, A., *Memorials of the Faculty of Physicians and Surgeons of Glasgow, 1599–1850: With a Sketch of the Rise and Progress of the Glasgow Medical School and of the Medical Profession in the West of Scotland* (Glasgow, 1896).

Dwyer, J., Mason, R. A. and Murdoch, A. (eds), *New Perspectives on the Politics and Culture of Early Modern Scotland* (Edinburgh, 1982).

Dyhouse, C., *No Distinction of Sex? Women in British Universities 1870–1939* (London, 1995).

Ellis, H., *A History of Bladder Stone* (Oxford, 1969).

Finlayson, G., *Citizen, State and Social Welfare in Britain 1839–1990* (Oxford, 1994).

Fraser, W. H. (ed.), *People and Society in Scotland Vol. II, 1839–1914* (Edinburgh, 1990).

Fry, M., *The Dundas Despotism* (Edinburgh, 1992).

Fry, M., *The Scottish Empire* (East Linton, 2001).

Gairdner, J., *Historical Sketch of the Royal College of Surgeons of Edinburgh* (Edinburgh, 1860).

Gardner, D. L., *Surgery Comes Clean. The Life and Work of Joseph Lister, 1827–1912* (Royal College of Surgeons of Edinburgh, 2002).

Geissler, P. R., *The Royal Odonto-Chirurgical Society of Scotland* (Edinburgh, 1997).

Gelfand, T., *Professionalising Modern Medicine. Paris Surgeons and Medical Science Institutions in the Eighteenth Century* (London, 1980).

Gentilcore, D., *Healers and Healing in Early-Modern Italy* (Manchester, 1998).

Geyer-Kordesch, J. and Ferguson, R., *Blue Stockings, Black Gowns, White Coats. A Brief History of Women Entering Higher Education and the Medical Profession in Scotland in Celebration of One Hundred Years of Women Graduates at the University of Glasgow* (Glasgow, 1994).

Geyer-Kordesch, J. and Macdonald, F., *Physicians and Surgeons in Glasgow. The History of the Royal College of Physicians and Surgeons of Glasgow, 1599–1858* (Oxford, 1999).

Gibson, T., *The Royal College of Physicians and Surgeons of Glasgow: A Short History Based on the Portraits and Other Memorabilia* (Edinburgh, 1983).

Gifford, J., McWilliam, C. and Walker, D. (eds), *The Buildings of Scotland. Edinburgh* (London, 1984).

Grant, A., *Story of the University of Edinburgh During its First Three Hundred Years*, 2 vols (Edinburgh, 1884).

Grant, J., *Cassell's Old and New Edinburgh*, 2 vols (London, 1884).

Guthrie, D., *Extramural Medical Education in Edinburgh and the School of Medicine of the Royal Colleges* (Edinburgh, 1965).

Habermas, J., *The Structural Transformation of the Public Sphere. An Inquiry into a Category of Bourgeois Society*, trans. T. Burger (Cambridge, 1989).

Hamilton, D., *The Healers. A History of Medicine in Scotland* (Edinburgh, 1981).

Hendrie, W. F. and Macleod, D. A. D., *The Bangour Story. A History of Bangour Village and General Hospitals* (Aberdeen, 1991).

Hook, A. and Sher, R. B., *The Glasgow Enlightenment* (East Linton, 1995).

Horn, D. B., *A Short History of the University of Edinburgh* (Edinburgh, 1967).

Houston, R. A., *Scottish Literacy and Scottish Identity. Illiteracy and Society in Scotland and Northern England 1600–1800* (Cambridge, 1985).

Houston, R. A. and Whyte, I. D. (eds), *Scottish Society 1500–1800* (Cambridge, 1989).

Hull, A. and Geyer-Kordesch, J., *The Shaping of the Medical Profession. The History of the Royal College of Physicians and Surgeons of Glasgow, 1858–1999* (Oxford, 1999).

Hutchison, I. G. C., *Scottish Politics in the Twentieth Century* (Basingstoke, 2001).

Innes-Smith, R. W., *English-Speaking Students of Medicine at the University of Leyden* (Edinburgh, 1926).

Jacyna, S., *Philosophic Whigs: Medicine, Science and Citizenship in Enlightenment Edinburgh* (Edinburgh, 1997).

Jenkinson, J. L. M., *Scottish Medical Societies 1731–1939* (Edinburgh, 1993).

Jenkinson, J. L. M., *Scotland's Health 1919–1948* (Bern, 2002).

Jenkinson, J. L. M., Moss, M. and Russell, I., *The Royal. The History of the Glasgow Royal Infirmary 1794–1994* (Glasgow, 1994).

Jordanova, L., *The Practice of History* (London, 2000).

Kaufman, M. H., *Surgeons at War: Medical Arrangements for the Treatment of the Sick and Wounded in the British Army During the Late 18th and 19th Centuries* (Westport, 2001).

Kaufman, M., *Medical Teaching in Edinburgh During the 18th and 19th Centuries* (Edinburgh, 2003).

Kaufman, M. H., *Musket-Ball and Sabre Injuries from the First Half of the Nineteenth Century* (Edinburgh, 2003).

Kaufman, M. H., *The Regius Chair of Military Surgery in the University of Edinburgh, 1806–55* (Amsterdam, 2003).

Lawrence, C., *Medical Theory, Surgical Practice. Studies in the History of Surgery* (London, 1992).

Lawrence, C., *Medicine in the Making of Modern Britain* (London, 2003).

Leneman, L., *In the Service of Life. The Story of Elsie Inglis and the Scottish Women's Hospitals* (Edinburgh, 1994).

Lockyer, R., *James VI and I* (London, 1998).

Loudon, I., *Medical Care and the General Practitioner, 1750–1850* (Oxford, 1986).

Loudon, I. (ed.), *Western Medicine. An Illustrated History* (Oxford, 1997).

Lynch, M., *Scotland. A New History* (London, 1991).

Lynch, M. (ed.), *The Early Modern Town in Scotland* (Edinburgh, 1987).

Lynch, M., Spearman, M. and Stell, G. (eds), *The Scottish Medieval Town* (Edinburgh, 1988).

McCullough, L. B., *John Gregory and the Invention of Professional Medical Ethics and the Profession of Medicine* (London, 1998).

McCullough, L. B., Jones, J. W. and Brody, B. A. (eds), *Surgical Ethics* (Oxford, 1998).

Macdougall, N., *James IV* (Edinburgh, 1989).

McHarg, J. F., *In Search of Dr John Makluire, Pioneer Edinburgh Physician Forgotten for Over 300 Years* (Glasgow, 1997)

Macintyre, I. M. C. and MacLaren, I. F., *Surgeons' Lives* (forthcoming).

McKean, C., *Edinburgh. An Illustrated Architectural Guide* (Edinburgh, 1992)

McLachlan, G. (ed.), *Improving the Common Weal. Aspects of Scottish Health Services, 1900–1984* (Edinburgh, 1987).

MacQueen, J. (ed.), *Humanism in Renaissance Scotland* (Edinburgh, 1990).

Maitland, W., *The History of Edinburgh from its Foundation to the Present Time* (Edinburgh, 1753).

Masson, A. H. B., *Portraits, Paintings and Busts in the Royal College of Surgeons of Edinburgh* (Edinburgh, 1995).

Masson, A. H. B., *A College Miscellany. An Illustrated Catalogue of Some of the Treasured Possessions of the Royal College of Surgeons of Edinburgh* (Edinburgh, 2001).

Mekie, D. E. C. and Fraser, J. (eds), *Colour Atlas of Demonstrations in Surgical Pathology* (London, 1983, 1986).

Menzies Campbell, J., *Dentistry Then and Now* (privately printed, 1981).

Miles, A., *The Edinburgh School of Surgery Before Lister* (London, 1918).

Mitchison, R., *Lordship to Patronage. Scotland 1603–1745* (London, 1983).

Mordaunt Crook, J., *The Greek Revival. Neo-Classical Attitudes in British Architecture 1760–1870* (London, 1995).

Nottingham, C., *The NHS in Scotland. The Legacy of the Past and the Prospect of the Future* (Aldershot, 2000).

Nutton, V. and Porter, R. (eds), *The History of Medical Education in Britain* (Amsterdam, 1995).

Parry, N. and Parry, J., *The Rise of the Medical Profession. A Study of Collective Social Mobility* (London, 1976).

Pelling, M., *The Common Lot: Sickness, Medical Occupations and the Urban Poor in Early-Modern England* (London, 1998).

Pelling, M., *Medical Conflicts in Early Modern London. Patronage, Physicians and Irregular Practitioners, 1550–1640* (Oxford, 2003).

Pennington, C., *The Modernisation of Medical Teaching at Aberdeen in the Nineteenth Century* (Aberdeen, 1994).

Pickstone, J. V. (ed.), *Medical Innovations in Historical Perspective* (Basingstoke, 1992).

Pitcairn, R. (ed.), *Criminal Trials in Scotland, from AD 1488 to AD 1624* (Edinburgh, 1833).

Porter, R., *The Greatest Benefit to Mankind. A Medical History of Humanity from Antiquity to the Present* (London, 1997).

Porter, R. and Teich, M. (eds), *The Scottish Enlightenment in its National Context* (London, 1981).

Poynter, F. N. L. (ed.), *The Evolution of Medical Education in Britain* (London, 1966).

Prebble, J., *The Darien Disaster* (Edinburgh, 1968).

Rhodes, P., *An Outline History of Medicine* (London, 1985).

Rintoul, R. F. (ed.), *Farquharson's Textbook of Operative Surgery*, eighth edn (Edinburgh, 1995).

Risse, G., *Hospital Life in Enlightenment Scotland. Care and Teaching at the Edinburgh Infirmary* (Cambridge, 1986).

Risse, G., *Mending Bodies. Saving Souls. A History of Hospitals* (Oxford, 1999).

Roberts, S., *Sophia Jex-Blake. A Woman Pioneer in Nineteenth-century Medical Reform* (London, 1993).

Robertson, E., *Glasgow's Doctor. James Burn Russell, 1837–1904* (East Linton, 1998).

Rodger, R., *The Transformation of Edinburgh. Land, Property and Trust in the Nineteenth Century* (Cambridge, 2001).

Rosner, L., *Medical Education in the Age of Improvement. Edinburgh Students and Apprentices 1760–1826* (Edinburgh, 1991).

Ross, J. A., *Memoirs of an Army Surgeon* (Edinburgh, 1948).

Ross, J. A., *The Edinburgh School of Surgery after Lister* (Edinburgh, 1978).

Rostowski, J., *History of the Polish School of Medicine at the University of Edinburgh* (London, 1955).

Rowe, N. L. and Killey, H. C., *Fractures of the Facial Skeleton* (Edinburgh, 1968).

Royal College of Surgeons of England, *Surgical Competence: Challenges of Assessment in Training and Practice* (London, 1999).

Rushman, G. B., *A Short History of Anaesthesia* (London, 1996).

Savile, R., *The Bank of Scotland. A History* (Edinburgh, 1995).

Schoemaker, R. and Vincent, M. (eds), *Gender and History in Western Europe* (London, 1998).

Short, A. I. and Lennard, T. W. J., *James IV of Scotland, Sovereign and Surgeon*, occasional paper (The Durham Thomas Harriot Seminar) no. 7 (Durham, 1992).

Smith, J., *The Origins, Progress and Present Position of the Royal College of Surgeons of Edinburgh* (Edinburgh, 1905).

Spece, R. G., Shimm, D. E. and Buchanan, A. E., *Conflicts of Interest in Clinical Practice and Research* (Oxford, 1996).

Stacey, M., *Regulating British Medicine. The General Medical Council* (Chichester, 1992).

Steedman, J. A., *History and Statutes of the Royal Infirmary of Edinburgh* (Edinburgh, 1778).

Stewart, M. A. (ed.), *Studies in the Philosophy of the Scottish Enlightenment* (Oxford, 1990).

Stiles, H. J., *Reminiscences of a Surgical Training* (Edinburgh, 1919).

Struthers, J., *Historical Sketch of the Edinburgh Anatomical School* (Edinburgh, 1867).

Sturdy, S. (ed.), *Medicine, Health and the Public Sphere in Britain, 1600–2000* (London, 2002).

Tait, H. P., *A Doctor and Two Policemen: The History of Edinburgh's Health Department, 1862–1974* (Edinburgh, 1974).

Tansey, V. and Mekie, D. E. C., *The Museum of the Royal College of Surgeons of Edinburgh* (Edinburgh, 1982).

Turner, A. L., *Story of a Great Hospital. The Royal Infirmary of Edinburgh, 1729–1929* (Edinburgh, 1937).

Wangensteen, O. H. and Wangensteen, S. D., *The Rise of Surgery: From Empiric Craft to Scientific Discipline* (Minnesota, 1979).

Webster, C., *The National Health Service. A Political History* (Oxford, 1998).

Whatley, C. A., *Bought and Sold for English Gold? Explaining the Union of 1707* (East Linton, 2001).

White, H., *The Content of the Form. Narrative Discourse and Historical Representation* (Baltimore, 1987).

Widdess, J. D. H., *The Royal College of Surgeons in Ireland and its Medical School 1784–1984*, third edn (Dublin, 1984).

Withers, C. J. and Wood, P. (eds), *Science and Medicine in the Scottish Enlightenment* (East Linton, 2002).

Wood, P. (ed.), *The Scottish Enlightenment. Essays in Reinterpretation* (Rochester, 2000).

Woodruff, M., *Nothing Venture, Nothing Win* (Edinburgh, 1996).

Wormald, J., *Court , Kirk and Community, Scotland 1470–1625* (London, 1981).

Young, S., *Annals of the Barber Surgeons of London* (London, 1980).

Youngson, A., *The Making of Classical Edinburgh* (Edinburgh, 1967).

Youngson, A., *The Scientific Revolution in Victorian Medicine* (London, 1979).

## Book chapters

Beier, L. M., 'Seventeenth-century English surgery: the casebook of Joseph Binns', in C. Lawrence (ed.), *Medical Theory, Surgical Practice. Studies in the History of Surgery* (London, 1982), pp. 48–84.

Blair, J. S. G., 'The Scots and military medicine', in D. Dow (ed.), *The Influence of Scottish Medicine* (Carnforth, 1988), pp. 17–30.

Buchanan, A. E., 'Is there a medical profession in the house?', in R. G. Spece, D. E. Shimm and A. E. Buchanan, *Conflicts of Interest in Clinical Practice and Research* (Oxford, 1996), pp. 105–36.

Collins, K. E., 'American Jewish medical students in Scotland 1925–40', in D. Dow (ed.), *The Influence of Scottish Medicine* (Carnforth, 1988), pp. 143–58.

Crowther, M. A., 'Poverty, health and welfare', in W. H. Fraser (ed.), *People and Society in Scotland Vol. II, 1839–1914* (Edinburgh, 1990), pp. 265–87.

Cunningham, A., 'Medicine to calm the mind: Boerhaave's Medical System and why it was adopted in Edinburgh', in A. Cunningham and R. French (eds), *The Medical Enlightenment of the Eighteenth Century* (Cambridge, 1990), pp. 40–66.

Emerson, R. L., 'Science and moral philosophy in the Scottish Enlightenment', in M. A. Stewart (ed.), *Studies in the Philosophy of the Scottish Enlightenment* (Oxford, 1990), pp. 11–36.

Girdwood, R. H., 'The influence of Scotland on North American medicine', in D. Dow (ed.), *The Influence of Scottish Medicine* (Carnforth, 1988), pp. 31–42.

Granshaw, L., '"Upon this principle I have based a practice": the development and reception of antisepsis in Britain, 1867–1900', in J. V. Pickstone (ed.), *Medical Innovations in Historical Perspective* (Basingstoke, 1992), pp. 17–46.

Hughes, F. E., 'Proficiency training for space flight', in Royal College of Surgeons of

England (ed.), *Surgical Competence: Challenges of Assessment in Training and Practice* (London, 1999), pp. 73–81.

Jackson, B., 'Why do we need to assess competence?', in Royal College of Surgeons of England, *Surgical Competence: Challenges of Assessment in Training and Practice* (London, 1999), pp. 6–16.

Lawrence, C. and Dixey, A., 'Practising on principle: Joseph Lister and the germ theories of disease', in C. Lawrence (ed.), *Medical Theory, Surgical practice. Studies in the History of Surgery* (London, 1992), pp. 153–215.

Loudon, I., 'Medical education and medical reform', in V. Nutton and R. Porter (eds), *The History of Medical Education in Britain* (Amsterdam, 1995), pp. 229–49.

Lynch, M., 'Continuity and change in urban society 1500–1700', in R. A. Houston and I. D. Whyte (eds), *Scottish Society 1500–1800* (Cambridge, 1989), pp. 85–117.

Lynch, M. and Dingwall, H. M., 'Elite society in town and country', in E. P. Denison, D. Ditchburn and M. Lynch (eds), *Aberdeen Before 1800. A New History* (East Linton, 2002), pp. 192–200.

Ouston, H., 'York in Edinburgh: James VII and the patronage of learning in Scotland 1673–1688', in J. Dwyer, R. A. Mason and A. Murdoch (eds), *New Perspectives on the Politics and Culture of Early Modern Scotland* (Edinburgh, 1982), pp. 133–55.

Sturdy, S., 'Introduction: medicine, health and the public sphere', in S. Sturdy (ed.), *Medicine, Health and the Public Sphere in Britain, 1600–2000* (London, 2002), pp. 1–24.

Sturdy, S., 'Alternative publics. The development of government health policy on personal health care, 1905–11', in S. Sturdy (ed.), *Medicine, Health and the Public Sphere in Britain, 1600–2000* (London, 2002), pp. 241–59.

Thomson, T. J., 'The Scottish Colleges – teaching and examining abroad', in D. Dow (ed.), *The Influence of Scottish Medicine* (Carnforth, 1988), pp. 159–70.

Torstendahl, R., 'Introduction: promotion and strategies of knowledge–based groups', in M. Burrage and R. Torstendahl (eds), *Professions in Theory and History* (London, 1980), pp. 1–10.

Vickery, A., 'Golden age to separate spheres? A review of the categories and chronology of English women's history', in R. Schoemaker and M. Vincent (eds), *Gender and History in Western Europe* (London, 1998), pp. 197–228.

Woodruff, M., 'Transplantation: a personal recollection', in P. Terasaki (ed.), *History of Transplantation: Thirty-five Recollections* (Los Angeles, 1991), pp. 184–98.

## Journal articles

Bell, J., 'Five years' surgery in the Royal Hospital for Sick Children', *Edinburgh Hospital Reports*, 1 (1893), pp. 1–10.

Bell, J., 'The surgical side of the Royal Infirmary, 1854–92', *Edinburgh Hospital Reports*, 1 (1893), pp. 1–10.

Bonner, T. N., 'Medical women abroad: a new dimension of women's push for opportunity in medicine, 1850–1914', *Bull. Hist. Med.*, 62 (1998), pp. 52–73.

Boog Watson, W. N., 'Early baths and bagnios in Edinburgh', *BOEC*, 24 (1979), pp. 57–67.

Bramwell, E., 'Postgraduate medical students and teaching in Edinburgh – the past, the present and the future', *University of Edinburgh Journal*, 9 (1937–8), pp. 116–23.

Broman, T., 'The Habermasian public sphere and "science" "in" the Enlightenment', *History of Science*, 36 (2) (1998), pp. 123–49.

Brunton, D., 'Practitioners versus legislators: the shaping of the Scottish Vaccination Act', *Proc. Roy. Coll. Phys. Edinb.*, 23 (1993), pp. 193–201.

Burnham, J. C., 'How the concept of profession evolved in the work of historians of medicine', *Bull. Hist. Med.*, 70 (1) (1996), pp. 1–24.

Cathcart, C. W., 'Some of the older Schools of Anatomy connected with the Royal College of Surgeons, Edinburgh', *EMJ*, 27 (1882), pp. 769–791.

Cathcart, C. W., 'Classification in Pathology', *EMJ*, 42 (1896), pp. 37–46, 141–8.

Chaudhry, A., Sutton, C., Wood, J., Stone, R. and McCloy, R., 'Learning rate for laparoscopic surgical skills on MIST VR, a virtual reality simulator: quality of human-computer interface', *Annals of the Royal College of Surgeons of England*, 81 (1999), pp. 281–6.

Chikwe, J., de Souza, A. and Pepper, J. R., 'No time to train the surgeons', *BMJ*, 328 (2004), p. 418.

Cohen, R. A., 'Lilian Lindsay 1871–1960', *British Dental Journal*, 131 (3) (1971), pp. 121–2.

Cook, H. J., 'Boerhaave and the flight from reason in medicine', *Bull. Hist. Med.*, 74 (2) (2000), pp. 221–40.

Cook, J., 'The changing pattern of surgical education 1955–1980', *J. Roy. Coll. Surg. Edinb.*, 25 (1980), pp. 293–8.

Cooter, R., 'The rise and decline of the medical member: doctors and Parliament in Edwardian and interwar Britain', *Bull. Hist. Med.*, 78 (1) (2004), pp. 59–107.

Craig, G. C., 'Fluorides and the prevention of dental decay: a statement from the Representative Board of the British Dental Association', *British Dental Journal*, 188 (12) (2000), p. 654.

Craig, S., Hamzah, M. and Walker, W. S., 'Video-assisted thoracoscopic pneumonectomy for bronchial carcinoid tumor in a 14-year-old girl', *Journal of Pediatric Surgery*, 32 (7) (1997), pp. 1724–6.

Cuschieri, A., 'The laparoscopic revolution', *J. Roy. Coll. Surg. Edinb.*, 34 (1990), p. 295.

Dean, A. C. B., 'Specialty Fellowship Examinations', *J. Roy. Coll. Surg. Edinb.*, 30 (2) (1985), pp. 141–2.

Dingwall, H., M., 'Original Fellowship Examination', *J. Roy.Coll. Surg. Edinb.*, 36 (1991), pp. 357–61.

Dingwall, H. M., '"General practice" in seventeenth-century Edinburgh: evidence from the Burgh Court', *Social History of Medicine* (6) (1993), pp. 125–42.

Dingwall, H. M., 'Making up the medicine: apothecaries in sixteenth- and seventeenth-century Edinburgh', *Caduceus*, 10 (3) (1994), pp. 121–30.

Dingwall, H. M., '"To be insert in the Mercury". Medical practitioners and the press in eighteenth-century Edinburgh', *Social History of Medicine*, 13 (1) (2000), pp. 25–42.

Driscoll, P., 'Challenges in Surgical training', *Surgeonsnews*, 3 (2) (2004), pp. 56–7.

'Editorial Notes', *EMJ*, 8 (1914), p. 292.

Emerson, R. L., 'The Philosophical Society of Edinburgh 1768–1783', *British Journal for the History of Science*, 18 (1985), pp. 255–303.

Forbes, E. G., 'The professionalization of dentistry in the United Kingdom', *Medical History*, 29 (1985), p. 169.

Forbes Gray, W., 'An eighteenth-century riding school', *BOEC*, 20 (1935), pp. 111–59.

Foster, J., 'The Forbes Laboratory', *Annual Report 2002–2003* (Royal College of Surgeons of Edinburgh, 2003), pp. 37–8.

Foster, J., 'Christine Evans – the Barbara Woodhouse of Urology', *Surgeonsnews*, January, 2004, pp. 94–5 (title of article by the editor, David Tolley).

Gardner, D. L., 'Early twentieth century surgical urology: the 1909–1939 experience of Henry Wade', *The Surgeon*, 1 (3) (2003), pp. 166–76.

Gow, I., 'Playfair: a northern Athenian', *Journal of the Royal Institute of British Architects*, May 1990, pp. 36–44.

Gow, I., 'Fittingly furnished', *Country Life*, 16 August 1990, pp. 58–9.

Guthrie, D., 'King James the Fourth of Scotland: his influence on medicine and science', *Bull. Hist. Med.*, 21 (1947), pp. 173–93.

Guthrie, D., 'The medical and scientific exploits of King James IV of Scotland', *BMJ*, 30 June 1953, p. 1195.

Herzfeld, G., 'Traumatic rupture of intestine without external injury', *Lancet*, 1 (1920), p. 377.

Herzfeld, G., 'Treatment of burns and scalds by tannic acid', *Practitioner*, 122 (1929), pp. 106–11.

Herzfeld, G., 'Injuries and malformations of the newborn', *Practitioner*, 164 (1950), pp. 52–60.

Holland, E., 'The Princess Charlotte of Wales. A triple obstetric tragedy', *British Journal of Obstetrics and Gynaecology*, 58 (6) (1951), pp. 905–19.

Jordanova, L., 'The social construction of medical knowledge', *Social History of Medicine*, 8 (3) (1995), pp. 361–83.

Kaufman, M. H., 'An early Caesarian operation (1800) performed by John and Charles Bell', *J. Roy. Coll. Surg. Edinb.*, 39 (1994), pp. 69–75.

Kaufman, M. H., 'Caesarian operations performed in Edinburgh during the eighteenth century', *British Journal of Obstetrics and Gynaecology*, 102 (1995), pp. 186–91.

Kaufman, M. H., 'Clinical case histories and sketches of gun-shot injuries from the Carlist War during the period between May 1836 and December 1837', *J. Roy. Coll. Surg. Edinb.*, 46 (2001), pp. 279–89.

Kaufman, M. H., McTavish, J. and Mitchell, R. 'The gunner with the silver mask: observations on the management of severe maxillo-facial lesions over the last 160 years', *J. Roy. Coll. Surg. Edinb.*, 42 (1997), pp. 367–75.

Kaufman, M. H., Purdue, B. N. and Carswell, A. L., 'Old wounds and distant battles: the Allcock-Ballingall collection of military surgery at the University of Edinburgh', *J. Roy. Coll. Surg. Edinb.*, 41 (5) (1996), pp. 339–50.

Kaufman, M. H. and Royds, M. T., 'Excision of a remarkable tumour of the upper jaw in 1834 by Robert Liston', *Scottish Medical Journal*, 45 (2000), pp. 158–60.

Keith, T., 'Cases of ovariotomy', *EMJ*, 12 (1866–7), pp. 493–509.

Lawrence, C., 'Alexander Monro *primus* and the Edinburgh manner of anatomy', *Bull. Hist. Med.*, 62 (1988), pp. 193–214

Lawrence, C., 'The Edinburgh Medical School and the end of the "Old Thing" 1790–1830', *History of Universities*, 7 (1988), pp. 259–86.

Levy, L. F., 'Personal view', *BMJ*, 285 (1982), p. 1271.

Lynch, M.,'Whatever happened to the medieval burgh? Some guidelines for sixteenth- and seventeenth-century historians', *Scottish Economic and Social History*, 4 (1984), pp. 5–20.

McCarthy, M. C., 'The Association of Women Surgeons', *Archives of Surgery*, 128 (6) (1993), pp. 633–6.

Macdonald, F., 'Vaccination policy of the Faculty of Physicians and Surgeons of Glasgow, 1801–1863', *Med. Hist.*, 41 (1997), pp. 291–321.

McGregor, J. S. and Buchan, A. C., 'Our clinical experience with the tensor fasciae latae myocutanous flap', *British Journal of Plastic Surgery*, 33 (2) (1980), pp. 270–6.

Macnicol, M. F., Penny, I. D. and Shephard, L., 'Early results of the Leeds-Keio anterior cruciate ligament replacement', *Journal of Bone and Joint Surgery*, 73 (3) (1991), pp. 377–80.

Maloco, A. and Dear, D., 'Symposium Hall for the Royal College of Surgeons of Edinburgh', *Edinburgh Architectural Association Review*, 12 (1984), pp. 105–15.

Maran, A. G. D., 'Revised Edinburgh Fellowship Examination', *J. Roy. Coll. Surg. Edinb.*, 35 (1990), pp. 137–9.

Miller, J. D. and Steers, A. J. W., 'Surgical neurology and clinical neurosciences in Edinburgh, Scotland', *Neurosurgery*, 39 (1) (1996), pp. 151–9.

Moffat, B., 'SHARP practice. The search for medieval medical treatments', *Archaeology Today*, 8 (1987), pp. 22–8.

Risse, G. B., 'Clinical instruction in Hospitals: the Boerhaavian tradition in Leyden, Edinburgh, Vienna and Pavia', *Clio Medica*, 21 (1987–8), pp. 1–19.

Rix, K. J. B., 'Alexander Wood (1725–1807): Deacon of the Incorporation of Surgeons, Surgeon-in-ordinary, Edinburgh Royal Infirmary, and "Doctor of Mirth"', *Scottish Medical Journal*, 33 (1988), pp. 346–8.

Roscoe, T. and Bacon, N., 'Why should surgeons use the internet?', *Surgeonsnews*, 3 (2) (2004), pp. 54–5.

Rosner, L., 'Thistle on the Delaware: Edinburgh medical education and Philadelphia practice, 1800–1825', *Social History of Medicine*, 5 (1) (1992), pp. 19–42.

Rowley, D., 'A vision for surgery – the future of UK surgical training', *Surgeonsnews*, 3 (1) (2004), p. 42.

Short, A. I. and Lennard, T. W. J., 'James IV of Scotland: monarchy and medicine', *Journal of Medical Biography*, 1 (1993), pp. 175–85.

Simpson, D. C., 'The Chairs of Surgery at Edinburgh 1777–1831', *J. Roy. Coll. Surg. Edinb.*, 22 (1977), pp. 91–102.

Stott, R., 'The library of Thomas Kincaid, a seventeenth-century Scottish surgeon', *Canadian Bulletin of Medical History*, 12 (2) (1995), pp. 351–67.

Taylor, D. W., 'The manuscript lecture notes of Alexander Monro *primus* (1697–1767), *Medical History*, 30 (1986), pp. 444–67.

Temple, J. G., 'MRCS', *Surgeonsnews*, 2 (1) (2003), pp. 74–5.

Thin, R., 'The Old Infirmary and Earlier Hospitals', *BOEC*, 15 (1927), pp. 135–63.

Thin, R., 'Medical Quacks in Edinburgh in the seventeenth and eighteenth centuries', *BOEC*, 12 (1938), pp. 132–59.

Wallace, W. A., 'Fortnightly Review: managing in-flight emergencies', *BMJ*, 311 (1995), pp. 374–5.

Watson, A., 'Report of the Edinburgh Eye Infirmary by Alexander Watson Esq., Fellow of the Royal College of Surgeons and Surgeon to the Institution', *EMJ*, 43 (1835), pp. 126–36

Watson-Jones, R., 'Honours to Sir Walter Mercer', *Journal of Bone and Joint Surgery*, 38B (1) (1956), p. 435.

Wilson, J., 'Training women for surgical leadership', *J. Roy. Coll. Surg. Edinb.*, 41 (3) (1996), pp. 212–14.

Wojcik, W. A., 'Time in context – the Polish School of Medicine and the Paderewski Polish Hospital in Edinburgh 1941 to 1949', *Proc. Roy. Coll. Phys. Edinb.*, 31 (2001), pp. 69–76.

Worling, P., 'The Edinburgh apothecaries', *Pharmaceutical Historian*, 33 (3) (2003), pp. 37–44.

## Unpublished works

El-Khalili, N. H., 'Surgical training on the world wide web' (unpublished Ph.D. thesis, University of Leeds, 1999).

Ross, J. A., 'Memoirs of an Edinburgh Surgeon' (unpublished, Royal College of Surgeons of Edinburgh, 1988).

Stott, R. M., 'The Incorporation of Surgeons of Edinburgh and medical education and practice in Edinburgh 1696–1755' (unpublished Ph.D. thesis, University of Edinburgh, 1984).

Watson, F., 'The role of virtual reality in surgical training in the UK' (unpublished MSc thesis, University of Sheffield, 2000).

Williams, M., 'A Report on the History of Old Surgeons' Hall, Edinburgh' (unpublished MA essay, University of Edinburgh, 2004).

# Index of names

# General index

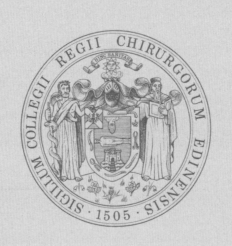